Core Topics in Op Practice

Anaesthesia and Crit

Recent developments to medical career structures and roles and responsibilities have raised the profile of operating department practitioners (ODPs). Required knowledge is vast, and exams must be sat in working towards statutory registration. This is the first in a series of three books providing comprehensive information for healthcare staff working in the operating department. Topics include anaesthesia, critical care, post-interventional care, enhancing care delivery, professional practice, leadership and resource management. The clear and concise format is ideally suited to study and qualification as well as continued reference during practice. Written by specialists with a wealth of knowledge and experience to offer, and incorporating problem-based learning from case studies, this book will be important for ODPs and theatre nurses throughout the UK, in Australia where the same structures have been adopted, and worldwide for all professionals working in operating departments.

Brian Smith is Senior Lecturer in Continuing Professional Development at Edge Hill University, Liverpool.

Paul Rawling is Senior Lecturer in Operating Department Practice at Edge Hill University, Liverpool.

Paul Wicker is Head of Operating Department Practice Programmes at Edge Hill University, Liverpool.

Chris Jones is Senior Lecturer in Continuing Professional Development at Edge Hill University, Liverpool.

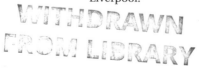

WITHDRAWN FROM LIBRARY

BRITISH MEDICAL ASSOCIATION

0847935

Core Topics in **Operating Department Practice**

Anaesthesia and
Critical Care

Brian Smith

Paul Rawling

Paul Wicker

Chris Jones

WITHDRAWN FROM LIBRARY

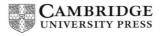
CAMBRIDGE
UNIVERSITY PRESS

CAMBRIDGE UNIVERSITY PRESS

Cambridge, New York, Melbourne, Madrid, Cape Town, Singapore, São Paulo

Cambridge University Press
The Edinburgh Building, Cambridge CB2 2RU, UK
Published in the United States of America by Cambridge University Press, New York

www.cambridge.org
Information on this title: www.cambridge.org/9780521694230

© Cambridge University Press 2007

This publication is in copyright. Subject to statutory exception and to the
provisions of relevant collective licensing ageements, no reproduction of any
part may take place without the written permission of Cambridge University Press.

Printed in the United Kingdom at the University Press, Cambridge

A catalogue record for this publication is available from the British Library

Library of Congress Cataloging-in-Publication Data

Core topics in operating department practice : anaesthesia and critical care / Brian Smith . . . [et al.].
    p. ; cm.
Includes bibliographical references and index.
ISBN-13:   978-0-521-69423-0   (pbk.)
ISBN-10:   0-521-69423-X   (pbk.)
1. Anesthesia. 2. Critical care medicine. I. Smith, Brian, 1965-II. Title: Anesthesia and critical care.
[DNLM: 1. Anesthesia. 2. Critical Care. 3. Perioperative Care. WO 200 C797 2007]
RD81.C693 2007
617.9′6–dc22

                            2006038564
ISBN-13 978-0-521-69423-0 paperback
ISBN-10 0-521-69423-X paperback

Cambridge University Press has no responsibility for the persistence or accuracy
of URLs for external or third-party internet websites referred to in this publication,
and does not guarantee that any content on such websites is, or will remain,
accurate or appropriate.

Every effort has been made in preparing this publication to provide accurate and
up-to-date information which is in accord with accepted standards and practice at
the time of publication. Although case histories are drawn from actual cases, every
effort has been made to disguise the identities of the individuals involved.
Nevertheless, the authors, editors and publishers can make no warranties that the
information contained herein is totally free from error, not least because clinical
standards are constantly changing through research and regulation. The authors,
editors and publishers therefore disclaim all liability for direct or consequential
damages resulting from the use of material contained in this publication.
Readers are strongly advised to pay careful attention to information provided by
the manufacturer of any drugs or equipment that they plan to use.

Contents

Acknowledgements

We would like to thank the publishers for their support and especially Mr Geoffrey Nuttall for being encouraging towards us.

A special mention must go to Dr Simon Bricker (Consultant Anaesthetist) for writing the foreword and above all a key critic in the development of this book.

Finally, a personal thank you to our colleagues who have given their time, dedication, and expertise to each unique chapter. Their strength and commitment to this book has been duly noted and appreciated.

Brian Smith, Paul Rawling,
Paul Wicker, Chris Jones
Liverpool 2006

Contributors

Toni Bewley
Royal Liverpool Children's NHS Trust and
Faculty of Health
Edge Hill University
Liverpool

Mark Bottell
St. Helens & Knowsley Hospital Trust
Whiston Hospital
Prescot, Merseyside

Robert Campbell
Liverpool Women's Hospital
Liverpool

Trish Finn
Aintree Cardiac Centre
University Hospital Aintree
Liverpool

Gill Hall
Respiratory Education UK
Liverpool

Teresa Hardcastle
Faculty of Health
Edge Hill University
Liverpool

Kevin Anthony Henshaw
Faculty of Health
Edge Hill University
Liverpool

Chris Jones
Faculty of Health
Edge Hill University
Liverpool

Helen McNeill
Faculty of Health
Edge Hill University
Liverpool

Martin Maguire
University Hospital Aintree
Liverpool

Jill Nolan
Intensive Care Unit
Royal Liverpool and Broadgreen Hospital
Liverpool

Maria Parsonage
Wirral Hospitals NHS Trust
Merseyside

Paul Rawling
Faculty of Health
Edge Hill University
Liverpool

Michael A. Sewell
Burnley General Hospital
Burnley

Brian Smith
Faculty of Health
Edge Hill University
Liverpool

Cheryl Wayne-Conroy
Faculty of Health
Edge Hill University
Liverpool

Paul Wicker
Faculty of Health
Edge Hill University
Liverpool

Tom Williams
Independent Academic Adviser
Alicante

Margaret Woods
Faculty of Health
Edge Hill University
Liverpool

Stephen L. Wordsworth
Division of Operating Department Practice
Faculty of Health
The University of Central England
Birmingham

Norman Wright
Faculty of Health
Edge Hill University
Liverpool

Foreword

Most senior consultant anaesthetists will be able to recall times during their early careers when anaesthetic assistance in theatre could be described at best as rudimentary. There was often willing help for the anaesthetists but it was provided largely by those whose training, through no fault of their own, was negligible. It is true, of course, that the early anaesthetic assistants did not have to contend with the complex range of anaesthetic equipment that is now available, and it comes as a surprise to many, for instance, to learn that the use of pulse oximetry did not become routine in the operating theatre until the late 1980s. That chapters in this book include accounts of topics such as perioperative myocardial infarction, mechanical ventilation and awareness during anaesthesia indicates just how much progress has been made since those often unsatisfactory times. Further chapters on the development of a personal portfolio and on the implications of professional accountability also serve notice that the era of the Anaesthetic Practitioner is nigh: an era that the ODAs of twenty-five years ago could never have envisaged. The modern reality, finally, is that the theatre orderly of two or more decades ago is now a degree student, ODP, of whom is required an understanding of the basic sciences which underpin the safe practice of sophisticated modern anaesthesia. This book is the first of a series which should go much of the way towards fulfilling that ambition.

Dr. Simon Bricker
Consultant Anaesthetist
The Countess of Chester Hospital

Preface

Healthcare in the UK has experienced intense change over the past few years, much of which has been focused on the perioperative environment. The NHS Plan, introduced by the Labour government in 2000, was at the forefront of the modernisation of the UK's National Health Service. Focusing on major areas of concern, such as modernisation of the workforce, increasing patient choice, and increasing the efficiency and effectiveness of patient care, the government strategy to rebuild the NHS has affected every segment of the care sector.

Perioperative practitioners have responded to these pressures by re-examining professional boundaries and roles within perioperative care. As practice has advanced to meet these new challenges, new roles have developed, including for example, the surgical care practitioner, anaesthesia practitioner, and non-medical prescribing practitioners. These roles have the potential to increase the quality of patient care, as well as offering an opportunity for perioperative practitioners to extend their skills, knowledge, and competencies.

The intention is to provide a series of books exploring all aspects of core practice in perioperative care. This book, the first of the series, focuses on developments in anaesthetic practice.

For many anaesthetic practitioners[1] the thought of further professional development can be

[1] The term 'anaesthetic practitioner' depicts the role of either an operating department practitioner or a nurse acting as assistant to the anaesthetist.

daunting. The increasingly specialist area of anaesthetic practice has been mirrored by an increasing need for specialist knowledge. Consider, for example, the differing needs of a patient undergoing major vascular surgery, an elderly patient requiring hip arthroplasty and a young mother undergoing caesarean section under spinal anaesthesia. The advanced anaesthetic techniques available in a modern operating department mean that care for these groups of patients is vastly different.

The purpose of this book is therefore to support anaesthetic practitioners in the crucial process of professional development.

Key learning points are included at the beginning of each chapter to focus the reader on the main topics discussed. The editors have developed the content of this book to reflect current concerns in anaesthetic practice. The book does not try to cover the vast area of anaesthetic practice, instead it focuses on areas of concern where practitioners are developing new roles. The reader should draw on this publication as a key resource for contemporary practice and use it where fitting to apply theory into practice.

The book commences with introductory chapters looking at the advancing role of the anaesthetic practitioner and risk assessment in the anaesthetic environment. Risk assessment is seen as a core area of concern for anaesthetic practitioners because of the high-risk environment where they deliver patient care.

The book continues by exploring core areas of developing practice, such as electrocardiogram monitoring, applying cricoid pressure, breathing systems, preventing awareness under anaesthesia and developments in resuscitation. The chapters offer knowledge and understanding of key clinical issues which affect practitioners' practice.

Later chapters of the book look at issues in advanced anaesthetic practice, for example, managing difficult intubations, understanding total intravenous anaesthesia and infusion pumps and anaesthesia for patients undergoing electroconvulsive therapy.

The last two chapters of the book explore professional anaesthetic practice in relation to continual professional development – accountability and learning from practice through reflection and portfolio development.

It is at this point of great changes in anaesthetic practice that we offer this textbook, developed by specialists, to support the ongoing professional development of the anaesthetic practitioner.

**Brian Smith, Paul Rawling,
Paul Wicker, Chris Jones**
Liverpool 2006

Introduction: anaesthetic practice. Past and present

Brian Smith and Paul Wicker

Key Learning Points

- Understand historical events in anaesthesia
- Explore the place of present-day changes in anaesthetic practice
- Recognise the importance of evidence in developing a body of anaesthetic knowledge
- Develop a reflective approach to anaesthetic practice

The past three centuries have brought many changes to the care of patients undergoing anaesthesia. Many of those changes have been at the hands of inspirational doctors who many now regard as pioneers of present-day anaesthesia.

Before anaesthesia, surgery was a traumatic event, full of pain and suffering of an unimaginable degree, which often led to patients' death. It is important to understand the horror and brutality of early surgery without anaesthesia, to understand the real value of anaesthesia today. It is hard to imagine how patients must have suffered under the knife when, for example, cutting through the perineum, opening the bladder, extracting a stone and then sewing up the wounds. Meanwhile the patient would have been in unbearable agony, suffering convulsions and muscle spasms, may have gone into deep shock and would have most probably died of the experience.

Joseph Priestly, in 1777, developed one of the most valuable contributions to present-day anaesthesia. Arguably the first anaesthetist, Priestly discovered the value of nitrous oxide for anaesthesia. The work of Humphrey Davy in 1800 described the analgesic action of nitrous oxide, thus confirming its use for anaesthesia. Nitrous oxide is an anaesthetic gas which anaesthetists still use today to aid the delivery of volatile agents and to control the patient's conscious level and pain.

Nitrous oxide does not, however, come free of controversy. Tramer *et al.* (1996) argue that nitrous oxide is an emetic and causes postoperative nausea and vomiting. Other case reports (Puri, 2001) suggest introducing nitrous oxide to a patient's anaesthetic can raise the Bispectral Index System (BIS) reading, which is a translated electroencephalogram (EEG) of the effects of the anaesthetic on the brain. Indeed Glass *et al.* (1997) found that nitrous oxide combined with propofol raised the BIS reading and patients failed to respond to verbal commands when compared with an anaesthetic without nitrous oxide.

Similarly, in 1847 Simpson suggested that chloroform was the ideal 'knock out' gas for obstetric patients. The discovery of chloroform may not have been an acceptable approach in today's conventional terms; nevertheless the experiments which Simpson carried out on himself, conducted by sniffing the solvents, did lead to the discovery of this early anaesthetic agent. Chloroform remained in practice for a few years but never became the 'single agent' for anaesthesia, because of its rather distressing side effects.

Core Topics in Operating Department Practice: Anaesthesia and Critical Care, eds. Brian Smith, Paul Rawling, Paul Wicker and Chris Jones. Published by Cambridge University Press. © Cambridge University Press 2007.

The search was on for other doctors to find the perfect anaesthetic agent. In 1846, William T. G. Morton gave the first ether anaesthetic. This was an exciting stage in anaesthesia and created a strong interest among many surgeons, including Robert Listen 'The showman surgeon', Professor of Clinical Surgery at University College London. Shortly after this news had reached Listen, he performed the first pain-free surgical procedure with the patient waking up to ask 'When will we begin?'.

In 1847 John Snow favoured inhaling ether and later designed a suitable machine for its delivery. He developed this equipment because he discovered that patients received unregulated levels of anaesthetic agent due to flaws in the anaesthetic administration technique. The new equipment resulted in much safer anaesthesia by regulating the depth of the patient's unconsciousness.

In present-day anaesthesia, the 'vaporiser' equipment has developed through a long line of improvements from Snow's original machine. Today we benefit from the interlocking mechanism on the back bar system to which a vaporiser is attached (Al-Shaikh & Stacey, 2002). This safety feature of preventing two vaporisers turning on simultaneously inhibits the delivery of potentially lethal mixtures of volatile agents. Also, the intricate mechanics of the vaporisers ensures the delivery of an accurate percentage of the volatile agent. The temperature-compensating bimetallic strip helps with this accuracy by detecting any deviations in temperature.

The idea of an 'anaesthetic machine' was developed from the work of these early pioneers and has resulted in the sophisticated, but safe and efficient, anaesthetic machines used today. Sir Frederic Hewitt, Elmer McKesson, and Robert Boyle's invention of the anaesthetic machine, and later improvements from 1898, have produced many advances for anaesthesia. Their early introduction of a machine that could deliver oxygen and volatile agents helped anaesthesia to develop into a precise science. With the advantages of anaesthesia recognised by many surgeons, and its increase in popularity, there became a pressing need to accurately control the delivery of anaesthetic agents. Anaesthetists required this control to prevent the deaths that occurred regularly with chloroform in 1886. Today the definition of an anaesthetic machine is clear, however, the role of the various pieces of anaesthetic equipment on the machine remain similar in many ways to the original Boyle's machine.

The original Boyle's machine delivered fresh compressed gas from cylinders attached to the machine by channelling the flow through the fine controls of a flowmeter. The journey of the fresh gas continued through the volatile agent (ether, chloroform and later halothane) and out the other side of the vaporiser, delivering a mixture to the patient. The patient would receive this mixture usually through an anaesthetic circuit that would have a face mask attached, known as 'a continuous flow apparatus'. The modern-day anaesthetic machine is also classified under this heading to show that the machine is dependent on a supply of compressed gas.

Another important comparison with past and present anaesthetic practice is the invention of the 'circle absorber system'. According to Ince and Davey (2000), 200 years before Brian Sword brought carbon dioxide absorption into anaesthetic practice, Joseph Priestly had described the absorption proprieties of alkalis.

Introducing the circle to anaesthesia in 1928 reduced atmospheric pollution and helped to recycle the patient's expired gas. Directing the expired gas in a unidirectional way passes the exhaled gas through soda lime to absorb carbon dioxide, thus filtering the mixture and making it suitable for recycling.

Today the principle use of the circle system has not changed and two of the key aims still include improved cost-effectiveness and reduced pollution. However there are many concerns about its use with some modern volatile agents. Moriwaki *et al.* (1997) discussed the known reaction of sevoflurane with carbon dioxide absorbents resulting in the 'generation of five degradation products'. Their studies have identified that sevoflurane with partially exhausted soda lime (carbon dioxide absorbent) produced less concentration of the degradation product compound A. The debate continues with the argument that it is unclear if low-flow sevoflurane anaesthesia can lead to renal injury. However, it is noted that a study mentioned by Moriwaki *et al.* (1997) suggests the possibility of compound A contributing to renal injury in the patient.

It is clear that anaesthesia methods, medication and monitoring have changed from the eighteenth century. However, there are also some areas that have not changed and are still taught today. For example, the traditional description of the stages or depth of anaesthesia (Figure 1.1) is still in use today. These stages have informed anaesthetic practice for several years, and have helped the anaesthetist to gauge the dosage of anaesthetic agent to give.

The first description of the stages of anaesthesia was in the days of ether and its delivery by inhalation. It was noted that the patient moves progressively through the analgesia and delirium stages to the surgical anaesthesia stage, enabling tracheal intubation or the surgical procedure to continue. In some unfortunate cases, the delivery of too much of the volatile agent resulted in stage four, medullary depressions, which eventually resulted in death.

This model has aided the anaesthetic team (AAGBI, 2005) to make clinical judgements about the dosage of anaesthetic agents each patient needs. With the increase in different methods of delivery of anaesthesia, for example, with intravenous and regional approaches, it may be fitting to consider Snow's stages of anaesthesia as applied to non-inhalational delivery.

The question arises of whether all the stages of anaesthesia are present during the use of modern intravenous induction agents. According to Drummond (2000), John Snow's stages of anaesthesia have changed and the emphasis now focuses more on the depth of anaesthesia. Initially, the hazards of overdosing concerned many anaesthetists, however, this focus has also shifted towards reducing underdosage, which can result in awareness under anaesthesia.

Equally, the patient and anaesthetic team should make a joint decision about the anaesthetic approach to use. Total Intravenous Anaesthesia (TIVA; without inhalation agents) might be a more suitable approach when considering each patient's medical history, surgical procedure, and recovery time. A randomised, double-blinded study by Ozkose *et al.* (2002) suggests TIVA can be a useful anaesthetic technique on patients who need to undergo a lumbar discectomy. It promotes rapid recovery without post-operative nausea and vomiting. These conditions offer the opportunity for the patient to have a neurological assessment post-operatively to identify the success of the procedure.

Pharmaceutical agents developed over the last 20 years, such as remifentanil and propofol have significantly contributed to anaesthesia as

---

Stages of Anaesthesia

Stage One – Analgesia: between induction of anaesthesia and ends at loss of consciousness.

Stage Two – Excitement or delirium: often sudden response to stimuli or uncontrolled movements.

Stage Three – Surgical anaesthesia – Plane 1
                                     Plane 2
                                     Plane 3
                                     Plane 4

Stage Four – Medullary depression: overdose of the patient.

Figure 1.1 Stages of anaesthesia.

alternatives to inhalational anaesthesia. Constant review and trials of different drugs draw new findings and continue to develop the scientific field of anaesthesia.

Evidence-based practice and quality is at the heart of the anaesthetic service. This in turn is dependent on those who invest time, knowledge and resources to increase the effectiveness and safety of anaesthetic provision.

At the time of writing this book, anaesthetists who have undertaken further training, after having qualified as a doctor, predominately deliver anaesthesia. The further training often takes six years or more working through the specialist qualification to become a consultant anaesthetist.

Developing the consultant anaesthetist role has been the result of trial and error by many influential doctors, such as John Snow, Sir James Young Simpson, William T. Morton, and others. According to the Association of Anaesthetists of Great Britain and Ireland (AAGBI) (2006), Dr Henry Featherstone founded the association in 1932 before the birth of the National Health Service (NHS). Before this time general practitioners (GPs) gave anaesthetics as an optional extra to their role. Pay was low for this role, and many saw it as being subordinate to the surgeons.

The main reason for founding the AAGBI was to promote and encourage anaesthetic advances through academic and clinical application. The AAGBI also supported the welfare of anaesthetists because of the pressures experienced by many in that role.

Concurrently, there have been several developments over the last century for the assistants to the anaesthetist. Before 1976, the group of staff referred to as theatre technicians adopted an alliance towards the anaesthetist. They often became skilled and reliable assistants to the anaesthetist with the main purpose of increasing the safety of the patient under anaesthesia.

Theatre technicians soon reached a key stage in their development with the publishing of the Lewin report. The report itself introduced some key changes for this group of staff. According to Wicker and Smith (2003), the Lewin report (DH, 1970) resulted in national training centres and the name change from technician to operating department assistant (ODA). Ince (2000) states that this report also introduced the City and Guilds of London Institute (CGLI) qualification 752 for Hospital Operating Department Assistants.

Throughout the two-year training scheme the ODA studied knowledge and skills in surgery, anaesthesia, and recovery and related subjects. Although the course prepared ODAs to work in all areas of the operating department, the presence of nurses in surgery created a natural opening in anaesthesia which ODAs migrated towards. The lack of uptake of surgical duties by the individual and the department resulted in a further report in 1989 (NHS Management Executive, 1989, the 'Bevan report').

Theatre nurses were also building on their experiences within anaesthesia. The English National Board (ENB) anaesthetic units of study gave nurses (in England) a nationally recognised qualification to practice as an anaesthetic nurse. The lack of a similar qualification in Scotland led to some confusion of the acceptability of locally developed anaesthetic courses, even when developed by Higher Education Institutes.

These two groups did not work in harmony, tensions arose between ODAs who were aspiring to become registered, and nurses who already had statutory registration. The differences in training led to further tensions as the two groups tried to understand each other's priorities for patient care. Professor P. G. Bevan (1989) identified the overlaps of roles and Wicker (1997) further commented on this area several years later.

Bevan's report identified opportunities for developing both professions through shared learning and management of the theatre service. Partly because of this report, partly the professions' internal changes in thinking, the ODA became an Operating Department Practitioner (ODP). The emphasis changed from 'assisting' to 'practicing', and the profession took another step in its long struggle towards statutory registration.

In 2006, 'The Anaesthetic Team' guidelines (AAGBI) identified the nationally accepted qualification for an ODP. The report recommended that ODPs should hold a Diploma of Higher Education in Operating Department Practice, gained from a two-year programme of study. The increased academic profile for the profession subsequently supported the acceptance on the statutory register with the Health Professions Council.

What is not clear from the AAGBI document is the relevant qualification for an anaesthetic nurse. Since the English National Board (ENB) dissolved in 2002, there has been increasing uncertainty about the accepted nationally recognised qualification for registered nurses wishing to practice in anaesthesia.

Previously the ENB (formerly Joint Board for Clinical Nursing Studies (JBCNS)) 182 units of learning had set out common objectives so the registered nurse could meet the needs of the patient undergoing anaesthesia. Those had encouraged and developed the registered nurse interested in anaesthetic care (ENB, 1994).

Today, *The Anaesthesia Team* (2005) recommends: 'Assistance for the anaesthetist may be provided by ODPs or nurses. Whatever the background, the training for all anaesthesia assistants must comply fully with national standards'. Judging from the activities of the Association for Perioperative Practice, the Association of Operating Department Practitioners and the British Association of Anaesthetic and Recovery Nurses, anaesthetic nursing is still of interest to the registered nurse and their employer. The former group's interest possibly takes its roots from the interesting scientific developments in anaesthetic care. The interest of the latter group may be credited to the national shortage of perioperative staff within the United Kingdom.

Employers seek new ways to staff the whole perioperative service and take action to advance many of their staff skills by crossing once traditional boundaries. Multi-skilling the individual is a long-standing term within the perioperative environment and draws with it the term 'Skill Mix'

as suggested by Mackenzie (1998). At the heart of this idea is the need to ensure that quality of care is affordable by ensuring flexibility across traditional divisions of labour.

It is no longer the historical case as mentioned by Pittaway (2004) that only perioperative nurses should have the opportunity for 'clinical experience and years of service' to progress their career. Instead, all perioperative practitioners today (registered nurses and ODPs) should be able to exercise their professional autonomy and choose which professional experiences would advance their career.

Practitioners may base their choice on the need to fulfil the requirements for registration with the Nursing & Midwifery Council or the Health Professions Council. Alternatively they may base their decision on a wish to undertake academic studies to develop their skills and knowledge in the area. Whatever approach the practitioner adopts, more opportunities for role improvement are available with the examples of the new roles emerging in the perioperative environment (Lipp, 2004).

The National Health Service Modernisation Agency (2004) recommended developing a select group of professionals with non-medical backgrounds to deliver anaesthesia. This development sits well with the two national agendas to reduce the doctors in training hours to a 58-hour week (DoH, 2004) and secondly with the NHS Career framework (Skills for Health) (Figure 1.2).

These two agendas offer opportunities for many perioperative practitioners to develop their knowledge and skills at higher levels to be able to progress their career to specialist practitioner, consultant practitioner and other levels. One possible new role for the perioperative practitioner will be to undertake both prescribing and administration of anaesthesia. Many other countries have set up the 'nurse anaesthetist' role. Within the United Kingdom the National Health Service Modernisation Agency (2004) is reviewing a pilot study looking at the non-medical anaesthetist role. When this role is firmly part of the anaesthetic

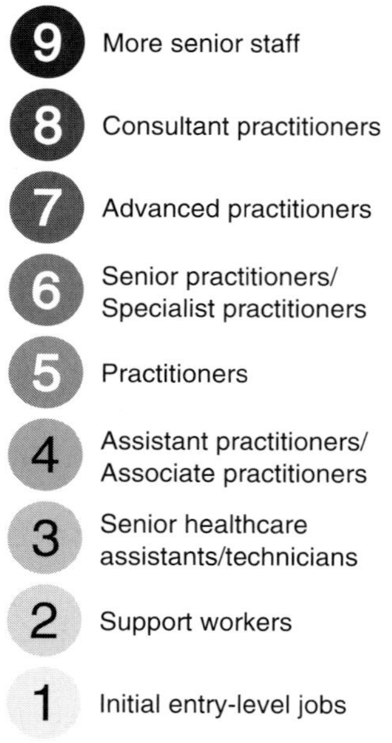

9 More senior staff

8 Consultant practitioners

7 Advanced practitioners

6 Senior practitioners/
Specialist practitioners

5 Practitioners

4 Assistant practitioners/
Associate practitioners

3 Senior healthcare
assistants/technicians

2 Support workers

1 Initial entry-level jobs

Figure 1.2 A Career Framework for Health. The Career Framework for Health is being developed by Skills for Health to support the introduction of flexible career opportunities for staff across the health sector and the concept of competence-based skills education. See: www.skillsforhealth.org.uk Skills for Health (2005).

team, then the nurse or ODP performing this role will be accountable in their own right for their performance (Hind & Wicker, 2000). Practitioners should not underestimate the scope of this undertaking, as careful reviewing of this role will be essential to address any accountability, autonomy, educational and registration issues that may arise.

This chapter has explored the long, sometimes torturous, development of anaesthesia, and in particular the role of practitioners working in this speciality. The result of many years of development, scientific investigation and trial and error, is a body of knowledge and skills which help to ensure the safest possible care for patients undergoing anaesthesia. Anaesthesia, on its own, is simply safer than driving a car, with a much lower mortality and morbidity rate.

It is on this foundation that the chapters of this book aim to support the advancing of practitioners' knowledge and abilities through their career progression. The breadth of knowledge from the core subjects will encourage others to continue to question, explore and contribute to the body of knowledge in anaesthesia and critical care.

The growing specialisation of anaesthetic practice, even within anaesthetic practice itself, means that practitioners have to develop skills and understanding far beyond those taught at preregistration level. The anaesthetic practitioner has a professional responsibility to advance patient care and to continue improving anaesthetic practice through developing the profession.

REFERENCES

AAGBI. (2005). *The Anaesthetic Team*. London: The Association of Anaesthetists of Great Britain and Ireland.

AAGBI. (2006). *The Association of Anaesthetists of Great Britain and Ireland*. Available at: www.aagbi. org/heritage/aagbihistory.htm (Accessed 12 October 2006.)

Al-Shaikh, B. & Stacey, S. (2002). *Essentials of Anaesthetic Equipment*, 2nd edn. London: Churchill Livingstone.

Department of Health. (2004). *A Compendium of Solutions to Implementing the Working Time Directive for Doctors in Training from August 2004*. London: HMSO.

Department of Health and Social Security, Welsh Office, Central Health Services Council. (1970). *The Organisation and Staffing of Operating Departments*. London: HMSO. (The Lewin Report.)

Drummond, J. C. (2000). Monitoring depth of anesthesia: with emphasis on the application of the bispectral index and the middle latency auditory evoked response to the prevention of recall. *Anesthesiology*, **93**(3), 876–82.

English National Board for Nursing, Midwifery and Health Visiting (ENB). (1994). *Creating Lifelong Learners: Preregistration Guidelines*. London: ENB.

Glass, P. S., Bloom, M., Kearse, L. *et al.* (1997). Bispectral analysis measures sedation and memory effects of propofol, midazolam, isoflurane, and alfentanil. *Anesthesiology*, **86**, 836–47.

Hind, M. & Wicker, P. (2000). *Principles of Perioperative Practice*. London: Harcourt.

Ince, C. S. & Davey, A. (2000). *Fundamentals of Operating Department Practice*. Greenwich: Greenwich Medical Media.

Lipp, A. (2004). New ways of working in anaesthesia. *British Journal of Perioperative Nursing*, **14**(9), 384–90.

Mackenzie, J. (ed.) (1998). *Ward Management in Practice*. Edinburgh: Churchill Livingstone.

Moriwaki, G., Bito, H. & Ikeda, K. (1997). Partly exhausted soda lime or soda lime with water added, inhibits the increase in compound A concentration in the circle system during low-flow sevoflurane anaesthesia. *British Journal of Anaesthesia*, **79**(6), 782–6.

National Health Service Modernisation Agency. (2004). *Changing Workforce Programme. Role Design: Review of Activities 2004*. London: HMSO.

NHS Management Executive. (1989). *The Management and Utilisation of Operating Departments*. London: VFM Unit. (The Bevan Report.)

Ozkose, Z., Yalcin, Cok O. *et al.* (2002). Comparison of hemodynamics, recovery profile, and early postoperative pain control and costs of remifentanil versus alfentanil-based total intravenous anesthesia (TIVA). *Journal of Clinical Anesthesia*, **14**(3), 161–8.

Pittaway, D. A. (2004). The changing role of the perioperative nurse. In M. Radford, M. Oakley and B. County, eds., *Advancing Perioperative Practice*. Cheltenham: Nelson Thornes, pp. 1–14.

Puri, G. D. (2001). Paradoxical changes in bispectral index during nitrous oxide administration. *British Journal of Anaesthesia*, **86**(1), 141–2.

Skills for Health. (2005). *A Career Framework for Health*. Available at: http://www.skillsforhealth.org.uk/careerframework/ (Accessed 8 March 2006).

Tramer, M., Moore, A. & McQuay, H. (1996). Omitting nitrous oxide in general anaesthesia: meta-analysis of intraoperative awareness and postoperative emesis in randomized control trials. *British Journal of Anaesthesia*, **76**, 186–93.

Wicker, P. (1997). Overlapping roles in the operating department. *Nursing Standard*, **11**(20), 44–5.

Wicker, P. & Smith, B. (2003). The changing workforce in the operating department: morphing the professions. Technic. *The Journal of Operating Department Practice*, **8–11**, 242.

2

Risk assessment

Toni Bewley

Key Learning Points
- Identification of hazards in the perioperative environment
- The principles of risk assessment
- Measures which practitioners can take to reduce risk
- Carrying out risk assessment

Few practitioners see the topic of health and safety as being relevant or interesting until they start to consider it in depth. As they explore the topic, the individual's anxiety heightens as the awareness of safe and unsafe practices grows. The reality is that any practitioner could, by act or omission, become involved in a critical incident. This awareness is especially important in the perioperative environment which by its nature is dangerous and full of many hazards which can harm patients or staff.

The motivating reasons that influence a practitioner's behaviour towards health and safety can be identified as:
- moral
- legal
- economic
- employment
- professional.

Moral reasons

It should be enough for all practitioners to always apply the principles of risk reduction and good adherence to health and safety practices, just because this is a moral responsibility to others. Nevertheless, if this is not reason enough to motivate practitioners, there is a wealth of health and safety legislation associated with the subject. As with any other Act, a breach of named regulations could result in the individual and/or the organisation receiving an enforceable punishment.

Legal reasons

Interestingly enough, most practitioners are aware of 'The Health and Safety at Work Act, 1974' (HSAWA). Why then, if perioperative practitioners have an awareness of their legal responsibilities about health and safety, do they often adopt seemingly complacent attitudes towards it?

This may occur because health and safety is a state of mind: practitioners believe they are as safe as they think they are. Therein lies the problem: practitioners may not be as safe as they think they are.

Mistakes happen, however the purpose of risk assessment is to identify set priorities and reduce risk. Proactive risk assessment enables there to be direct and justifiable decision-making. A ranking of risks with suitable financial and staff resource allocation raises staff awareness of a range of outcomes, protects the patient, prevents negative publicity and improves staff morale.

In 2000, the Chief Medical Officer reported on:
- the scale and nature of serious failures in the UK's National Health Service (NHS) care

Core Topics in Operating Department Practice: Anaesthesia and Critical Care, eds. Brian Smith, Paul Rawling, Paul Wicker and Chris Jones. Published by Cambridge University Press. © Cambridge University Press 2007.

- how the NHS could learn from its mistakes in care delivery
- measures which could minimise future risk.

This report, 'An Organisation with a Memory' (DH, 2000), written by an expert group learning from adverse events in the NHS, found that, although uncommon, when serious failures happen they:

- have devastating effects on patients and their families
- cause extreme distress to staff
- undermine public confidence in healthcare.

During a recent discussion involving the author, practitioners reflected on a 'near miss' incident involving a patient. In this case the patient arrived in theatre for surgery on her left arm, however written consent stated the surgery was on the right arm.

The theatre list was running late, tempers were frayed, practitioners did not check the case notes correctly and nobody marked the arm. Only when the patient was anaesthetised and in theatre, and the X-rays were checked, was the error spotted.

In this case no harm was done but an 'adverse incident investigation' followed. The investigating team examined policies and procedures, highlighted individual responsibilities, and introduced clear pathways for all staff to follow. The report highlighted a catalogue of errors which included wrong consenting procedures, failure to check documentation, and omissions in double-checking procedures.

The purpose of risk assessment however is to minimise risk to the lowest level reasonably practicable. When undertaking an 'adverse incident investigation' or 'root cause analysis' it becomes obvious that no single cause decides the outcome of events. There is often a chain or sequence of failings that leads to a poor outcome and ultimately lessons need to be learned from this to prevent the risk of a similar incident reoccurring. If there are robust procedures in place that are practicable and workable in the environment, and staff are trained to act under these procedures then risks can be minimised.

The main focus of the HSAWA is to provide for securing the health and safety and welfare of anyone at work as well as protecting others against risks to health and safety during work activities. Section 3 of the Act states that every employer is under a duty to conduct their undertaking in such a way to ensure, so far as is reasonably practicable, that all employees are not exposed to risks to their health and safety. This applies as well to anyone not in their employment, but who may be affected by the employer's activities. For healthcare providers this includes visitors to NHS property such as members of the public.

Employers with five or more employees must produce a written statement of general policy for health and safety and must point out the current arrangements in place for meeting the policy. The way in which employers should structure, review and monitor policies has been significantly changed by the need to comply with regulation 3 of the Management of Health and Safety at Work Regulations, 1999a (MHSWR). This regulation introduces risk assessment in its broadest sense. It points out that significant risks must be recorded; and the approved code of practice applied. The department should only approve a change of policy where circumstances (such as the findings of a risk assessment) show the proposed change is suitable and necessary.

Economic reasons

Economic pressures can be the drivers to force individuals and or organisations to comply with health and safety guidance. This compliance is sometimes only reached following a critical incident. It is perhaps a sad reflection on a twenty-first-century society when advertisements are displayed in healthcare settings advising of firms who will represent individuals following accidents. If all practitioners adopted a proactive approach to health and safety these advertisements may become something of the past.

Employment pressures

Contracts of employment state that employees have a duty to obey the reasonable orders of the employer. They also have a duty to act with care and skill and to support any policies, procedures and guidance that employers issue to protect the health, safety and welfare of employees and others.

Professional pressures

Specific professional standards of proficiency for operating department practitioners (HPC, 2004: 3a3) highlight the practitioner's requirement to 'understand the need to establish and maintain a safe practice environment'. This includes specifically the need to be able to work safely, being able to select suitable hazard control and risk management, and to carry out techniques safely under health and safety legislation.

Likewise the Nursing and Midwifery Council (NMC) states that there is both a legal and a professional duty to care for patients and clients. Indeed within the NMC code of professional conduct, standards for conduct performance and ethics (2004) professionals are required to 'Act to identify and minimise risks to clients'.

Lord Atkin defined the duty of care when he judged the case of *Donoghue* v. *Stevenson* (House of Lords, 1932). He said that 'You must take reasonable care to avoid acts or omissions which you can reasonably foresee would be likely to injure your neighbour'. Who then is your neighbour? Your neighbour is 'persons who are closely and directly affected by your acts, and accordingly you should have thought about them possibly being affected as a result directly of your acts or omissions' (NMC, 2005).

It is important to understand the term 'reasonable' for a professional to decide whether their actions would always be viewed as being so. To determine this, the case of *Bolam* v. *Frien Hospital Management Committee* (1957) is still used. This test, the 'Bolam Test' is often used to examine the actions of any professional person; it refers to 'the test being the standard of the ordinary skilled man exercising and professing to have a special skill. The man need not possess the highest expert skill at the risk of being found negligent, it is sufficient if he exercises the skill of an ordinary competent man exercising that particular art'.

This definition is supported and clarified in the case of *Bolitho* v. *City and Hackney Health Authority* (1988). One of the judges in this case discussed 'the appropriate standard of care' and commented that 'the experts have directed their minds to the question of comparative risks and benefits and have reached a defensible conclusion on the matter'.

The case of *Wilsher* v. *Essex AHA* (1986) set the standard of reasonable care to that which patients can expect of students and junior staff. It highlighted that the standard is that of a reasonably competent practitioner and not of a student. Therefore professionals have a duty to ensure that any care that they may delegate is carried out to a reasonably competent standard. The professional remains therefore accountable for the care, the delegation of the work and for ensuring that the person to whom the work is delegated is able to undertake it.

The possible outcomes of failure to manage health and safety within organisations include:
- prosecution, fines and imprisonment
- compensation claims for damages
- loss of service or output
- replacement costs
- retraining
- loss of reputation.

Risk assessment in clinical practice

It is therefore obvious that there are many reasons why it is in both the individual's and employer's best interests to develop robust methods of detecting hazards and therefore plan risk reduction. Mandelstam (2005) recognises that the term 'risk' is stamped all over health and social care.

A hazard is something which has the potential to cause harm. A risk is the likelihood of that harm happening. Risk occurs in:
- facilities
- equipment
- procedures
- organisations.

The Manual Handling Operations Regulations (1992, updated in 1998) (MHOR) highlight three major responsibilities for employers:
- The requirement to avoid hazardous handling as far as is reasonably practicable.
- The duty to assess the risk of injury from any hazardous handling (that cannot be avoided).
- The requirement to reduce the risk to the lowest level reasonably practicable and regularly review the risk reduction measures in place.

Consider how this would apply in a day surgery unit in a paediatric hospital. In this unit, unsafe handling would have been identified since anaesthetised patients are unable to move themselves independently and therefore need help. Patients may be able to walk into the anaesthetic rooms and even climb on to surgical trolleys independently, therefore some handling risks are minimised preoperatively. This would have been identified by a standard risk assessment, covering the day-to-day operation of this unit. Nevertheless, post-operatively potentially unsafe handling will be present as the patients will be highly dependent on the perioperative staff and therefore pose risks.

To comply with the MHOR, a risk assessment must be undertaken, and a planned course of action written with the sole objective of reducing identified risks to the lowest level reasonably practicable. Caution must be used when performing standard risk assessments. In manual handling risk assessment judgements are supposed to be based on the individual need, risk and circumstances. Standard assessments and recommendations should not be used when individual situations differ from those referred to in the standard assessment. Standardised risk assessments are often unsatisfactory, individual cases must be considered, and suitable plans made (Mandelstam, 2005).

Nevertheless, in areas such as a day surgery unit in a paediatric hospital with predictable levels and activities, it is essential to identify risk prevention measures. These measures may include buying specialised lifting and handling equipment to comply with legislative requirements and reduce the risk of injury to staff and patients. Risk reduction measures must be appropriate, highlight the potential need for equipment and must also identify the need for staff training to enable them to use any equipment provided for their health and safety.

It is unlikely that the report would identify the need for this unit in a paediatric hospital to be equipped with specialised handling equipment for bariatric patients. There is no standard agreement on a definition for 'bariatric', however, the body mass index (BMI), from a practical perspective, is often the measurement of choice. Voelker (2004: 12) identified that the BMI is the most common internationally accepted standard used to measure the weight and height of people. People with a BMI greater than 40 are considered bariatric.

Nevertheless the position would be different in a theatre in a general adult hospital that regularly performed 'gastric bypass procedures' on bariatric patients. It is reasonably foreseeable that the risk of injury to both patients and perioperative staff (without acceptable risk control measures in place) would be considerable. Acceptable risk prevention measures must be suitable to meet the needs of each identified situation. Risk prevention measures include documented risk assessment plans, specialised equipment and acceptable training for staff in the area.

Risk reduction is therefore achieved by planning: identifying potential hazards and reducing these risks to the lowest level reasonably practicable. For some time, courts have stated that the term 'reasonably practicable' balances risks against costs. In the paediatric day surgery unit described above, it would be ridiculous to invest large sums of money buying specialised bariatric lifting equipment and invest significant time buying this equipment. Nevertheless in areas where high risks are identified, for example in an adult hospital, there is an associated expectation that an investment in time and finance would be substantial, suitable and sufficient to reduce identified risks.

Risk assessment in emergencies

NHS establishments normally have emergency plans in place. A cardiac arrest for example is foreseeable in a healthcare setting. Robust risk assessments therefore need to be in place to minimise risks associated with caring for patients and staff during emergencies. Neglecting to reduce risks by planning is not defensible.

Healthcare is an area that is fraught with financial constraints and the main thrust of risk management is the avoidance or reduction of risk as far as is reasonably practicable.

NHS organisations are regularly assessed against a series of specifically developed risk management standards which reflect issues arising in NHS negligence claims. Standards are laid down by Clinical Negligence Schemes for Trusts (CNST) and include those of clinical and non-clinical risk.

The Health Care Commission (HCC) exists to promote improvement in the quality of the NHS and independent (private and voluntary) healthcare across England and Wales. This Commission has introduced 'Standards for Better Health' (HCC, 2004) for NHS Trusts to replace the current system of star ratings and Trusts will be assessed against these standards instead.

The need to manage risk is well established within the NHS and introducing clinical governance provides a framework to enable this to happen.

Risk management is one of the main components of clinical governance. Clinical governance is 'a framework through which NHS organisations are accountable for continuously improving the quality of their services and safeguarding high standards of care by creating an environment in which excellence in clinical care will flourish' (Donaldson & Scally, 1998).

Risk management aims to meet the objectives of continuous improvement in the delivery of safe care as highlighted by clinical governance. To achieve this, risk assessment should encourage effective systems to develop, including policies, procedures and training for staff in reducing both clinical and non-clinical risk. Another essential ingredient is to ensure that lessons are learned from both good and poor practices.

Critical incidents

A critical incident is any unintended event which reduced or could have reduced the margin of safety for the patient (Simpson, 2000). Causes of critical incidents include areas such as lack of staff, training needs, equipment failure, and resource implications. Management of these include audits of adverse incidents to enable there to be an early identification of trends and allow resultant remedial actions to be put in place to cancel any identified risks.

In the report 'An Organisation with a Memory' specific findings included those of a patchy and incomplete picture of drug errors and/or drug reactions, with staff under-reporting incidents involving medication (DoH, 2000). As a response to this report, the National Patient Safety Agency (NPSA) was set up in 2001. The purpose of this agency is to improve the safety and quality of care for NHS patients. This was to be achieved by thorough reporting and analysing critical incidents and near misses involving patients. The NPSA suggests that assessments of risk should regularly take place in NHS organisations to prevent reoccurrences of accidents and incidents.

Carrying out risk assessments

It is important there are clear policies, procedures and local guidance which are available and cascaded to all within the workplace. For example, there are standard risk assessments that need to be conducted annually to include issues such as, heating, lighting, ventilation, floor covering and storage areas. Templates and guidance as well as being available in the workplace may be obtained directly from the Health and Safety Executive.

Risk assessment is not just a 'paper' exercise but one that will enable planning of resources both for staff time and finances to minimise any risk identified. This is not as surprising as it may first seem – people identify risk and make associated plans to reduce them in their daily lives, for example, when driving cars, walking up and down stairs or crossing roads.

The HSAWA states that a competent person must carry out risk assessments. To enable this in the workplace specialised training is often available to allow individual staff to undertake specific risk assessments in certain areas.

Nevertheless as safety is not just confined to risk assessors it is everyone's responsibility and all are required to play a part.

In the 1970s perioperative practitioners used gluteraldehyde extensively. Even though it is still used, adverse health warnings and reporting from the Health and Safety Executive have resulted in a radical decline and control of its use.

Cooper (2002) stated 'that it is common practice within NHS hospitals to use chemicals such as gluteraldehyde to disinfect medical devices such as flexible endoscopes, and some surgical instruments where the devices cannot be decontaminated by conventional methods which employ steam at high temperature.'

As gluteraldehyde falls under 'The Control of Substances Hazardous to Health Regulations 1999' (COSHH), it is subject to rigorous controls and monitoring locally. Systematic risk assessment plans will dictate how, when, where and by whom it is used.

Where operating procedures suggest there is a high exposure risk from inhalation, HSAWA guidance states that environmental monitoring must take place. A suitably qualified person must carry out this monitoring. Following this, corrective action must follow if necessary. For gluteraldehyde this includes its use being restricted to areas where identified replacement substitutes have not been found.

Within any risk assessment the objectives are to reduce the risk to the lowest level possible. For example, using a substance that requires the worker to use protective clothing should never be a first choice. A suitable risk assessment may require the staff to identify a better product which, regardless of cost, poses less risk of potential harm to the worker.

If this cannot be done, other risk reduction procedures must be adopted. For example, risk assessment may identify the need for practitioners to use the product in a well-ventilated environment. The assessment may also require the department to identify practitioners who are at high risk of harm because of their exposure or because of their state of health.

Under these circumstances, the risk assessment may recommend that staff must only be in direct contact with the product for minimum periods of time and require them to rotate into areas where the product isn't used regularly.

It is important that practitioners review all risk assessments regularly with the objective of reducing risk by either using safer products as they come into the healthcare market or by adopting safer practices.

COSHH risk assessments are integral to risk management procedures within the perioperative environment and practitioners should be aware of individual roles and responsibilities. Each employer has a statutory duty under MHSAW and the COSHH regulations to ensure there is a safe working environment for their employees.

Employer responsibilities include those of:
- assessing health and safety risks
- deciding on precautions to prevent ill health

- preventing or controlling exposure
- ensuring controls are used and maintained
- monitoring exposure
- providing information, training and supervision for staff.

Employee responsibilities are straightforward and include:

- following the rules and safe systems of work
- co-operating with monitoring and health surveillance.

Specific questions which need to be asked when performing a COSHH risk assessment are aimed at identifying who, what, where, when and why. Who is doing the assessment? Do they have the necessary skills and experience? What is being assessed? Have you the product information? Where is the assessment taking place? Are there any specific environmental issues to consider? When is the assessment to be done? Have you enough time? Finally, why is the assessment taking place? Is it to assess existing control measures or to decide on new risk prevention methods?

Always refer to local policy and procedures, seek help from risk management departments, pharmacy departments, trade union safety representatives and/or the Health and Safety Executive.

Some of the questions required to perform a COSHH risk assessment are listed below although usually many more areas of concern may be identified before adopting safe procedures.

- *Storage* – Where can the product be stored? In what container? Dark or light? What temperature is correct and suitable for storage?
- *Effects* – How is the product used, in what quantities, with what other substances may it be used?
- *Environment* – What type of environment? Does it support combustion and if so what precautions need to be taken with this? Does heat or cold affect the product, if so, how? Does the product have to be used in a well-aired area?
- *Adverse reactions* – Are there any contra-indications to the use of the product? What are the symptoms that may suggest an adverse reaction?
- *First aid* – In case of accidental ingestion, or splashes into the eye, what emergency treatment is recommended?
- *Handling issues* – Does the product need staff to wear protective clothing, or take any other special precautions, if so, what are they?

It is important to realise that personal protective clothing for an employee should be recommended only after all other risk reduction methods have been evaluated and safer products or practices have not been discovered.

Latex allergy

Natural rubber latex (NRL) is a natural substance produced by the *Hevea brasiliiens* (rubber tree). Latex, although harmless to most people, has the potential to cause ill health to susceptible individuals. A major group of people at risk from latex allergy are healthcare workers, especially staff working in operating departments. This is mainly because of the length of time that they may be exposed to latex through the use of latex gloves and other equipment in the environment which contains latex.

The use of gloves has increased significantly over the past decade, mainly because of a growing concern over infection control and personal protection.

In 1996, The Medical Devices Agency (now part of The Medicines and Healthcare Product Regulatory Agency) stated that powdered latex gloves have higher extractable protein levels. They recommended that gloves should have the lowest levels possible of these extractable proteins. Following this and other guidance, Trusts are required to ensure that exposure to latex is limited and control measures taken from both national and local guidance must be adopted.

In May 2005, the National Patient Safety Agency also advised all NHS organisations in England to take better steps to protect patients with latex allergy. Control measures associated with the use of NRL involve a multifaceted team approach which includes staff from occupational health departments, infection control departments, clinical procurement and supplies departments as well as departmental employees and representatives from patient 'user groups'. The objectives of a team approach are to produce protocols that aim to minimise risks to employees and patients to the lowest levels possible. As with all other risk control measures it is important that any risk assessments and plans are reviewed regularly to see if the plans can be adapted and risks negated completely.

Conclusion

In conclusion and in line with all recommended guidance made to improve our own safety and that of others, practitioners need to adopt the following:

- Collect and analyse information on adverse incidents.
- Adopt a 'safety' as opposed to a 'blame' culture.
- Learn lessons from past experiences.
- Ensure that where risks exist, control measures are in place, national goals specified and mechanisms are put in place to monitor risk reduction outcomes.

In 2001 the National Patient Safety Agency estimated that 850 000 incidents and errors occurred every year. Practitioners need to recognise that this figure is unacceptable. Elcoat (2000) has stated that dissatisfaction with the present is the engine of change; with due care and attention to all aspects of risk reduction and prevention all practitioners can be part of that change.

REFERENCES

Bolam v. *Frien Hospital Management Committee*. (1957). All ER 118.

Bolitho v. *City and Hackney Health Authority*. (1988). AC 232.

Cooper, Y. (2002). *House of Commons Hansard Written Answers for 31st January 2002*. Available at: www.parliament.the−stationery-office.co.uk/pa/cm200102/cmhansrd/vo020131/text. . .(Accessed 24 January 2006).

Department of Health. (1974). *Health and Safety at Work Act*. London: HMSO.

Department of Health. (1998). *Manual Handling Operations Regulations*. London: HMSO.

Department of Health. (1999a). *Management of Health and Safety at Work Regulations*. London: HMSO.

Department of Health. (1999b). *Control of Substances Hazardous to Health*. London: HMSO.

Department of Health. (2000). *An Organisation with a Memory: Report of an Expert Group on Learning from Adverse events in the NHS*. London: HMSO.

Donaldson, L. J. & Scally, G. (1998). *Clinical Governance: Quality in the New NHS*. London: HMSO.

Donoghue (or *McAlister*) v. *Stevenson*. (1932). All ER Rep 1; (1932) ac 562; House of Lords.

Elcoat, C. (2000). Unpublished presentation delivered at The Institute of Child Health, Royal Liverpool Children's NHS Trust, Liverpool.

Health Care Commission. (2004). *Standards for Better Health*. London: Commission for Healthcare Audit and Inspection.

Health Professionals Council. (2004). *Standards of Proficiency − Operating Department Practitioners*. London: Park House.

Mandelstam, M. (2005). Risk, law and professional good practice and the avoidance of blanket policies. *The Column*, **17.3**, 2005.

Nursing and Midwifery Council. (2004). *Code of Professional Conduct: Standards for Conduct, Performance and Ethics*. London: NMC.

Nursing and Midwifery Council. (2005). *Duty of Care*. Available at: www.nmc-uk.org/nmc/main/advice/dutyOfCare.html (Accessed 24 January 2006).

Simpson, M. (2000). *Audit of Critical Incident Reporting − Raising the Standard*. London: The Royal College of Anaesthetists.

The Medical Devices Agency. (1996). *May Bulletin* (now renamed Medicines and Health Care Products Regulatory Agency). Available at: http://www.mhra.gov.uk (Accessed 24 January 2006).

The National Patient Safety Agency. (2001). Cited in Section 8, Risk Management Liverpool, National Prescribing Centre.

The National Patient Safety Agency. (2005). *Protecting People with Allergy Associated with Latex* (26th May bulletin). Available at: www.npsa.nhs.uk (Accessed 24 January 2006).

Voelker, M. (2004). Quality of life in gastric bypass patients. Unpublished presentation at the Madigan Army Medical Centre, Tacoma, WA.

Wilsher v. *Essex Area Health Board*. (1986). All ER 801.

3

ECG monitoring in the recovery area

Chris Jones and Trish Finn

Key Learning Points
- Understand the reasons why a patient's heart may develop rhythm problems in theatre
- Understand the reason for the correct positioning of ECG leads
- Appreciate the causes of intra-operative changes in ECG
- Understand the nature and ECG signatures of major rhythm problems
- Understand the nature and ECG signatures of changes in cardiac perfusion

When a patient is recovering from an anaesthetic, careful observation is required in order to note developing problems at an early stage.

Meticulous clinical observation of the patient can distinguish early problems associated with respiration and with circulation. One of the most important pieces of equipment to assist in patient assessment is the electrocardiograph (ECG) monitor.

The ECG was a breakthrough in the assessment of patients which we often take for granted. As a non-invasive and painless observation tool its information is crucial to the safe delivery of patients from surgery and anaesthetic.

This chapter will look at the nature of ECG monitoring, what the monitor can tell you about the patient and what it cannot.

Some common problems of cardiac function will then be described and their ECG signature discussed.

The information that ECG gives us

An ECG gives a graphic description of electrical events in the heart – an electrical signature of cardiac function, if you will. It does not measure any mechanical function of the heart, such as the pumping action. Mechanical function will mostly result from the electrical events, but there are circumstances where it may not.

This leads us to the first conclusion about interpreting information from the monitor. As an adjunct to your thinking about and observing your patient, ECG monitoring is extremely useful. As a replacement for your observation and careful thought, the ECG is next to useless. Intelligent observation of the patient is paramount and the information from the ECG is an invaluable component of that observation, but it is not the only information.

You should always observe your patient in the round and use the ECG as another piece of information on which to base your thinking. If you are worried about your patient, you ought not to wait until an abnormality in the ECG exists before drawing attention to it. This then is the first lesson

Core Topics in Operating Department Practice: Anaesthesia and Critical Care, eds. Brian Smith, Paul Rawling, Paul Wicker and Chris Jones. Published by Cambridge University Press. © Cambridge University Press 2007.

of ECG interpretation: *treat the patient and not the monitor.*

The relevance of ECG information to the patient in theatre

There can hardly be a more appropriate place than a theatre recovery area for an ECG monitor. Patients are waking up from surgery which is often prolonged. They will have been given large doses of anaesthetic gases and drugs. They may have lost some blood. Their breathing may have been commandeered by the anaesthetist and they may have undergone a prolonged period of mechanical ventilation. Their treatment in theatre might have resulted in shifts in electrolyte concentration like potassium, sodium and calcium. They might have become cold while on the operating table.

All of these events may cause changes in the pattern of the patient's ECG. As the patient re-emerges into consciousness these changes may signal danger and may require intervention at an early stage to protect the wellbeing of the patient.

Special patients

It goes without saying that all patients are at risk following surgery and all should be closely observed. Nevertheless, some patients should make the wary recovery practitioner especially careful. Among these patients will be the very elderly patient or the very young patient. Also on the list will be the patient who has been deemed an anaesthetic risk due to respiratory or cardiac insufficiency. Likewise extra attention should be paid to the patient who has a pre-existing medical condition such as hypertension or especially diabetes. Patients who look as though they lack physiological reserve such as the cachectic patient will be of special concern. As will the patients who are operated on as an emergency measure. All of these patients should be given extra attention.

Attaching the patient to the monitor

Most monitors have three or sometimes five leads which are attached to sticky pads which are placed on the patient's chest (Figure 3.1). Hairy chests or a wet surface on the chest caused, for example, by sweat may well cause a problem with adhesion. Most modern pads have a rough pad to remove skin debris and give a better grip.

The cables leading to the pads are colour coded and often have on them the location of their placement:

Red – RA – Right arm
Yellow – LA – Left arm
Green – LL – Left leg (though often placed around the area of the cardiac apex).

In the centre of the pads is a small amount of gel, which improves the electrical contact.

If the connection of the cables to the pad or the pad to the skin is compromised, the monitor might indicate some alarming but insignificant changes. The trace may wander or go flat and the monitor might alarm. This situation can be annoying to the patient and must be resolved by proper placement of pads and leads.

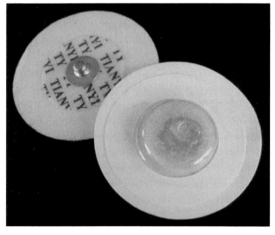

ECG lead electrodes

Figure 3.1 ECG lead electrodes.

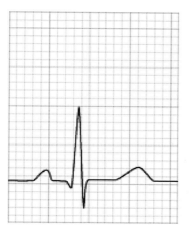

Normal ECG lead II

Figure 3.2 Normal sinus complex.

When the leads are properly fixed the monitor will generally offer the option of lead I, II or III for observation.

Most recovery staff prefer lead II as the individual elements of the ECG; the P, the QRS and the T waves can be clearly seen from this perspective. This is because the average angle of flow of electricity in a normal heart is towards lead II. This gives the complex a positive appearance. This means that the ECG complex points up from the flat baseline. In lead II it is predominantly upright. (See Figure 3.2.)

Setting the alarms on the monitor

Monitors are usually supplied with alarm systems which will alert you to any changes in the patient's trace. These are very useful devices but they again should carry a caution. Despite the fact that the alarms will alert you to alterations in the patient's ECG this should not encourage you to observe the patient less. Rather it should encourage you to observe the patient more. If the alarm is frequently reacting to insignificant changes caused by, for example, the patient moving, then the noise

might disturb and worry the patient unnecessarily. On the other hand it could alert you to the first changes in the patient's condition which could mean deterioration.

Reasons a patient's heart may develop rhythm problems

The patient might be old and have an underlying subclinical heart condition. The strain of surgery may be enough to reveal it and cause problems.
- Stimulation of the sympathetic or parasympathetic nervous system might speed or slow the heart
- Ischaemic heart disease
- Hypotension or hypertension
- Anaesthetic agents might cause changes
- Catecholamine release such as adrenaline might speed the heart up
- The patient may be hypoxic or hypercarbic
- The patient's electrolyte balance might be disturbed
- The patient might be on drugs which speed or slow the heart such as beta-blockers or digoxin.

Clinical assessment of the patient in recovery

A constant assessment should be kept on the patient's airway. If the patient is still drowsy they might not be able to protect it. Excess salivation or nausea may further threaten it. The patient must be protected from inhaling fluid.

Their breathing should also be under constant review. This should include observations of the patient's respiratory rate, the volume of gas entering the lungs, the pattern of the patient's breathing and the noises which the patient is making.

The feel of a patient's pulse is also a useful observation. The strength of the patient's pulse will give information that the monitor alone will not, such as how full the circulation is.

Interpreting the ECG

The ECG charts the language of the heart. Like learning all languages reading ECGs is a matter of exposure, time, patience, practice and not being ashamed of asking for assistance when you are unsure.

Before we begin to analyse what might be abnormal on an ECG, let us review what the components of a normal complex look like. There are innumerable textbooks and websites which describe the normal ECG but a brief recap here will be worthwhile.

The first thing to say is that the ECG is a graphical representation of an electrical event which is occurring in the heart. As such it is a graph with different axes. Along the horizontal axis is measured time in seconds.

On the vertical axis the ECG measures voltage. Heart muscle generates voltage in direct proportion to the amount of muscle in the corresponding chamber's wall. The taller the peak of the graph, the more voltage the chamber is generating and therefore the more muscle is in that chamber.

For traditional reasons which go back to the origins of ECG recording, the ECG complex is divided into components which correspond to electrical events going on inside the heart. These are listed as P, Q, R, S and T. Going back to our original picture of a normal complex (Figures 3.3 and 3.4):

The P wave represents electrical activity in the atria which usually precedes atrial contraction. It is not very high in voltage because the muscle walls of the atria are thin.

The Q, R and S waves represent ventricular electrical activity which usually precedes ventricular contraction. This is a high-voltage phenomenon because the muscle walls of the ventricles are relatively thick.

The T wave represents ventricular repolarisation: the resetting of the ventricle ready for the next firing.

In addition to the waves formed by the heart's activity, it is also important to understand that the spaces between the waves can be of significance. Let us look at the complex once more.

The **P-R interval** represents the length of time (measured on the horizontal axis) that atrial electrical activity takes to be conducted down to the ventricles. In various conditions, notably in atrioventricular dissociation (or 'heart blocks') this interval can extend and look abnormal.

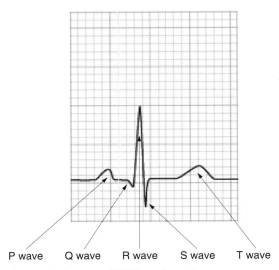

P wave   Q wave   R wave   S wave   T wave

Figure 3.3 Elements of PQRS configuration.

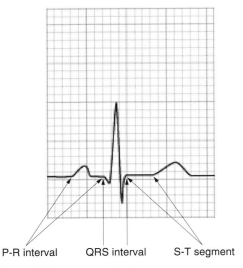

P-R interval   QRS interval   S-T segment

Figure 3.4 Intervals and timings.

The **QRS interval** represents the time taken for conduction within and between the ventricles. Damaged intraventricular conduction pathways, drugs or congenital conditions can extend this time, and in these circumstances the QRS interval will lengthen.

The S-T segment can start to look abnormal where there are problems with the perfusion of ventricular muscle. It may start to look depressed, that is to say it may fail to come back to its baseline after the S wave (see below) or it may elevate. In this latter case it will appear to 'balloon' up between the S wave and the T wave (see below).

Classifying ECG disturbance

A couple of general classifications might be a good place to start.

   Problems of rhythm
   Problems of perfusion.

Problems of rhythm

The more practice with ECGs the easier they become. But to start one off you should ask a series of standard questions and adhere to a system.

How does the patient appear?

This might seem like a strange question to ask, but it goes to the heart of ECG monitoring. If the person is recovering well from anaesthetic and is sitting up talking to you, it is unlikely that a flat ECG trace is asystole! Remember at all times, the machine is only there to help you think.

What is the ventricular rate?

The monitor will mostly count this for you and will display the rate as a numerical value on the screen. Nevertheless it is useful not to take this for granted. There may well be occasions where the ventricular rate is not the same as that shown on the ECG screen. An abnormally high T wave for instance might cause the machine to double count the ECG rate because it perceives the T wave as another R wave. Taking the patient's pulse will reveal the real rate of the patient's heart and listening with a stethoscope will confirm the finding. *Treat the patient not the monitor.*

Sudden changes in the patient's heart rate – speeding or slowing, should always be given very serious attention especially where other haemo-dynamic effects become apparent such as falling blood pressure or patient distress. Even gradual changes in the trend of a patient's heart rate should be noted. Pain and discomfort may first come to the attention of the recovery staff by alterations in heart rate. Tachycardia and sweating are classic signs that a patient's pain control is slipping.

Are the complexes regular or irregular?

If there is an irregularity, is it a regular irregularity or is it an irregular? This might seem like a strange question to ask, but the answer to this question will reveal several interesting points.

The heart rate may speed up and slow down in time to the patient's respirations. This is quite normal.

A rhythm might be regular, but with occasional missed beats.

If the patient has fibrillating atria, the result may be a rhythm that seemingly has no regularity.

Do P waves precede all QRS complexes?

Absent P waves might suggest ectopic beats which may be atrial or ventricular in origin. With atrial ectopics the QRS would be narrow and the P wave may be abnormally shaped (Figure 3.5). With ventricular ectopics the P wave is absent and the complex is broad and bizarre.

Are there more P waves than QRS complexes?

If not it may be the case that some P waves are not being conducted to the ventricles because the atria's impulses are being blocked on the way along the conduction pathway.

Problems of rhythm can be further subdivided into narrow complex rhythm disturbance and broad complex rhythm disturbance.

Problems of perfusion can be further subdivided into changes suggesting ischaemia and changes suggesting infarction.

Is the QRS broad or narrow?

By and large, if a rhythm has a narrow QRS it is likely that it originates from a point above the ventricles.

If the impulse originates further down in the ventricles the QRS will take on a broader shape.

The fact that the impulse is emerging from the ventricle means that something very abnormal is going on.

Narrow complex rhythm disturbances

The fact that a QRS complex is narrow strongly suggests that it originates from above the level of the ventricle, at the SA mode, from within the atrium or at the junction of the atrium and the ventricle.

Slow rates

The problem might be that the patient's heart has slowed down to an extent that compromises his circulation. A slow heart beat can be a normal finding in a person who is young and/or fit.

A person whose rate has dropped suddenly or from a normal pre-operating rate should be further examined and have attention drawn to this event.

It could be that pre-operative drugs or anaesthetic agents have reduced the heart rate to an alarming extent.

Fast rates

If the problem is a heart rate which is too fast, then a different set of problems might be at play. Pain alone might speed up the heart rate, and the increase in speed on the ECG monitor may be the heart's way of requesting assistance and pain relief (Figure 3.6).

The problem might also be more severe. If the heart rate dramatically increases then circulatory disturbance might precipitate a critical drop in blood pressure.

Causes of narrow complex tachycardia might include re-entry tachycardias, where the atria stimulate their own acceleration due to backward flow of impulse. This is often described as supraventricular tachycardia, that is to say it emerges from above the ventricle. Here are examples of such a rhythm:

• Atrial flutter: where the atria depolarise at a rate faster than the ventricles can respond (Figure 3.7). This cardiac problem is characterised by a 'saw

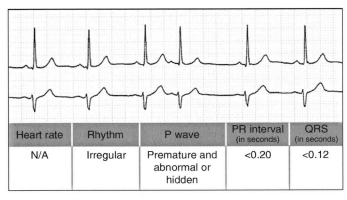

Heart rate	Rhythm	P wave	PR interval (in seconds)	QRS (in seconds)
N/A	Irregular	Premature and abnormal or hidden	<0.20	<0.12

Figure 3.5 Premature atrial contraction.

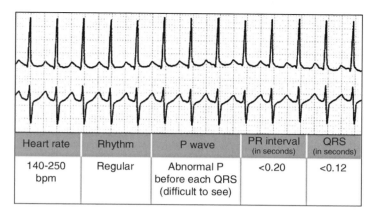

Heart rate	Rhythm	P wave	PR interval (in seconds)	QRS (in seconds)
140-250 bpm	Regular	Abnormal P before each QRS (difficult to see)	<0.20	<0.12

Figure 3.6 Atrial tachycardia.

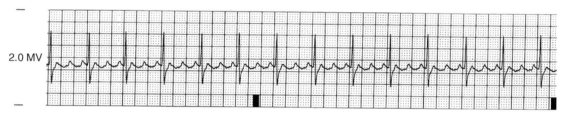

Figure 3.7 Atrial flutter.

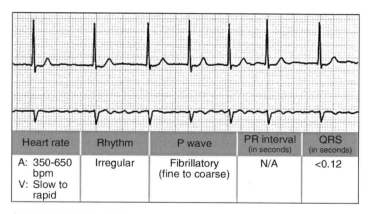

Heart rate	Rhythm	P wave	PR interval (in seconds)	QRS (in seconds)
A: 350-650 bpm V: Slow to rapid	Irregular	Fibrillatory (fine to coarse)	N/A	<0.12

Figure 3.8 Atrial fibrillation.

toothed' appearance of the space between the complexes which comprises of the extra P waves.

• Atrial fibrillation: this is a very irregular rhythm which can be very rapid (Figure 3.8). It results from the disorganised fibrillation of the atria and the absence of any organised atrial depolarisation. The fact that there is no organised depolarisation means that there is an absence of P wave and the fibrillation of the atria can give the ECG baseline a curious wrinkled appearance. These arrhythmias might look somewhat similar on the screen and require further investigations to distinguish the differences between the compacted QRS complexes, but where the patient's blood pressure drops because of a compromised cardiac function cardio-version might be considered as a matter of urgency.

Other treatments that might be used to control tachycardias of atrial origin are:-
* β blockers
* Verapamil
* Adenosine.

Broad complex rhythm disturbances

If you observe nestled among a screen of sinus rhythm a broad, bizarre complex which has no pre-ceding P wave and a pause afterwards, you might infer that a ventricular event has taken place, because of the broad nature of the complex (Figure 3.9).

If there is just one complex then this is likely to be a ventricular ectopic or premature beat.

Often these are normal and need raise little more interest than a raised eyebrow. The causes of ectopic beats are what concern the recovery staff. These can be:
* hypokalaemia: this could be a problem where the patient has been given a dose of potassium depleting diuretic
* hypoxia: if the patient's lungs are not taking in enough oxygen or if oxygen is not being delivered to cardiac muscle in enough quantity
* blood pH abnormalities: even if the patient is taking in enough oxygen there may be a problem with the lungs failing to excrete enough carbon dioxide. This could result in alterations in the blood's acidity which could in turn result in the formation of ectopics.

Where ectopics start to come in clusters, or to space normal beats at the rate of 1:3 or 1:2 or where they change shape indicating a change in the origin of this activity on the ventricular wall, then curiosity should turn to concern, and the problem should be reported and investigated (Figures 3.10 and 3.11).

Where one broad and bizarre beat follows another in rapid succession and where no P wave is visible then the patient has developed ventricular tachycardia (Figure 3.12).

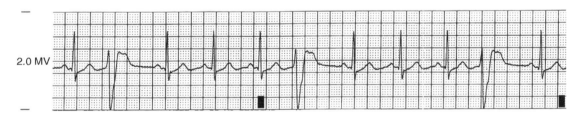

Figure 3.9 Premature ventricular contraction.

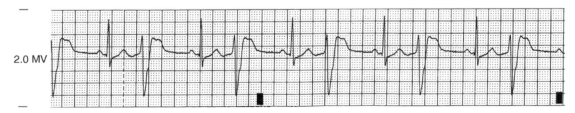

Figure 3.10 Ventricular bigeminy.

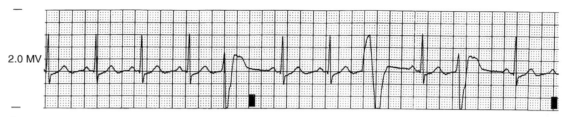

Figure 3.11 Multi-focal premature ventricular contractions.

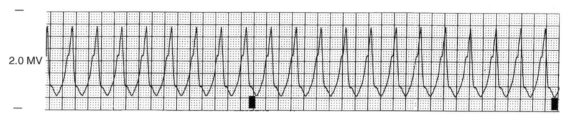

Figure 3.12 Ventricular tachycardia.

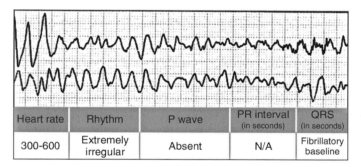

Heart rate	Rhythm	P wave	PR interval (in seconds)	QRS (in seconds)
300-600	Extremely irregular	Absent	N/A	Fibrillatory baseline

Figure 3.13 Ventricular fibrillation.

This is a life-threatening arrhythmia and should be treated as an emergency.

Draw attention to any case of broad complex tachycardia as a matter of the highest urgency. Often, though not always, the patient will lose consciousness and blood pressure. Left untreated, this rhythm may degenerate into ventricular fibrillation (Figure 3.13).

Ventricular fibrillation
This is almost the complete absence of any rhythm and represents the heart in a state of electrical chaos. Cardiac output will have fallen to nothing and the patient will lose consciousness. The patient will be without any pulse. Unless the heart is restarted, the patient will die. All observation of the patient should be aimed at preventing this state of affairs. If it does happen, then prompt and efficient resuscitation should be administered, according to your hospital's policies and Advanced Life Support guidelines.

Conduction problems which might lead to rhythm changes
The heart has a sophisticated system of conduction pathways which orchestrate the unified contraction of the heart's muscle. Sometimes this conduction system can dysfunction and produce symptoms

ranging from the trivial to the catastrophic. All of these problems can be precipitated by surgery or the drugs used in anaesthesia, and they can all be clearly seen on an ECG monitor. Traditionally, because the conduction system does not pass on the conduction of impulse, these failures to conduct are called heart blocks. A more scientific description might be atrioventricular (AV) dissociation.

These are divided into types or degrees of AV dissociation. How are these degrees of AV dissociation classified?

First degree AV dissociation

If the AV node takes too long to conduct an impulse from the atria to the ventricle it produces an abnormality of ECG. The gap between the P wave and the QRS is too long and produces the type of abnormality shown in Figure 3.14.

Here we can see that the P wave is too far from the QRS. This abnormality is usually symptom free and is of little clinical significance.

Other examples of AV dissociation are not so innocent. Second degree AV dissociation can be more serious. This type of conduction problem is further divided into two types (Figures 3.15 and 3.16):

Second degree AV dissociation (Wenkebach phenomenon)

This conduction disorder describes a situation where there is a progressive widening of the gap between the P wave and the QRS. When the gap has become pronounced a QRS complex will be dropped and the gap between the P wave and the QRS goes back to normal.

Second degree AV dissociation (Mobitz type II)

In this conduction abnormality, there is a normal relationship between the P wave and the QRS, however it sometimes or consistently requires more than one P wave to trigger a QRS.

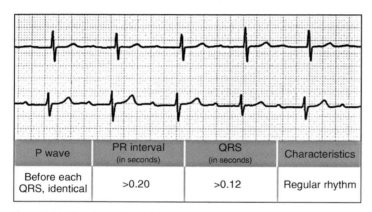

P wave	PR interval (in seconds)	QRS (in seconds)	Characteristics
Before each QRS, identical	>0.20	>0.12	Regular rhythm

Figure 3.14 First degree heart block.

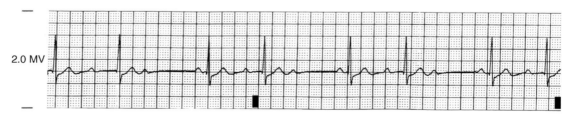

Figure 3.15 Wenkebach phenomenon. Mobitz type I atrioventricular dissociation.

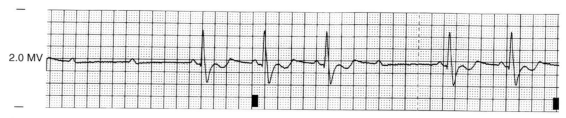

Figure 3.16 Mobitz type II atrioventricular dissociation.

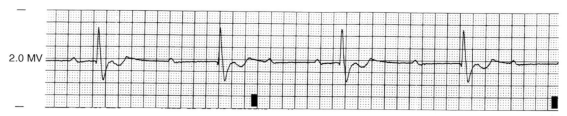

Figure 3.17 Complete atrioventricular dissociation.

Third degree AV dissociation

In this instance there is a complete breakdown of communication between the atria and the ventricles (Figure 3.17). This gives rise to an ECG where the P waves bear no relationship to the QRS and seem to be scattered across the ECG baseline randomly. The QRS also often has a broad appearance because the impulse may originate from low in the ventricles. The P wave rate will be regular and the QRS may also be regular, but the heart rate will be very slow.

Problems of perfusion

Inadequate perfusion of the myocardium with oxygenated blood due to ischaemia, anaemia or hypoxia may cause a characteristic change in the ECG complex on the screen.

The T wave may become inverted or the space between the S wave and the T wave can develop a curious sagging appearance (Figure 3.18).

This can suggest that the heart is struggling because its oxygen supply is inadequate and this must be brought to attention. Extra oxygen may be required in the form of high-flow

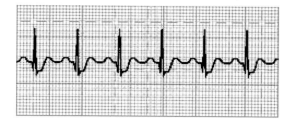

Figure 3.18 ST segment depression.

supplements of high-concentration oxygen. Oxygen-carrying capacity might be required in the form of blood transfusion. Drugs such as nitrates might be needed to dilate the coronary arteries.

If on the other hand, the patient's coronary arteries have been completely blocked rather than just partially occluded, this will leave its own signature on the patient's ECG picture.

Instead of the patient's ST segment coming down to the baseline it may exhibit a bizarre ballooning up of the ST complex called ST elevation (Figure 3.19).

Neither of these ECG changes should be ignored and should be reported as soon as possible,

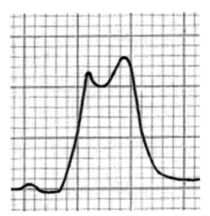

Figure 3.19 ST segment elevation.

especially where circulatory disturbance is suspected due to alterations in blood pressure or where the patient develops a pale, clammy or shocked appearance.

This could herald the development of myocardial infarction and should be treated with urgency. If this is a developing infarction, then delay could mean that the heart muscle dies and the heart's function is irredeemably compromised. It could even mean that the patient dies.

The first requirement will be a formal 12-lead ECG to locate the source of the problem and to confirm the monitor's findings. While this is performed the doctor who administered the anaesthetic should be informed of this turn of events.

Conclusion

Clinical staff who work in a recovery area have a legal and moral duty to develop a familiarity with the basics of monitoring the patient through an ECG machine. This will help staff to anticipate and deal with developing problems in the patient.

Perseverance and dedication are required to develop a working knowledge of rhythm disturbances, but this will be amply rewarded in terms of patient safety and comfort.

Acknowledgements

The authors would like to express their thanks to the following who very kindly allowed their images of ECGs to be used in the preparation of this chapter:
- GE Health Care, Hatfield, Herts., England
- Dr Dusan Staier of the University Medical Centre, Ljubljana
- BMJ publishing Group Ltd 2006 for the use of their ECGs found at www.besttreatments.co.uk
- Johan Van Schalkwyk at www.anaesthetist.com

BIBLIOGRAPHY

In this chapter we have relied on many sources for information. There are many texts we found particularly useful but the one we found most informative is:

The Only EKG Book You Will Ever Need by Malcolm S. Thaler (2002). Lippincott Williams and Wilkins.
For the rest, the most useful resources we found were, inevitably, on the Web. Here are some of the most useful links:
1. www.skillstat.com/Flash/ECG_Sim_022505.html
   This short programme permits you to familiarise yourself with ECGs and then to test yourself.
2. medstat.med.utah.edu/kw/ecg/animations/ecg.html
   This programme allows you to look at the normal ECG from the perspective of different leads.
3. medlib.med.utah.edu/kw/ecg/image_index/index.html
   This website gives innumerable pictures of different ECGs and the problems caused by different conditions.
4. www.blaufuss.org/
   On this website is a short demonstration of the effect on the ECG of changes in cardiac axis. This is the quickest way we have discovered to understand the concept. There is also a tutorial on atrial tachycardias which has excellent graphics.

The use of cricoid pressure during anaesthesia

Cheryl Wayne-Conroy

Key Learning Points

- Related anatomy and physiology of the upper respiratory tract
- Managing regurgitation and vomiting during anaesthesia
- The technique for applying cricoid pressure during anaesthesia
- Training practitioners to apply cricoid pressure

Sellick's Manoeuvre involves 'pressure being externally exerted on the cricoid cartilage during anaesthetic induction in an attempt to prevent regurgitated stomach contents entering the lungs. This is effective due to the cricoid cartilage being a circular structure and when depressed occludes the oesophagus. Utilised during emergency situations when the patient may not have been fasted, even with fasting still has the potential to have maintained gastric contents (Smith & Williams, 2004: 204)

Dr Brian Sellick first defined this technique for applying cricoid pressure during general anaesthesia in 1961.

In 1950 the Association of Anaesthetists of Great Britain and Ireland (AAGBI) examined deaths caused by pulmonary aspiration of gastric contents, which had long been recognised as a risk during anaesthesia. Forty-three deaths had been caused by regurgitation and aspiration. By 1956, there were a further 110 deaths attributable to aspiration of gastric contents (Sinclair & Luxton, 2005).

According to Owen *et al.* (2002), pressing on the lower part of the larynx to occlude the oesophagus was reported in medical literature as far back as the eighteenth century. In 1774, a doctor named Alexander Monro described an early form of cricoid pressure during experiments on cadaver subjects. The more modern technique still used today was described in 1961 by Dr Brian Sellick, an anaesthetist working in London. Dr Sellick described using a 'simple manoeuvre' to prevent regurgitation of stomach contents into the larynx during induction of anaesthesia and intubation (please refer to Chapter 11). Before this technique was developed, anaesthesia was induced in an upright position to help provide airway protection (Sinclair & Luxton, 2005).

Anatomy and physiology

The close relationship between the anatomy of the upper respiratory and the gastrointestinal tracts aids the employment of this technique. Figure 4.1 shows the anatomical position of the trachea and the oesophagus.

The trachea is the tube-like portion of the respiratory tract that connects the larynx (voice box) with the bronchial parts of the lungs. The oesophagus is the tube-like portion that carries food from the oropharynx (mouth) to the stomach;

Core Topics in Operating Department Practice: Anaesthesia and Critical Care, eds. Brian Smith, Paul Rawling, Paul Wicker and Chris Jones. Published by Cambridge University Press. © Cambridge University Press 2007.

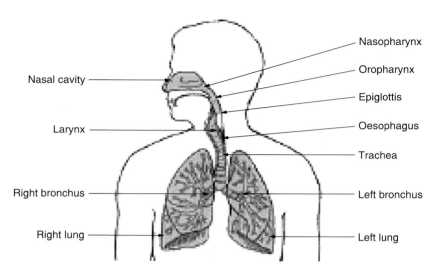

Figure 4.1 The anatomical position of the trachea and the oesophagus.

it lies just behind the trachea and the larynx. The openings of the oesophagus and the larynx are close together in the throat (Amersham Health Medical Dictionary, 2005).

The specialised junction between the oesophagus and the stomach, the oesophagogastric junction, acts as a sphincter or valve to prevent stomach contents from returning to the oesophagus after entering the stomach. When the conscious level is lowered this junction works less efficiently and if the pressure within the stomach – the intragastric pressure – is greater than the closing pressure of the sphincter then regurgitation may occur (Mijumbi, 1994).

Regurgitation is different from the act of vomiting. Regurgitation is passive and occurs because of a reduced or altered level of consciousness and awareness. Vomiting however is active and usually occurs at a normal or near-normal level of consciousness. When the vomiting centre in the human brain (which is found within the brain stem) detects a variation from 'normal', for example, a feeling of dizziness, it launches the vomiting sequence. The trachea automatically closes and the abdominal wall and diaphragm muscles tighten suddenly and forcefully.

Acidic stomach contents entering the lungs can prove to be fatal. Death usually results from pneumonitis, an inflammation and infection of the lungs otherwise known as Mendelson's syndrome. This was initially recognised during anaesthesia for obstetric surgery but is now generally used to describe all incidences involving gastric aspiration.

Mendelson's syndrome was first described by Curtis Lester Mendelson, a twentieth-century American obstetrician and gynaecologist. Mendelson described aspiration of gastric contents occurring during periods of altered consciousness. The patient develops symptoms of a cough, wheezing, cyanosis (blue colouring around the lips, ear lobes and nail beds), dyspnoea (difficulty in breathing) and tachypnoea (fast shallow breathing). The pathological changes that occur consist of a chemical tracheobronchitis and pneumonia because of gastric acid. Secondary bacterial infection also manifests itself following aspiration.

Regurgitation is an increased risk where emergency inductions and intubations are required, where the patient may not have been fasted adequately before surgery. Reasons which increase the risk of aspiration even further include, for example:

- patients who have a hiatus hernia (where part of the stomach pushes up into the lower chest through a defect in the diaphragm leading to an increased potential for gastric reflux into the oesophagus)
- patients in the late stages of pregnancy (where the position of the foetus causes gastric reflux)
- patients who have suffered traumatic injury (traumatic injury slows digestion and stomach emptying)
- cases of severe head injury (unconscious patients have no natural ability to protect their airway from regurgitated stomach contents)
- patients who are intoxicated with drug or alcohol use (deeply unconscious patients through misuse of alcohol and drugs are unable to protect their own airway naturally from regurgitated stomach contents)
- any other clinical situation where gastric emptying is delayed.

There are also emergency situations where the use of cricoid pressure is not advised, including for example, active vomiting, unstable cervical spine injury and cricotracheal injury. Cricoid pressure is a part of an anaesthetic technique known as Rapid Sequence Induction (RSI). RSI is often carried out where gastric emptying is delayed. Conditions such as these present difficulties for anaesthetists and healthcare providers and wherever possible alternatives to general anaesthesia may be sought.

Applying cricoid pressure

When applying cricoid pressure, the cricoid cartilage (the only complete ring of cartilage in the trachea) is manually pushed back against the cervical spine at the level of the C5/C6 vertebrae to occlude the oesophagus, which lies directly beneath the trachea. All other cartilage rings contained in the trachea are made up of semicircles and are therefore not suitable for use in this technique. The manoeuvre is achieved by using the thumb and index finger usually of the right hand to compress the cricoid cartilage (Figure 4.2). The right hand is normally used because of the design of many anaesthetic rooms in the UK. The anaesthetic equipment is usually located on the patient's right or at the head end of the patient trolley/bed and the anaesthetic assistant is mainly positioned to the right side of the patient, making use of the right hand naturally more effective than the left. Nevertheless, dependent on the situation, the use of either hand is equally effective.

A formally qualified and experienced anaesthetic practitioner is required to apply 'effective' cricoid pressure. According to Anaesthesia UK (2004), the following components are essential for undertaking RSI:

- Tilting table/trolley
- Full monitoring of blood pressure, ECG, pulse oximetery and End Tidal CO_2 monitor
- Suction ready (switched to the ON position and placed under the patient's pillow)
- Fully trained assistant
- IV access
- Pre-oxygenation for 3 minutes

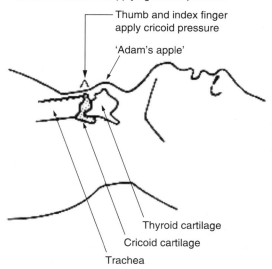

Sellick's manoeuvre, applying cricoid pressure

Thumb and index finger apply cricoid pressure

'Adam's apple'

Thyroid cartilage

Cricoid cartilage

Trachea

Figure 4.2 Applying cricoid pressure.

- Suitable sleep dose of induction agent
- Cricoid pressure
- Suxamethonium®
- Laryngoscopy and intubation
- Check position
- Secure tube.

If conscious, the practitioner should tell the patient about the procedure before induction. The practitioner must firstly find and identify the anatomy of the cricoid cartilage and position fingers lightly over the correct area, telling the patient the reasons for these actions.

The patient is pre-oxygenated for a full 3 minutes, to create a reservoir of oxygen in the lungs. This provides the anaesthetist with the maximum time available to intubate the patient without compromising the patient's oxygen saturation. Forced ventilation using a Bag Valve Mask (BVM) technique is contraindicated in patients who are at high risk of gastric aspiration as there is a risk of forcing air into the stomach (causing possible gastric distension) thus increasing the likelihood of regurgitation. Cricoid pressure is also recommended for mask ventilation during cardio pulmonary resuscitation (CPR), if there are two or more rescuers, to reduce gastric distension and consequent regurgitation (MERCK, 2004).

The anaesthetist then gives Thiopentone® or Etomidate® – depending on the patient's cardiovascular stability. Etomidate® may be an alternative if the patient is losing large volumes of blood, or has underlying cardiovascular problems, as it does not drop the blood pressure as rapidly as Thiopentone®. Both these drugs act to induce narcosis (sleep). Cricoid pressure is applied gradually as the patient closes their eyes and the patient's 'lash reflex' has decreased. The lash reflex is used by anaesthetists to decide if the patient is unconscious, by gently touching the eyelash and establishing if the patient's eyes blink. When blinking is absent, the anaesthetist will then give the depolarising muscle relaxant Suxamethonium® to achieve total muscle paralysis in readiness for intubation. Suxamethonium® is a short-acting muscle relaxant which has a rapid

onset of about 45 seconds, the effects of which last about 2–5 minutes (Yentis *et al.*, 2004).

Cricoid pressure should not be removed until the anaesthetic practitioner is directed to do so by the anaesthetist. Removal of pressure usually occurs once the patient has been intubated, the cuff of the endotracheal tube is inflated and the anaesthetist is satisfied that the tube is in the correct position. If pressure is removed too early the patient could be at risk of regurgitation and aspiration.

The practitioner should be ready to release the pressure if the patient shows signs of vomiting. During vomiting the patient may be prone to oesophageal rupture if cricoid pressure is not removed immediately. The stomach is normally relaxed, but when squeezed forcefully by the abdominal wall, it ejects any food or fluid up through the oesophagus and vomiting occurs. A pressure over 60 cm of H_2O can develop which may tear the oesophagus at the oesophagogastric junction if the oesophagus is occluded because of cricoid pressure. Oesophageal rupture is normally fatal to the patient. If vomiting occurs during induction of anaesthesia and the use of cricoid pressure, the pressure should be removed and the patient should be tilted head down or turned to the left lateral position. Suction is then applied to remove the vomit from the oropharynx.

Training the technique of cricoid pressure

The technique used to apply cricoid pressure varies from practitioner to practitioner. The force of pressure required to be exerted on the larynx is estimated at between 20 and 40 Newtons – where 10 Newtons equal about 1 kilogram of pressure.

As with many clinical skills, there are good and poor techniques, several contraindications for its use and few signs, apart from the absence of regurgitation, of whether the manoeuvre has been carried out successfully. Most healthcare providers were, in the past, often taught the technique 'in-house' and told to 'just put your hand there and press'. Nevertheless, this is not enough training for what is a difficult technique to perfect, which is frightening for both the patient and the practitioner when first encountered.

Patients are at risk of harm from practitioners who fail to apply cricoid pressure consistently or correctly. Death from Mendelson's syndrome can result from applying cricoid pressure inefficiently, not applying cricoid pressure at all, or relaxing the pressure before intubation has been successfully established (Murray *et al.*, 2000).

Cricoid pressure also has the potential to cause anatomical distortion to the upper airway. Failed intubations using conventional laryngoscopy can sometimes be increased during the use of cricoid pressure. Nevertheless, pressure can be adjusted slightly, to aid the view of the vocal cords if requested by the anaesthetist. Other useful items of equipment such as the Gum-Elastic Bougie (see Figure 4.3) can be employed to aid airway management during intubation if the view of the larynx is in anyway distorted either due to the cricoid pressure or pre-existing anatomical difficulties (The Ambulance Service Association, 2001).

There are now simulation manikins or task trainers available in most clinical skills training environments (see Figure 4.4) which students and health professionals can use to practise and learn this technique successfully, without compromising patient safety.

The manikin contains an electronic monitor which displays the correct and incorrect hand placement and continuously shows the force being applied to the cricoid cartilage. When using the task trainer, many healthcare providers are surprised by the force required and the difficulty in maintaining that force correctly.

Various research studies into the use of cricoid pressure during RSI raise questions about the effectiveness of the technique in preventing regurgitation and the practical application of this manoeuvre. A recent magnetic resonance

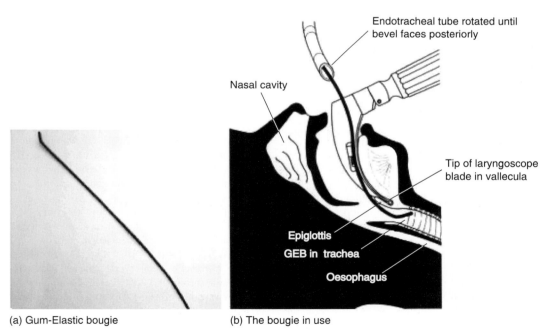

(a) Gum-Elastic bougie   (b) The bougie in use

Figure 4.3 Sample picture on right
Left – the Gum-Elastic Bougie. **Right** – the Bougie in use.

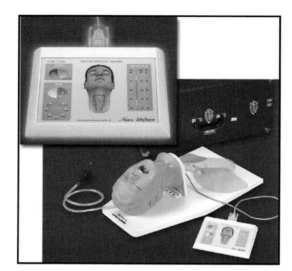

Figure 4.4 Life/form® Cricoid Pressure Trainer 2005.

imaging (MRI) study carried out in Texas in the United States on healthy volunteers suggests that the cricoid cartilage and oesophagus are not always anatomically aligned in the same axis and that application of cricoid pressure further displaced both the oesophagus and larynx laterally.

The researchers suggested that gastric content aspiration may occur during the induction of anaesthesia despite the application of cricoid pressure (Hernandez *et al.*, 2004).

Much debate will undoubtedly remain among the medical profession about the use of cricoid pressure. All patients who present for emergency surgery, especially patients who require intestinal surgery, where there is suspicion of delayed gastric emptying, should be induced using RSI technique. For example, even a patient requiring an appendicectomy, who has been a hospital inpatient for a week or more and fasted of oral solids and fluids and was showing no signs of recent vomiting, should not undergo general anaesthetic induction without the use of cricoid pressure.

No definite alternative has currently been devised or developed to replace the use of cricoid pressure during rapid sequence induction. Therefore, the priority for health professionals is to standardise the use and technique of cricoid pressure and start training programmes for those who teach and practise this technique. This would help to reduce errors and poor techniques and ensure future patient safety throughout the procedure.

REFERENCES

Amersham Health Medical Dictionary. (2005). Available at: www.amershamhealth.com (Accessed 6 April 2005).

Anaesthesia UK. (2004). *The Components for Rapid Sequence Induction.* Available at: www.frca.co.uk (Accessed 4 April 2005).

Hernandez, A., Wolf, S. W., Vijayakumar, V., Solanki., D. R. & Mathru, M. (2004). *Sellick's Manoeuvre for the Prevention of Aspiration...Is It Effective?* Available at: www.asaabstracts.com/strands (Accessed 9 April 2005).

MERCK Manual. (2004). *Cardiopulmonary Resuscitation.* Available at: www.merck.com/mrkshared/mmanual/section16 (Accessed 30 March 2005).

Mijumbi, C. (1994). *Anaesthesia for the Patient with a Full Stomach.* Available at: www.nda.ox.ac.uk (Accessed 5 April 2005).

Murray, E., Keirse, M., Neilson, J. *et al.* (2000). *A Guide to Effective Care in Childbirth and Pregnancy.* Available at: www.maternitywise.org (Accessed 6 April 2005).

Owen, H., Follows, K., Reynolds, J., Burgess, G. & Plummer, J. (2002). Learning to apply effective cricoid pressure using a part task trainer. *Continuing Education in Anaesthesia, Critical Care & Pain,* **5**(2), 45–8.

Sinclair, R. C. F. & Luxton, M. C. (2005). Rapid sequence induction. *Continuing Education in Anaesthesia, Critical Care and Pain,* **5**(2), 45–8.

Smith, B. & Williams, T. (eds.) (2004). *Operating Department Practice A–Z.* London: Greenwich Medical Ltd.

The Ambulance Service Association. (2001). *Difficult Intubation Protocol: Use of the Endotracheal Tube Introducer (Gum-Elastic Bougie).* Available at: www.asancep.org.uk/Endotrachealtubeintroducer.htm (Accessed 9 April 2005).

Yentis, S., Nicholas, P. H. & Smith, G. B. (2004). *Anaesthesia and Intensive Care A–Z – An Encyclopaedia of Principles and Practice,* 2nd edn. Edinburgh: Elsevier Ltd.

5

Anaesthetic breathing circuits

Norman Wright

Key Learning Points

- Discuss the basic design of breathing circuits
- Describe the evolution of breathing circuits
- Identify the benefits and disadvantages of each circuit

An anaesthetic breathing circuit is an assembly of parts, which connects the patient's airway to the anaesthetic machine creating an artificial atmosphere, from and into which a patient breathes (Ravi Shankar, 2004).

Shankar also states that a breathing circuit mostly consists of:

- a tube through which fresh anaesthetic gases are delivered from the anaesthetic machine to the patient
- a method of connecting the circuit to the patient's airway
- a rebreathing bag or corrugated rubber tubing (used in the early circuits) which acts as a gas reservoir, which would meet the peak inspiratory flow requirements
- an expiratory valve which allows the expired gases to pass into the scavenging circuit
- a carbon dioxide absorber for total rebreathing, and tubing to connect all the parts; as stated earlier in the early stages the tubing was composed of corrugated rubber. (Ravi Shankar, 2004).

Even though the design and materials used for breathing circuits have developed over the years, the individual component's roles have remained almost unchanged.

Since introducing ether as an anaesthetic in 1846, many improvements in the design of breathing circuits have occurred. Initially, inventors developed apparatus to deliver a single anaesthetic agent, such as nitrous oxide. Nitrous oxide fell from favour as a single-agent anaesthetic but was reintroduced in 1868, stored in cylinders, as part of a combination of anaesthetic agents. Barth, in 1907, developed a method of delivering nitrous oxide to patients using a valve, a reservoir bag and a Clover's inhaler. A Clover's inhaler consists of a black triangular mask attached to one side of a central silver drum with a flattened black rubber elliptical bag attached. By changing the lever's position in the valve, Barth could allow patients to either completely rebreathe the anaesthetic gases, or alternatively breathe completely from the atmosphere.

The Boyle's machine was developed in 1917. This development coincided with Magill and Rowbotham mastering endotracheal intubation using a single-lumen red rubber tube. Following from this, a simple anaesthetic delivery circuit called the 'Magill's Circuit' was developed.

The next 20 years saw many of the core advances in anaesthetic technology:

- 1929 – Cycloprane (C_3H_6): a flammable colourless gas which was used as an anaesthetic.
- 1931 – Cuffed endotracheal tubes: the cuff sits beyond the vocal chords to form a seal within the trachea to prevent anaesthetic gases escaping

Core Topics in Operating Department Practice: Anaesthesia and Critical Care, eds. Brian Smith, Paul Rawling, Paul Wicker and Chris Jones. Published by Cambridge University Press. © Cambridge University Press 2007.

and to prevent gastric contents from entering the lungs.

- Water's 'to and fro' circuit for closed circuit anaesthesia: this is a complete circuit consisting of tubing, a soda lime canister and a swivel connector.
- 1936 – Sword's circle circuit: this circuit was similar to earlier circle circuits but required smaller amounts of fresh gas each minute.
- 1937 – Ayre's T piece: used for paediatric anaesthesia, later modified by Jackson Rees.
- 1941 – The EMO inhaler: an early version of a vaporiser using the 'drawover' method.
  (Online Medical Dictionary, 1997).

The fifties and sixties saw breathing circuits develop at an increased rate, which was due in part to the new methods of providing anaesthesia. The ether 'open drop' method was no longer used and modern anaesthetic machines had vaporisers. The classification of anaesthetic machines depended on the whim of the developer, however, most developers agreed that breathing circuits should essentially deliver gases from the machine to the alveoli in the concentration that was set by the user and in the shortest possible time. The circuit also has to effectively eliminate dead-space (areas in the circuit where no movement of gases occurs), provide minimal apparatus dead-space and have a low resistance to the inspiration and expiration of air, to and from the patient's lungs.

There are also several other requirements when developing breathing circuits, which include economy of fresh gas, conservation of heat and the ability to humidify fresh gas adequately. The circuits should also be lightweight, which was not possible in the days of corrugated rubber tubing, but is now possible because of modern plastics. They should be efficient during both spontaneous and controlled ventilation, to ensure good CO_2 elimination and fresh gas use. They also need to be adaptable for adult, paediatric and mechanical ventilation. One of the most important developments of breathing circuits is the provision for scavenging (collecting, reusing and expelling from the operating department) waste anaesthetic gases,

thus reducing theatre pollution. This followed the introduction of CO_2 absorbers which used soda lime to absorb the exhaled CO_2.

The purpose of breathing is to maintain a supply of oxygen to the lungs for the blood to transport to the tissues and to remove CO_2 and other waste products from the body. A breathing circuit must enable a patient to breathe satisfactorily without significantly increasing the work of breathing or increasing the physiological dead-space, caused by the resistance to airflow in the air passages of the respiratory system. It must also conduct inhalational anaesthetic agents. The volume of gas expired with each breath is called the tidal volume (normally 6–10 ml/kg). The total volume breathed in a minute is the minute volume and the volume of gas in the lungs at the end of normal expiration is the functional residual capacity (FRC).

There are several breathing circuits commonly in use in anaesthesia today. W. W. Mapelson classified the circuits in 1954 as A, B, C, D and E, later adding the Mapelson F system to the list (Figure 5.1).

The Mapleson A system

Sir Ivan Magill designed the Mapleson A system (Figure 5.2) in the 1930s. This is an ideal circuit for spontaneous respiration. The expiratory (Heidbrink) valve reduces dead-space by positioning it close to the patient. During spontaneous respiration this circuit has a three-phase cycle; inspiration, expiration and respiratory pause. The patient inhales the gas from the reservoir bag during inspiration. The reservoir bag is also a visual indicator that breathing is taking place, as it partially collapses during inspiration.

During the early part of expiration the pressure does not increase, because the bag is not full. The exhaled gas of which the first portion is dead-space gas passes along the tubing to the bag, which is also filled with gas from the anaesthetic machine. As shown in Figure 5.2 the bag fills during expiration, which increases the pressure within the circuit,

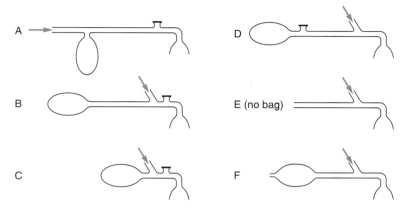

The arrow indicates entry of fresh gas to the system

Figure 5.1 The Mapleson classification of anaesthetic breathing circuits (Milner, 2004).

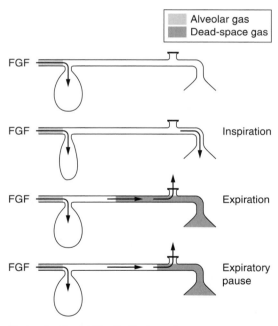

Mode of action of Magill attachment
during spontaneous ventilation

Figure 5.2 The Mapleson A circuit (Milner, 2004).

the Heidbrink valve opens thus allowing alveolar gas, which contains CO_2, to leave the circuit.

The expiratory pause allows more fresh gas to enter the circuit, thus forcing any remaining alveolar gas back along the tubing and out through the valve.

If used effectively this circuit can provide a respiratory cycle in which no rebreathing takes place. This requires a high fresh gas flow rate, which drives all the alveolar gas from the circuit before the next inspiratory phase takes place. With careful adjustment, the anaesthetist can reduce the fresh gas flow, which would allow only fresh gas and dead-space gas to be in the breathing circuit at the start of inspiration.

In practice the fresh gas flow would be near to the patient's total minute volume. A patient weighing 75 kg would therefore need a fresh gas flow of around 6 l per minute to prevent rebreathing. This figure is obtained from the formula for an average person's minute volume being 80 ml/kg/min.

This circuit is efficient for spontaneous respiration where no CO_2 absorption is available. Nevertheless, it is inefficient for controlled ventilation because a fresh gas flow rate of 2.5 times a patient's minute volume is required to minimise rebreathing resulting in a fresh gas flow rate of 12–15 l/min. This high flow rate would be exhausting for the patient and would result in the use of high quantities of anaesthetic agent.

Therefore, the Mapleson A (Magill) circuit should not be used for positive pressure ventilation.

The Lack system

The Lack circuit (Figure 5.3) is a variation of Mapleson A. A four-way block is attached to the fresh gas outlet (F). This block is connected to an outer reservoir tube (R) attached to the patient (P), an inner exhaust tube (E), a breathing bag (B) and a spring-loaded expiratory valve (V).

The Lack circuit is essentially similar in function to the Magill circuit, except that the expiratory valve is placed at the machine-end of the circuit,

being connected to the patient adaptor by the inner coaxial tube.

The valve's location is more convenient, helping intermittent positive pressure ventilation and scavenging of expired gas.

In common with other coaxial circuits, if the inner tube becomes disconnected or breaks, the entire reservoir tube becomes dead-space. This situation can be avoided by use of the 'parallel Lack' circuit, which replaces the inner and outer tubes by conventional breathing tubing and a Y-piece (Figure 5.4).

The Mapleson B system

The Mapleson B circuit (Figure 5.5) features the fresh gas inlet near the patient, distal to the expiratory valve. The expiratory valve opens when

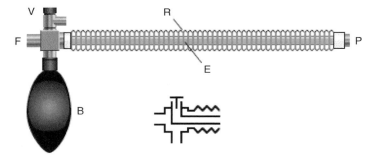

Figure 5.3 The Lack system (Anaesthesia UK, 2005).

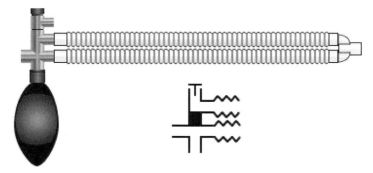

Figure 5.4 The parallel Lack circuit (Anaesthesia UK, 2005).

Gas flow during inspiration and expiration in the Lack circuit

Inspiration: the valve closes and the patient inspires fresh gas from the outer reservoir tube.

Expiration: the patient expires into the reservoir tube. Towards the end of expiration, the bag fills and positive pressure opens the valve, allowing expired gas to escape through the inner exhaust tube.

Expiratory pause: fresh gas washes the expired gas out of the reservoir tube, filling it with fresh gas for the next inspiration.

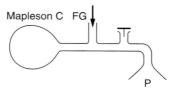

Figure 5.6 The Mapleson C system (Anaesthesia UK, 2005).

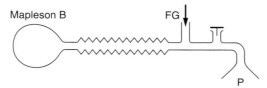

Figure 5.5 The Mapleson B System (Anaesthesia UK, 2005).

pressure in the circuit increases, and discharges a mixture of alveolar gas and fresh gas. During the next inspiration the patient inhales a mixture of retained fresh gas and alveolar gas. Using fresh gas flow rates of greater than twice the minute ventilation for both spontaneous and controlled ventilation avoids the problems of rebreathing waste anaesthetic gases.

The Mapleson C system

The Mapleson C circuit (Figure 5.6) is also known as the Water's circuit, but without an absorber. It is similar in construction to the Mapleson B circuit, but the main tubing is shorter. The prevention of rebreathing requires a low fresh gas flow, equal to twice the patient's minute ventilation.

Carbon dioxide builds up slowly with this circuit when compared with the Mapleson A and B systems. This is because both Mapleson A and B systems mix alveolar and fresh gas during spontaneous or controlled ventilation, leading to a fairly high chance of rebreathing expired gases and

therefore increasing CO_2 intake. The shorter main tubing of the Mapleson C circuit makes rebreathing less of a risk and easier to control using lower gas flow rates.

The Mapleson C system is an ideal circuit to use during resuscitation and when transferring patients because the valve and the rebreathing bag are close to the patient (Gwinnutt, 1996).

The Mapleson D system

The Mapleson D system (Figure 5.7) may be described as a coaxial modification (an inner tube to deliver the fresh gas and an outer tube for the waste gases) of the basic T-piece circuit, developed to help scavenging of waste anaesthetic gases.

The Bain circuit is a modification of the Mapleson D system. It is a coaxial circuit in which the fresh gas flows through a narrow inner tube within the outer corrugated tubing. The Bain circuit therefore works in the same way as the T-piece, except that the tube supplying fresh gas to the patient is placed inside the reservoir tube.

During spontaneous ventilation, normocarbia requires a fresh gas flow of 200–300 ml/kg. During controlled ventilation, a fresh gas flow of only 70 ml/kg is required to produce normocarbia.

J. A. Bain and W. E. Spoerel have recommended the following:

- 2 l/min fresh gas flow in patients weighing less than 10 kg
- 6–9 l/min fresh gas flow in patients weighing between 10 and 50 kg

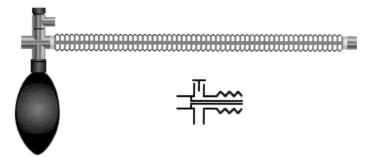

Figure 5.7 The Mapleson D system (Anaesthesia UK, 2005).

- 70 ml/kg fresh gas flow in patients weighing more than 60 kg.

The recommended tidal volume is 10 ml/kg and respiratory rate is 12–16 breaths per minute.

The advantage of this circuit is the reduced volume of dead-space, low resistance to breathing and efficient scavenging of waste gases.

The disadvantages of the circuit are that it needs a high fresh gas flow rate which may cause problems when using the oxygen emergency flush valve and that it may also cause barotraumas (i.e. trauma to the airways or sinuses).

Another major problem with coaxial circuits is that if the inner gas supply tube becomes disconnected or breaks, the entire breathing tube becomes dead-space, which leads to severe alveolar hypoventilation. The practitioner can check for broken or disconnected tubes in circuits fitted with a bag, by closing the valve and pressing the oxygen emergency flush button. If the inner tube is intact, the force of the rapid stream of gas leaving the inner tube will empty the bag of gas. Conversely, if there is inner tube damage the gas flows into the bag, which will fill.

As with the Lack circuit, the so-called 'parallel Bain circuit' removes these disadvantages. This circuit replaces the inner and outer tubes with conventional circle absorber tubing and a Y-piece. This circuit can also be used in the Humphrey ADE circuit.

> **Gas flow during inspiration and expiration in the Mapleson D system**
>
> Inspiration: the patient inspires fresh gas from the outer reservoir tube.
>
> Expiration: the patient expires into the reservoir tube. Even though fresh gas is still flowing into the circuit at this time, it is wasted as it is contaminated by expired gas.
>
> Expiratory pause: fresh gas from the inner tube washes the expired gas out of the reservoir tube, filling it with fresh gas for the next inspiration.

The Mapleson E system

The Mapleson E system (Figure 5.8) is a modification of Ayre's T-piece which Phillip Ayre (a Newcastle anaesthetist) developed in 1937 for use in paediatric patients undergoing cleft palate repair or intracranial surgery.

The circuit comprises a three-way T-tube whose limbs are connected to (F) the fresh gas supply from the anaesthesia machine, (R) a length of corrugated reservoir tube and (P) the patient connector. It has minimal dead-space, no valves and minimal resistance. Jackson Rees further varied the circuit (described later in this chapter) (Gwinnutt, 1996).

During spontaneous ventilation the fresh gas and exhaled gas flow down the expiratory limb. Peak expiratory flow occurs early in exhalation.

Table 5.1 Fresh gas flow requirements appropriate to patient body weights

Body weight (kg)	Fresh gas flow (l/min)
5	1.4–1.8
10	2.4–3.2
20	4.1–5.4
40	7.2–9.6

Source: Anaesthesia UK, 2005.

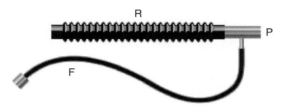

Figure 5.8 The Mapleson E system (Anaesthesia UK, 2005).

Gas flow during inspiration and expiration in the Mapleson E system

Inspiration: the patient inspires fresh gas from the reservoir tube.

Expiration: the patient expires into the reservoir tube. Even though fresh gas is still flowing into the circuit, it is wasted, as it is contaminated by expired gas. An expiratory limb volume greater than the patient's tidal volume prevents entrainment of room air (which would dilute anaesthetic gases and oxygen).

Expiratory pause: fresh gas washes the expired gas out of the reservoir tube, filling it with fresh gas for the next inspiration.

A fresh gas flow greater than three times the minute ventilation prevents rebreathing.

Thus, the proportion of fresh gas added to the exhaled gases increases. During the next breath, the patient draws fresh gas from the fresh gas inlet and the expiratory limb.

The original analysis of the Mapleson E circuit suggested that a gas flow rate of 2.5–3 times the minute volume was required to prevent rebreathing of expired gas. However, this assumed a square-wave respiratory pattern, and investigations using a more realistic breathing pattern have suggested that 1.5–2 times the minute volume is acceptable in spontaneously breathing patients (Table 5.1).

Again, these values are guidelines only – if there is evidence of rebreathing (i.e. build-up of CO_2), the flow rate should be increased.

Controlled ventilation

In contrast with Mapleson A circuits, Mapleson D and E circuits are more efficient during controlled ventilation. This is because the tidal volume must be supplied during the expiratory pause. With the almost sinusoidal respiratory pattern of spontaneous respiration, there is relatively little time for this volume to be supplied, so the fresh gas flow rate must be high. The pattern of controlled ventilation, however, is usually one of a rapid inspiration, expiration and a relatively prolonged expiratory pause. This long expiratory pause gives enough time for the tidal volume requirement to be supplied, even with a low fresh gas flow rate. Thus, during controlled ventilation, the recommended fresh gas flow rate is similar to that of the Mapleson A circuits during spontaneous ventilation (see above). Intermittent positive pressure ventilation may be performed by intermittently occluding the end of the reservoir tube.

The use of the T-piece

Figure 5.9 shows the most commonly used T-piece circuit known as the Jackson-Rees' modification of the Ayre's T-piece (sometimes also known as the Mapleson F circuit). This circuit connects an open-ended bag to the expiratory limb of the circuit; gas escapes through the 'tail' of the bag.

The bag allows respiratory movements to be more easily seen and allows intermittent positive ventilation if necessary. The bag is, however, not essential to the circuit functioning as it would operate in the same way as the original Ayre's T-piece. Nevertheless, anaesthetists had to tape a feather or a piece of tissue paper to the end of

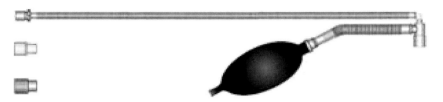

Figure 5.9 The Jackson-Rees' modification of the Ayre's T-piece (Mapleson F circuit).

the tubing to discover whether the patient was breathing. This practice is considered unacceptable today.

Intermittent positive pressure ventilation (IPPV) may be performed by occluding the tail of the bag between the ring finger and the little finger squeezing the bag. Alternatively, a 'bag-tail valve', which employs an adjustable resistance to gas flow, may be attached to the bag tail. This causes the bag to remain partially inflated and so helps one-handed performance of IPPV.

Several different designs of T-piece are available, which work in essentially the same way. Modern T-pieces incorporate 15-mm fittings for the reservoir tube and endotracheal adaptor.

The advantages of the modern T-piece circuit are that they are compact, inexpensive and have no valves. This circuit produces minimal dead-space, minimal resistance to breathing and is economical for controlled breathing.

A major disadvantage with this circuit is that the bag may become twisted and impede breathing. The circuit also needs a high flow rate and it is therefore only suitable for children who weigh less than 20 kg.

Humphrey ADE

David Humphrey designed a single circuit that can be changed from a Mapleson A to a Mapleson D by moving a lever on the block which connects the circuit to the fresh gas supply on the anaesthetic machine (see Figure 5.10).

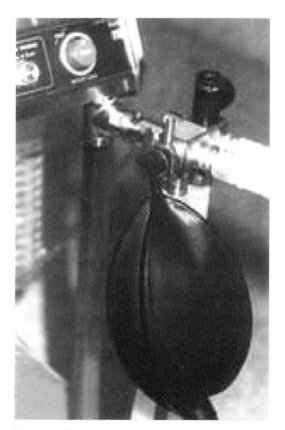

Figure 5.10 The Humphrey ADE circuit.

Humphrey Block

The Humphrey Block circuit (Figure 5.11) can be used for spontaneous or controlled ventilation. It consists of two lengths of tubing with a Y connector at the patient end: one for the fresh

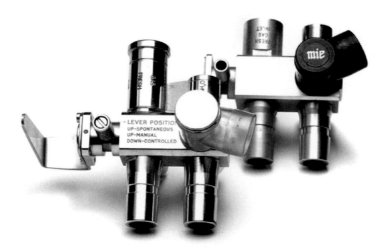

Figure 5.11 The Humphrey Block.

gas and one for the exhaled gas. In addition it consists of an APL valve, a lever to select controlled or spontaneous respiration, a reservoir bag, a port to connect to the ventilator and a safety pressure relief valve.

Conclusion

Breathing circuits have undergone major changes from the days of the heavy corrugated rubber tubing, which practitioners had to sterilise regularly, to the modern circuits which are plastic, single use and lightweight.

The modern-day emphasis on safety and efficiency of use has resulted in several different types of breathing circuits developing. It is essential for the anaesthetic practitioner to be familiar with the most common of these circuits to provide the best patient care. The misuse of circuits can severely affect the patient's respiration and breathing pattern and could eventually lead to harm or even death. The practitioner should check the anaesthetic circuit before each patient and the circuits should be changed in accordance with the manufacturer's guidelines, in line with trust policy. These days with the new lightweight circuits

the chances of disconnection or dislodging the endotracheal tube are much reduced, but practitioners must always take great care to ensure the highest level of patient safety.

REFERENCES

Anaesthesia UK (2005) is available at www.frca.co.uk.

Gwinnutt, C. (1996). *Clinical Anaesthesia*. Oxford: Blackwell Science Ltd.

Milner, Q. (2004). *Anaesthetic Breathing Systems*. Available at: www.nda.ox.ac.uk/wfsa/html/u07/u07–012.htm (Accessed February 2005).

Online Medical Dictionary. (1997). Available at: http://cancerweb.ncl.ac.uk/omd/index.html (Accessed March 2006).

Ravi Shankar, M. (2004). *Anaesthetic Breathing Systems*. Available at: www.capnography.com/Circuits/Breathingsys/ravi.htm (Accessed January 2005).

Further Reading

Aitkenhead, A.R., Rowbotham, D.J. & Smith, G. (2001). *Textbook of Anaesthesia*, 4th edn. London: Elsevier Science Ltd.

Al-Shaikh, B. & Stacey, S. (2002). *Essentials of Anaesthetic Equipment*, 2nd edn. London: Churchill Livingstone.

Clarke, P. & Jones, J. (1998). *Brigden's Operating Department Practice*. Edinburgh: Churchill Livingstone.

Davey, A. & Ince, C. (2000). *Fundamentals of Operating Department Practice*. London: Greenwich Medical Media Ltd.

Kumar, B. (1998). *Working in the Operating Department*. New York: Churchill Livingstone.

Robson, N. (2004). *Anaesthesia Breathing Systems*. Available at: www.usyd.edu.au/su/anaes/lectures/breathing-sys-nr.html (Accessed February 2005).

6

Deflating the endotracheal tube pilot cuff

Martin Maguire

Key Learning Points
- Understanding the literature behind safe deflation of the ET tube cuff
- Implications of non-deflated pilot tubes
- Review of manufacturers' ET guidelines

Introduction

Tracheal extubation of patients following anaesthesia is a complex and skilled procedure that carries potential risks of various complications. These risks range from minor, such as a sore throat, to major life-threatening complications, such as airway obstruction. Minimisation of these risks is essential if recovery from anaesthesia is to be smooth and trouble free. There are many different methods employed by anaesthetists and perioperative staff for the extubation of post-operative patients within theatre or in the recovery room. The deflation of the endotracheal tube cuff with a syringe is generally advocated, but there are times when the cuff is deflated by snapping or cutting off the pilot tube apparatus. This practice infringes all guidelines and advice given in textbooks, journals and by endotracheal tube manufacturers. There is evidence that this practice could lead to, or aggravate, some potentially harmful post-anaesthetic complications.

Defining the problem

Asai *et al.* (1998) studied respiratory problems associated with both intubation and extubation and found the incidence of complications associated with extubation were significantly higher than during the induction of anaesthesia ($p < 0.001$). They therefore implied that 'the incidence of respiratory complications associated with tracheal extubation may be higher than that during tracheal intubation' (Asai *et al.*, 1998). Even though their list of factors that could contribute to post-extubation complications does not include the snapping of pilot tubes, other studies (notably Grap *et al.*, 1995 and Hartley & Vaughan, 1993) do suggest that unplanned tracheal extubation, where there is no deflation of the endotracheal tube cuff, can lead to respiratory problems such as airway spasm, oedema and trauma.

Few would recommend the removal of an endotracheal tube without first deflating the cuff. Unplanned extubation has been associated with many complications including: trauma, laryngeal spasm, bronchospasm, coughing and pain. Maguire and Crooke (2001) showed that snapping of the pilot tube causes the tracheal tube cuff to deflate more slowly and less predictably than deflation using a syringe. Sometimes the cuff has failed to deflate at all (see Figure 6.1) therefore snapping of the pilot tube is often tantamount to extubating a patient without deflating the cuff. The resultant complications seen in the recovery room are comparable to those seen following unplanned extubation. Patients may experience stridor because of laryngeal trauma or laryngeal spasm. They may cough or suffer varying degrees of

Core Topics in Operating Department Practice: Anaesthesia and Critical Care, eds. Brian Smith, Paul Rawling, Paul Wicker and Chris Jones. Published by Cambridge University Press. © Cambridge University Press 2007.

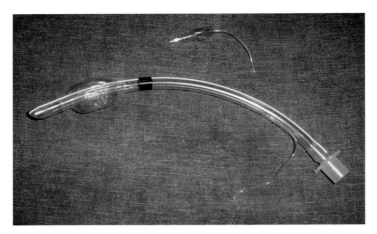

Figure 6.1 Endotracheal tube showing snapped pilot tube and undeflated cuff.

respiratory distress. They may also complain of sore throat or suffer hoarseness of voice. The increased stimulation of the laryngeal and pharyngeal mucosa may precipitate excess secretions, which would further aggravate coughing or laryngeal spasm. Rare but significant complications include arytenoid dislocation and recurrent laryngeal nerve paralysis.

The two arytenoid cartilages are pyramidal in shape and attach to the vocal cords. Their movement (rocking and sliding) enables the adduction and abduction of the vocal cords leading to the activation of the main functions of the larynx – airway protection, respiration and voice production (see Figure 6.2).

The recurrent laryngeal nerves branch from the vagus nerve and innervate the intrinsic muscles of the larynx. They are vulnerable to damage during surgery in the neck, particularly thyroid surgery. Minor damage to the recurrent laryngeal nerves results in changes in vocal tone, usually causing hoarseness. Major damage (e.g. severing) can lead to total obstruction of the airway because of the vocal cords becoming totally adducted.

Confounding issues

There is however some controversy about the causes of these post-extubation complications.

There are several confounding issues that may contribute to the problems associated with difficulty in extubation. It sometimes seems there are as many different techniques for extubation as there are anaesthetists! They will all favour their own particular method as the best. Within what might be described as the *correct* method there can be several variations. For example, some will stress the importance of timing of extubation. 'Deep' versus 'light' has long been debated. Some prefer to extubate patients while they are still deeply anaesthetised, especially if the patient is undergoing intracranial or intra-ocular surgery, because this is claimed to lessen the incidence of coughing, straining or cardiovascular effects. Dyson *et al.* (1990) showed increases of over 20% in the heart rate and arterial pressure of 70% of patients during or immediately following extubation. Lowrie *et al.* (1992) identified a significant increase in plasma concentrations of adrenaline after tracheal extubation in a small group of patients who had undergone major elective surgery. These cardiovascular effects can undoubtedly be minimised by deep-plane extubation, but there are problems associated with early extubation. Asai *et al.* (1998) found the incidence of other respiratory complications following extubation will be greater when the trachea is extubated when the patient is still deeply anaesthetised. Deep-plane anaesthesia

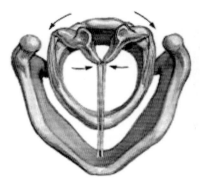

Action of lateral cricoarytenoid muscles
Adduction of vocal ligaments

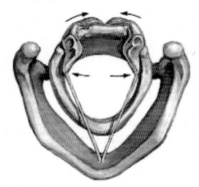

Action of posterior cricoarytenoid muscles
Abduction of vocal ligaments

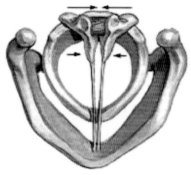

Action of transverse cricoarytenoid muscle
Adduction of vocal ligaments

Figure 6.2 Action of the cricoarytenoid joint.

extubation can avoid cardiovascular stimulation, but may lead to subsequent difficulty in management of the airway. The current thinking is that extubation should be carried out when the patient's defensive airway reflexes have returned. The possible adverse effects of late extubation are a small price to pay for ensuring that protective mechanisms for the patient's airway are fully functional before removing an endotracheal tube.

Some would advise suctioning of the upper airway above the cuff before extubation. Others would suggest passing a suction catheter down the lumen of the endotracheal tube and applying

suction while removing both the tube and the suction catheter at the same time. Some say that if you extubate the patient when the cough reflex has already returned then there is no need to suction before extubation, as the patient will cough or swallow to protect their own airway from possible aspiration. Some anaesthetists recommend the use of positive pressure by a Mapleson C breathing circuit or similar to force out foreign material from the larynx at the time of extubation. The removal of secretions during extubation should reduce the risk of laryngeal spasm developing. Many more variations of *correct* technique exist, and the possibility of deflating the tracheal cuff with a syringe or by snapping the pilot tube further confuses the issue regarding the causes which contribute to post-extubation complications.

Manufacturers' recommendations

Endotracheal tube manufacturers provide training manuals and video or DVD recordings which give very precise and detailed guidance on intubation techniques, but little instruction on how best to extubate. Each box of endotracheal tubes contains an advice insert, which provides users with suggested directions for use. One manufacturer, Malinckrodt, includes an advice insert that contains the following:

9. Prior to extubation, deflate the cuff by inserting a syringe into the valve housing and removing the air until a definite vacuum is noted in the syringe and the pilot balloon is collapsed.

10. Extubate the patient, following currently accepted medical techniques.

Under the heading: 'Warnings/Precautions' it also states:

Deflate the cuff prior to repositioning the tube. Movement of the tube with the cuff inflated could result in patient injury.

Another manufacturer, Rusch, states in its directions for use:

10. Extubate the tube only after complete deflation . . . with a luer tip syringe . . .

When approached, representatives from both of these companies made it clear that they in no way condoned the practice of snapping of pilot tubes to deflate tracheal cuffs. There is no reason to assume that any other manufacturers of endotracheal tubes would advise differently.

Medical education

Anaesthetists and anaesthetic practitioners learn the difficult skill of extubation 'on-the-job'. No formalised standardised method for teaching the skill exists. Junior anaesthetists learn their technique (good or bad) from whichever consultant they happen to be working with at the time. This in itself causes a problem, because juniors are assigned to different consultants daily and what one consultant tells them one day could be contradicted the next day by another. The age-old principle of 'see one, do one teach one' may persist within many hospitals. The added problem of junior staff having to learn several different 'correct' techniques leads to a very unsatisfactory way of learning a difficult skill that, if done wrongly could lead to potentially devastating complications. Since clinical governance, the standardisation of practices should be aimed to ensure patients' safety. That standardisation must include training skills such as intubation and extubation.

The theory related to intubation and extubation is accessed from recommended texts and/or anaesthetic journals. *Lee's Synopsis of Anaesthesia*, which describes itself as 'a summary of current teaching and practice', contains less than one page on extubation, in which it states that 'difficulty in extubation is unusual, but may be caused by the cuff failing to deflate'.

The Textbook of Anaesthesia, edited by Smith, G. and Aitkenhead, A. R. does describe a method for extubation, but again takes barely more than half a page to do so. Both of these texts are among those most often recommended to those entering the anaesthetic speciality, and neither devotes much space to the practicalities and problems of extubation. Considering the findings of Asai *et al.* (1998) that more complications occur at or just following extubation than intubation, the relative importance granted to each in the texts seems paradoxical.

Examples of 'snapping of pilot tubes'

Very little literature exists relating to the snapping of pilot tubes to deflate tracheal cuffs. Much has been written on the post-anaesthetic complications of intubation and/or extubation, and there is some literature on the problems associated with unplanned extubation. The lack of literature on the subject of snapping of pilot tubes could be because the practice is known to be incorrect, against manufacturers' guidelines, and may be looked on as poor practice. There may be legal concerns to think about. If it is known that a certain action carries risks for the patient (that can be avoided by using a different method), that action could be considered negligent if a patient suffered harm because of that action. The following two cases deal directly with the issue of snapping the pilot tube. The first is a case report and the second is a letter. Both describe a failure of the cuff to deflate following snapping of the pilot tube. In each case a method is described for the subsequent deflation of the cuff to simplify safe extubation.

Brock-Utne et al. (1992) describe a patient who became alert in the post-anaesthetic care unit, and attempted to extubate herself. In an effort to deflate the cuff rapidly, the pilot balloon and valve assembly were pulled off the pilot tube. In the process, the pilot tube was stretched and the remaining stump of the pilot tube was occluded. The endotracheal tube could not then be removed. Direct laryngoscopy confirmed the tracheal cuff was still inflated. A 25-gauge needle attached to a 1-ml syringe was inserted into the pilot tube and air was withdrawn from the tracheal tube cuff. The patient was awake and reassured throughout. She was subsequently extubated easily and made an uneventful recovery from anaesthesia. Brock-Utne et al. go on to describe various other causes of difficult extubation. These include: tracheal tubes inadvertently wired to facial bones; tubes sutured to the pulmonary artery; tubes transfixed by screws or drill bits, or entangled with nasogastric tubes; and one case of a tube being stuck below the cords by folds in a large deflated cuff. They claim that their report is the first to present a complication at extubation directly attributable to pulling off the pilot balloon to deflate the cuff. Literature searches would seem to support their claim, but it is hardly something to boast about! They also concede that this is an increasingly common practice, and the justification for it appears to be in the difficulty in

quickly finding a syringe with which to deflate the tube cuff. They advise that this practice should be 'strongly discouraged' for two reasons: the first is the risk of the tube cuff not deflating and the second is the importance of having a functional endotracheal tube of the correct size should reintubation become necessary in an emergency. If the pilot tube and valve assembly have been snapped off, then the choice of reusing the existing tube is no longer available.

The second case is a letter from Singh et al. (1995). They describe how the inflating tube was detached in an attempt to deflate the tracheal cuff rapidly. As with the Brock-Utne case, the pilot tube stretched and the endotracheal tube could not be removed. Laryngoscopy revealed the failure to extubate was because of the tracheal cuff remaining inflated. As in the previously described case, the stretched pilot tube had become occluded. Nevertheless, Singh et al.'s management was different. They describe how a small V-shaped cut was made through the wall of the endotracheal tube across the pilot tube just beyond the attachment of the pilot tube. The cut segment was then lifted to allow air to escape. The tube was subsequently removed easily. They claim that this method is quick, easy and safer than other methods described in the literature. Unlike Brock-Utne et al. they do not warn against the practice of snapping pilot tubes. Had a syringe been used to deflate the cuff in both cases, the complication would not have arisen and the solutions described would not have become necessary. In both cases the reason given for snapping the pilot tube was to extubate quickly, and in both cases extubation was delayed more than if a syringe had been obtained.

Incidence

Perioperative staff working in recovery rooms will no doubt identify with finding the evidence of snapping of pilot tubes. All too often the pilot balloon and valve assembly is found lying next to a patient's head, having been left there following extubation. It is difficult to establish with any certainty the incidence of snapping within the anaesthetic and allied professions, because there is bound to be reluctance to admit taking part in an incorrect activity that may lead to harmful consequences. Any audit would undoubtedly lead to change in practice once it was known what the audit entailed, but this should not deter those wishing to carry out such an audit as the resultant change in behaviour can only be to the benefit of future patients. From a North West of England hospital, Aintree Hospitals, study where an anonymous questionnaire was completed by 24 senior anaesthetists, Figure 6.3 shows 18 out of 24 (75%) admitted to snapping of the pilot tube at some time. One third snapped the pilot tube at least 50% of the time.

Some anaesthetists and theatre practitioners refuse to accept the practice of snapping of pilot tubes can cause problems. They point out that they have snapped the pilot tubes for a long time without facing any difficulties. They might even refuse to use a syringe that has been offered to them for cuff deflation. One argument put forward by those who continue to snap pilot tubes is the cuff is always deflated when the endotracheal tube is removed; therefore, there is no difference from when a syringe is used. This may be because as the cuff is slowly deflating, the act of pulling it through the vocal cords has the effect of squeezing out any residual air from the tracheal cuff. This partially deflated cuff could still have the potential to cause laryngeal trauma and post-extubation airway problems.

The mechanics of the problem

Maguire and Crooke (2001) carried out a bench test to prove that snapping the pilot tube was less reliable than use of a syringe for the deflation of the tracheal cuff. They used a model trachea and timed the deflation of the cuff when a syringe was used and when a snapping technique was used. Fifty cuffs were deflated using a syringe and 50 pilot tubes were snapped to deflate the cuffs. They found the deflation of the cuff using a syringe was significantly quicker and more predictable than when the pilot tube was snapped ($p < 0.001$).

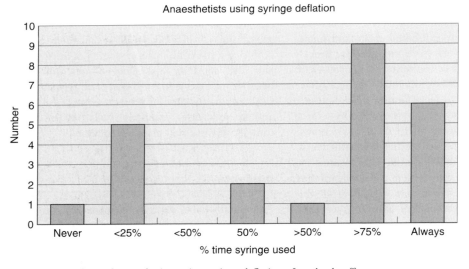

Figure 6.3 Numbers of anaesthetists using syringe deflation of tracheal cuff.

As this is due to the small internal diameter of the pilot tube, air escaping passively from the cuff will do so more slowly than when negative pressure is applied using the suction effect of a syringe. As the pilot tube is stretched, the internal diameter of the tube is reduced even further and the pilot tube can become occluded as discussed earlier. If the cuff fails to deflate during attempted extubation of a patient, then the extubation is either impossible or could lead to trauma of the vocal cords. If the cuff deflates slowly, then the risk of trauma is lessened but still remains, because it is usual that the endotracheal tube is removed almost immediately following deflation of the tracheal cuff.

Conclusion

Snapping pilot tubes could be a widespread practice despite lack of evidence for best practice within any relevant text, literature or manufacturers' guidance. There is some evidence to suggest the snapping of pilot tubes leads to slow, unpredictable deflation of the tracheal cuff and may result in a failure of the cuff to deflate at all. There is also support for the belief that extubation of a patient when the tracheal cuff is not deflated can lead to complications in the early post-operative period. Some would argue the new high volume, ~ressure cuffs are unlikely to cause trauma to ~nx, but the vocal cords and associated ~nsist of highly sensitive and fragile ~s accepted that anaesthetists and ~s are autonomous practitioners, ~ps his or her own strategies ~ce. Nevertheless, in areas ~ausing harm, there is a ~d training and the ~rect' technique.

This way junior anaesthetists can be certain they are given the right advice. If they choose not to follow that advice, they do so at their peril. In areas such as theatres, where patients are vulnerable to many risks, the first priority must always be to uphold patients' safety and wellbeing. This is impossible if we allow practices to continue which we know to be unsafe and potentially harmful to those patients. The rarity of a complication does not justify actions, which could lead to that complication arising.

REFERENCES

Asai, T., Koga, K. & Vaughan, R. S. (1998). Respiratory complications associated with tracheal intubation and extubation. *British Journal of Anaesthesia*, **80**, 767–75.

Brock-Utne, J. G., Jaffe, R. A., Robins, B. & Ratner, E. (1992). Difficulty in extubation. A cause for concern. *Anaesthesia*, **47**, 229–30.

Dyson, A., Isaac, P. A., Pennant, J. H., Griesecke, A. H. & Lipton, J. M. (1990). Esmolol attenuates cardiovascular responses to extubation. *Anaesthesia and Analgesia*, **71**, 675–8.

Grap, M. J., Glass, C. & Lindamood, M. O. (1995). Factors related to unplanned extubation of endotracheal tubes. *Critical Care Nurse*, **15**(2), 57–65.

Hartley, M. & Vaughan, R. S. (1993). Problems associated with tracheal extubation. *British Journal of Anaesthesia*, **71**, 561–8.

Lowrie, A., Johnston, P. L., Fell, D. & Robinson, S. L. (1992). Cardiovascular and plasma catecholamine responses at tracheal extubation. *British Journal of Anaesthesia*, **68**, 261–3.

Maguire, M. P. & Crooke, J. (2001). Pilot tubes: to snap or not to snap. *British Journal of Anaesthesia*, **86**(2), 308–9.

Singh, B., Gupta, M. D. & Sham, L. S. (1995). Difficult extubation: a new management. *Anaesthesia and Analgesia*, **81**, 433.

7

How aware are you? Inadvertent awareness under anaesthesia

Paul Rawling

Key Learning Points
- Potential causes of awareness under general anaesthesia
- Introduce what the incidence of awareness is believed to be
- Monitor methods used to detect awareness
- Appreciate the possible patient outcomes

Have you ever tried to imagine what it may feel like to be awake, yet paralysed? Have you ever experienced a dream where an event was happening to you but you were unable to respond in any way and the screams are only in your mind?

Awareness during anaesthesia is widely accepted as being defined as the spontaneous recall of events by a patient that took place during an episode of general anaesthesia. Inadvertent awareness during anaesthesia is not a new occurrence but one which has attracted increased media attention in recent years. Some 159 years ago Dr John Snow commented that:

the advent of the third degree of narcotism is marked by the cessation of all voluntary motion . . . . . . as there are no signs of ideas in this degree, I believe that there are none, and the mental faculties are completely suspended: consequently the patient is perfectly secured against mental suffering from anything that may be done (Snow, 1847 cited in Power, 1998).

Snow's comment clearly shows that in the early days of anaesthesia the issue of awareness during surgery was given consideration. In more recent times patients have become more inclined to report episodes of awareness following anaesthesia and surgical interventions, due partly to the increase in popular media reporting.

The problem is undergoing re-evaluation because of recent studies suggesting that awareness is a relatively common event of greater proportion than was previously believed. Inadvertent awareness during anaesthesia has considerable potential for patient morbidity including severe emotional distress. More importantly, the extreme psychological insult and trauma experienced by patients who have been aware and sometimes in pain have been likened to post-traumatic stress disorder (PTSD). Bailey and Jones (1997) asserted that because of the 'profound physical and psychological trauma' experienced by patients who experience awareness episodes, successful litigation is almost certain. Also suggested is thorough investigation to ensure that fraudulent claims are not made. It must be remembered that situations of intra-operative awareness n only involve the patient but can also be potenti damaging to the anaesthetist and the entire who contribute to the patient's care. A pote more disturbing issue as Gravenstein suggests is that awareness under genera thesia may occur without spontaneous intra-operative events, which has the be just as psychologically destructive to

Core Topics in Operating Department Practice: Anaesthesia and Critical Care, eds. Brian Smith, Paul Rawling Chris Jones. Published by Cambridge University Press. © Cambridge University Press 2007.

Every patient who receives general anaesthesia is at risk of experiencing an inadvertent awareness event. The nature of awareness under general anaesthesia may be more difficult to identify in clinical practice than other anaesthetic-related problems.

It is widely believed possible that as many as 1–2 patients per 1000 (0.1–0.2%) have some degree of recall of events which occurred during perioperative procedures involving general anaesthesia, which rises to as many as 3 patients per 1000 (0.3%) or greater in cardiac surgery, obstetric surgery and trauma surgery (Myles *et al.*, 2003). Placing the problem into a local context of an average district general hospital of moderate size, it is likely that 30 patients out of 15 000 undergoing perioperative procedures involving general anaesthesia might experience awareness under anaesthesia. Between 2001 and 2002, over 6 million surgical procedures were carried out in the United Kingdom, many of which would have involved general anaesthesia (National Statistics, 2003). The simple mathematical calculation shows that if 3 million general anaesthetics took place a very significant number, potentially 3000–6000 cases of inadvertent intra-operative awareness may have taken place during this period. Many will have been reported by the patients, others will not.

Much of the research into this subject has been carried out in Australia and Scandinavia over a number of years. Myles *et al.* (2004) published findings from a large randomised controlled trial using Bispectral Index (BIS) monitoring as a potential monitor for detecting awareness in patients undergoing general anaesthesia which included the use of muscle relaxant drugs. Of 1225 patients in the BIS-monitored group two cases of awareness were reported, though in the standard anaesthetic care group of similar but not identical size, 11 cases were identified. It was found that patients in the BIS-monitored group recovered faster than the standard anaesthetic care group to a predetermined point of eye opening. In this study of almost 2500 patients the use of BIS monitoring reduced the incidence of awareness by 82% in adult patients who were described as being at risk of potential intra-operative awareness under general anaesthesia involving muscle relaxant drugs. The definitive identification and interpretation of potential awareness cases remains extremely problematic. This may be due to the difficulty of differentiation between the possibility of patients dreaming, and experiencing awareness and recollection in the early post-operative stages of recovery.

A recent Anaesthetic Incidence Monitoring Study (AIMS), a voluntary incident reporting system used widely in Australia that reviewed 8372 incidents, identified 81 cases of definite or highly probable incidents of awareness between 1998 and 2001. Most of the cases included in the study were believed to be preventable by the researchers but 13 had no obvious cause (Bergman *et al.*, 2002). The 81 cases were subsequently divided into those without any obvious cause, those due to low inspired volatile agent and those because of drug error. The largest part of these cases was attributed to drug error at the beginning of anaesthesia resulting in inadvertent paralysis and recall of intubation during the induction phase of the procedure. Within the study, there was no suggestion of labelling of syringes, which would aid the elimination of this hazard.

Pederson and Johansen (1989) (cited in Bailey and Jones, 1997) studied 5926 non-obstetric patients reporting an incidence of 0.1% episodes of awareness under general anaesthesia. This study however was later criticised for relying purely on patient reporting rather than using a structured interview technique post-operatively as a more scientific and true alternative. A controlled trial conducted by Moerman *et al.* (1993) involved experienced anaesthetists who were shown anaesthetic records of patients, some of whom had been previously proven to experience an awareness episode. Of the patients who had experienced an awareness episode none were accurately identified using routine autonomic parameters (increasing pulse rate and blood pressure, tear formation and sweating).

The research carried out in Scandinavia was primarily prospective, using historical data and controlled cohort trials. Ekman *et al.* (2002) used a large cohort of 4945 patients monitored with standard monitoring techniques with the addition of BIS and 7826 patients using a standard form of monitoring. The incidence of awareness appears statistically significant; the BIS monitored group in this study returned results of 0.04% and in routine standard monitored patients 0.18%. Myles *et al.* (2003) have produced a few studies the most interesting of which was a survey of randomly selected anaesthetists who were asked for their personal opinions of awareness and depth of anaesthesia monitoring in current clinical practice. A high response rate of 85% was recorded in this survey indicating significant interest in this subject area. Unreliability of accurate data provided by the monitor appeared to be the major drawback for most anaesthetists surveyed and the cost of the monitoring equipment was high on the agenda. The overall cost was estimated at approximately $4000 per incident of awareness in Australia. An interesting point in the survey however, was the anaesthetists who had previously experienced awareness cases were less concerned with the cost of the monitoring equipment.

The majority of the evidence found in the studies was relevant to the subject area and may be of potential benefit to patients of the future. The overarching outcome for the patient is significant from the studies explored, although now the benefit to the individual organisation would need to be balanced against the initial cost of buying and running this equipment in the clinical arena. The samples used tended to be large but appeared to be representative of the population and the data tended to be collected from historical databases or survey methods. It was evident from the findings of the studies the results fit with what may be described as common knowledge.

Awareness may occur during general anaesthesia for a multitude of reasons which should not be viewed in isolation. They include human error, equipment failure and failure to carry out pre-use equipment checks, individual patient variation and in certain cases and types of surgery justified risk taking (Cobcroft, 1994). This view is supported by Domino (1996) who suggests that recall occurred in the majority of closed-claims cases in the United States because of the failure to provide a volatile anaesthetic agent, incorrect labelling of syringes and a lack in anaesthetic practitioner vigilance.

In an age of technological advancement and innovation, an accurate monitor that would ensure the patient was unconscious during general anaesthesia and the surgical procedure must surely be close to availability in mainstream medicine. The surgical patient will experience stimulation significant enough to produce awareness during the perioperative period. Some types of surgery are universally believed to carry a higher risk of awareness than others, these being caesarean section, cardiac and trauma surgery. The reasoning behind the differing levels of recorded incidence within these types of surgery is potentially that in caesarean section surgery the unborn baby should be protected as far as possible from noxious volatile anaesthetic agents and opiate drugs (Kumar, 2002; Chin & Yeo, 2004), thus reducing the requirement for prolonged active resuscitation of the baby following birth. In trauma surgery, the patient may be significantly haemodynamically unstable requiring reduced doses of drugs and anaesthetic agents, which can have a significant effect on the cardiovascular status of the patient. Within cardiac surgery, Tempe and Siddiquie (1999) suggest drugs and anaesthetic agents have less efficacy during cardiopulmonary bypass and the rewarming period.

The almost universal use of neuromuscular blocking agents during general anaesthesia leads to the belief that patients may experience awareness yet they may not be able to communicate the fact until after the event. As suggested by Simpson and Popat (2002), Yentis *et al.* (2004) and Aitkenhead *et al.* (2001) conscious or unconscious awareness would occur only if the anaesthetic became lightened, yet the muscle relaxant in use remained effective. It must be remembered the sense of hearing is the last sense to disappear on induction and may be affected by prolonged attempts at intubation of the airway, and it is the first sense to return on reversal and awakening from anaesthesia. This point clearly fits with the notion that reported incidents of awareness mainly involve conversations that may have taken place at these periods of the anaesthetic episode. Awareness could be associated with defects in the anaesthetic technique including low volatile agent concentrations and equipment faults as alluded to by Aitkenhead *et al.* (2001) including inadvertent malpositioning of vaporisers on anaesthetic machines leading to leakage of volatile agent and a harmful effect on the patient from lower inhaled concentrations.

Adequate levels of intravenous and/or inhalational drugs towards the surgical stimulus are essential (Gravenstein, 1991) to increase the likelihood that patients will not experience awareness of intra-operative events, yet may be difficult to provide as each individual patient will react differently to the drugs actually being used. This would include patients who may be less able to tolerate many of the drugs commonly used in general anaesthesia for a wide variety of reasons ranging from pre-existing disease to acute surgical need.

Due in part to the assumption that some patients who experience intra-operative awareness do not report the fact (Bailey & Jones, 1997) it is difficult to ascertain a true level of proven numbers of these adverse events from any previous study. To discover an accurate figure a large study involving the interviewing of all patients would potentially be required. Awareness can be defined as the experiencing of events happening around us and recall is the ability to remember something, which has previously occurred (Plourde, 2002). Explicit recall suggests a conscious understanding and spontaneous recollection of events that can be described and implicit recall means the recall of events that are not supported by conscious recognition by the patient. As Aitkenhead *et al.* (2001) suggest, the

brain can continue to process stimuli and information and retain memories even during general anaesthesia which should therefore be considered by all in clinical practice who may be tempted to verbally misbehave for any reason.

As Sice (2005) suggests, implicit memory occurs where recollection of events ceases to exist but the patient's behaviour is modified in some way by information given during anaesthesia. These definitions are supported by Pain (2002) who argues that post-operative structured interviews would identify most cases of explicit recall, though implicit recall of awareness events would potentially only be identified from in-depth psychological interviews and testing.

Patients have reported the experience of conscious intra-operative awareness as causing feelings of great distress and even of impending doom or death (Pain, 2002). Most patients reporting awareness incidents experience auditory sensations, which may not be discernible from events taking place on induction and recovery from anaesthesia. Many patients have reported seeing light and being touched though few have reported feelings of pain, probably due to the use of powerful opiate analgesics in the anaesthetic technique (Bailey & Jones, 1997). Anaesthetists and anaesthetic practitioners must keep caution within their practice, as the processing of auditory stimulus during the perioperative period may continue despite a perception of an adequate level of general anaesthesia (Pain, 2002). This may lead to 'fear conditioning' which would mean the patient would associate certain stimuli with the described unpleasant and potentially damaging events and feelings.

Studies have shown that recall of intra-operative awareness episodes may not be identified until some time post-operatively. Symptoms may however include post-operative distress, anxiety, restlessness, anger and other forms of changed and uncharacteristic behaviour which may begin as early as in the recovery phase of the patient's perioperative journey and may lead to more serious sequelae such as PTSD requiring prolonged medical and psychological treatment. Post-traumatic stress disorder causes altered behaviour states in the patients who suffer from this disorder. Patients may interpret awareness episodes, if experienced, as dreams or nightmares leading often to none reporting of actual incidents agreeing with Yentis *et al.* (2004) who claim that unpleasant dreams may mark a subconscious phase within awareness, although this notion is not supported with evidence. Sandin (2001) infers that some patients may not realise or understand exactly what is happening at the time, but may go on to suffer PTSD. Behaviour changes and sleep disturbance as referred to by Kenny (2001) and Pain (2002), could mean the patient might become reluctant to talk about their experience, which may have serious consequences regarding future health issues. Bailey and Jones (1997) allude to anecdotal evidence suggesting that early counselling may reduce the incidence of PTSD in perioperative awareness patients.

Awareness is a significant cause of anxiety about modern anaesthesia and raises concerns of dissatisfaction with the quality of care being provided for the patient (Myles *et al.*, 2004) and the potential for long-lasting and serious morbidity as suggested by Osterman *et al.* (2001). Post-traumatic stress disorder as stated by Osterman *et al.* (2001) is characterised by 're-experiencing, avoidance, and physiological hyper arousal'. The re-experiencing of the awareness event including the patient's surgery may occur as flashbacks or nightmares about pain, paralysis, or conversations between the theatre team. Osterman *et al.* (2001) explain that traumatised patients had reported smells, sounds, images, and other physical sensations in detail, which occurred when the traumatic event initially took place, which sometimes was a decade or more years previously.

Cobcroft (1994) reminds everyone involved in anaesthetic practice that apart from the potential experiencing of pain and feelings of being totally paralysed and helpless, patients can also feel extremely distressed. This is caused through the act of not being believed by healthcare professionals when a potential awareness incident is reported, and an explanation of possible causes of this report may go some way to alleviating the problem. Cobcroft (1994) goes on to suggest that preoperative explanation of awareness, as a potential major hazard would be useful in patients who are identified as being high risk. Every patient who is distressed enough to disclose potential awareness recollections of perioperative events must therefore be treated with care (Pain, 2002).

Today, depth of anaesthesia has been monitored using signs such as tachycardia, sweating, hypertension, lacrimation, pallor, and dilated pupils, though during awareness episodes these signs may not be present (Aitkenhead *et al.*, 2001; Yentis *et al.*, 2004). This may be the result of unreliable information (Bergman *et al.*, 2002; Myles *et al.*, 2004) because of some anaesthesia drug effects on the patient (McCarthy, 2000). Clinical signs of arterial blood pressure and heart rate are normally used to estimate the depth of anaesthesia by anaesthetists though these values are not capable of predicting if the patient is aware or not, at any given stage of the perioperative procedure. Sweating and tear formation indicate sympathetic nerve activity and as suggested by Kenny (2001) these clinical indicators are not reliable enough to detect episodes of awareness under general anaesthesia.

As suggested by Bailey and Jones (1997) many possible monitoring methods are available to the practice of anaesthesia. These methods could include clinical signs and anaesthetist and anaesthetic practitioner experience and lower oesophageal contractility, frontalis electromyogram, respiratory sinus arrhythmia and electroencephalogram (EEG). Within the latter suggested method (EEG) there are further potential options of BIS analysis and midlatency auditory evoked potential (MLAEP).

The Tunstall method of limb isolation (Hughs & Griffiths, 2002) involves inflating a tourniquet cuff above the level of the systolic blood pressure on an upper limb before induction of anaesthesia begins. This allows the limb to move if anaesthesia becomes too light by excluding the chosen limb from muscle relaxant drugs (Aitkenhead *et al.*, 2001). Nevertheless, this method may simply indicate a potential awareness episode after it has occurred but not necessarily explicit awareness and recall (Sice, 2005). Russell (1993) states that in a study carried out on major gynaecology patients receiving Midazolam and Alfentanyl and the isolated forearm technique, 72% of patients were able to perform limb movements on command during general anaesthesia and 63% reported experiencing pain.

Lower oesophageal contractility is known to increase at times of stress in conscious patients and may behave similarly when the patient is anaesthetised. Bailey and Jones (1997) suggest that individual patient variability may render this technique unreliable in a similar fashion to that of the frontalis electromyogram measurement. The frontalis muscle is less sensitive to muscle relaxant drugs than many other muscles and has decreased activity during anaesthesia, though patient variability dictates that this method of measurement may again be unreliable. Respiratory sinus arrhythmia is described as the variation of heart rate during the phases of respiration and is a clear indicator of vagal tone, which diminishes during anaesthesia using propofol and isoflurane. The pharmacological effects of anaesthetic drugs on the brainstem mediate this method of monitoring potential inadvertent awareness.

Depths of anaesthesia monitors use a variety of electrophysiological techniques to monitor patient response to given stimuli. Monitors currently in the UK are the BIS and the auditory evoked potential (AEP). The BIS monitor is an electronic monitor designed to measure EEG signals and calculate a dimensionless number which indicates the current depth of anaesthesia as stated by Aitkenhead *et al.* (2001) and Plourde (2002). The BIS is not well known among perioperative practitioners. The BIS algorithm was originally designed for use with single anaesthetic agent anaesthesia such as total intravenous anaesthesia (TIVA). The numerical range of BIS monitors is 85–100 representing awake and 40–65 representing general anaesthesia, however it is accepted that no single value is applicable to every individual patient as stated by Crippen (2004). Artefacts during monitoring as suggested by Sice (2005) have caused false readings and include cardiac pacemakers, electro surgery equipment, intravenous fluids, patient-warming devices and patient movements.

Kenny (2001) suggests that favourable results have been found using AEP for monitoring depth of anaesthesia, which works on the analysis of EEG signals from an active auditory stimulus, usually high-frequency clicks and suggests that auditory response appears to be responded to by anaesthetised patients appropriately. This suggestion is supported by Aitkenhead *et al.* (2001). The high-frequency sounds stimulate auditory cortical activity, which may then be measured as a brainstem response by the monitor. The AEP also uses a dimensionless arbitrary number scale, which is 60–100 awake and 20–30 general anaesthesia. Kenny (2001) goes on to suggest that this method of monitoring may improve accuracy of drug delivery. AEP however is clearly limited in its use on patients who suffer from hearing difficulties, which may be a problem with the ageing population in the United Kingdom. Kenny (2001) discusses the possible control of anaesthetic agent delivery to a predetermined level as in target-controlled infusion (TCI) via a computerised feedback connection between AEP monitor and portable computer. This system is capable of altering the depth of anaesthesia and is known as a closed-loop system in patients breathing spontaneously during surgery, a method of monitoring supported by Bailey and Jones (1997). Morley *et al.* (2000) dispute that closed-loop control of TCI has any advantage over a conventional method of drug delivery. This method of monitoring is therefore limited in its use when surgery requires access to the ear and the surrounding area or the patient has a pre-existing hearing disorder.

Monitoring of end-tidal anaesthetic gas concentration is a further method which allows the anaesthetist to estimate depth of anaesthesia in current clinical practice using the mean alveolar concentration (MAC) value as discussed by Gravenstein (1991) and Sandin *et al.* (2000) which may prevent some cases of inadvertent awareness. The use of low-end tidal anaesthetic gas concentration alarms did not make a significant difference in identifying potential awareness events. The MAC value of a volatile agent is the concentration at (a pressure of 1 atmosphere) which 50% of patients make a purposeful movement in response to a standard painful stimulus, usually surgical, but there is no recall of this stimulation taking place. The MAC value in practice is known to reduce under certain conditions including decreased body temperature, hypoxia, and age, sedative drugs and systemic and epidural opiate drugs (Sice, 2005). It has to be considered that EEG monitoring of any kind would not be effective as a measure of awareness in episodes of inadvertent paralysis (Bergman *et al.*, 2002) which may occur before the patient is connected to the monitor, for example in the anaesthetic room, the cause of which may be the inadvertent mislabelling of syringes.

In conclusion, there are myriad studies, all with similar outcomes. The monitors currently being used and tested do appear to make a difference but due to the perceived relatively low incidence of awareness in the first place, the cost of the monitors would appear to be prohibitive for acquisition and ongoing outlay. Smith *et al.* (2003) suggest that it may not simply be the use of monitoring which makes modern anaesthesia relatively safe but the interpretation of the information provided by the monitors by the anaesthetist and anaesthetic practitioners. Nevertheless, if litigation costs continue to increase, and coverage of reported adverse anaesthetic incidents is delivered to the public through the mass media, can this technology be ignored for much longer? Nowak (2004) argues that the use of depth of anaesthesia monitoring or some form of brain activity monitor in future clinical practice may be taken by legal departments.

Leslie and Myles (2001) suggest that as many as 54% of patients are concerned about awareness during anaesthesia and a study by Myles *et al.* (2003) into anaesthetist attitudes towards awareness under general anaesthesia highlighted that anaesthetists in Australia only regard awareness under general anaesthesia as a moderate problem. Integration of an awareness monitoring device in clinical practice rests with the anaesthetist's perception of the importance of inadvertent awareness under general anaesthesia (Myles *et al.*, 2004). It would be interesting to ascertain the attitude among anaesthetists in the UK in a similar fashion. Healthcare practitioners must be prepared to acknowledge that this problem does occur and treat the patients who report being affected by it, with dignity and compassion.

Anaesthetists who are faced with a patient who claims to have had an episode of awareness under general anaesthesia must be prepared to discuss the event openly and honestly and be prepared to refer the patient for professional psychological support if further treatment is deemed necessary. The diagnosis of inadvertent intra-operative awareness remains problematic for all concerned. The lack of universal agreement on monitoring methods and the lack of substantive evidence that monitors under development achieve an acceptable level of accuracy, remains a major issue. The anaesthetist and anaesthetic practitioner must rely on their skills of thorough preparation, checking procedures of all equipment outlined in the guidelines prepared by the Association of Anaesthetists of Great Britain and Ireland (AAGBI, 2004) and observation during procedures including full monitoring and a continuous presence of an anaesthetist and anaesthetic practitioner throughout the perioperative period (Bailey & Jones, 1997). It should never be assumed the anaesthetist has sole responsibility for the observation of patients undergoing anaesthesia; the anaesthetic practitioner also has a duty of care towards the patients.

The American Society of Anesthesiologists (ASA) House of Delegates (2005) have accepted and implemented a 'practice advisory for intra-operative awareness and brain function monitoring' which includes the use of a BIS or other brain activity monitor for patients who are clinically assessed and believed to be at risk of a potential inadvertent awareness event during the perioperative period. Bispectral index monitoring has been used in the United States since 1996 onwards. Further research and clear evidence of significant improvements in accuracy of depth of anaesthesia monitors is required, if acceptance of these monitors is to be gained within current UK operating theatre departments. Until this occurs, vigilance and caution within clinical practice must be encouraged from all staff engaged in anaesthetic practice.

REFERENCES

Aitkenhead, A.R., Rowbotham, D.J. & Smith, G. (2001). *Textbook of Anaesthesia*. London: Churchill Livingstone.

Association of Anaesthetists of Great Britain and Ireland. (2004). *Checklist for Anaesthetic Equipment*. Available at: http://www.aagbi.org/pdf/checklistA4.pdf (Accessed 10 May 2006).

Bailey, A.R. & Jones, J.G. (1997). Patients' memories of events during general anaesthesia. *Anaesthesia*, **52**, 460–76.

Bergman, I.J., Kluger, M.T. & Short, T.G. (2002). Awareness during general anaesthesia: a review of 81 cases from the Anaesthetic Incidence Monitoring study. *Anaesthesia*, **57**, 549–56.

Chin, K.J. & Yeo, S.W. (2004). A BIS-guided study of sevoflurane requirements for adequate depth of anaesthesia in Caesarean section. *Anaesthesia*, **59**, 1064–8.

Cobcroft, M.D. (1994). *Awareness Under General Anaesthesia. WFSA Distance Learning: (On Line) Paper 5*. Available at: http://www.nda.ox.ac.uk/wfsa/dl/html/papers/pap005.htm (Accessed 12 October 2003).

Crippen, D.W. (2004). *Bispectral Index: is it Ready for Prime Time in the ICU?* Available at: http://www.medscape.com/viewarticle/471955?src=search (Accessed 16 January 2006).

Domino, K.B. (1996). Closed malpractice claims for awareness during anaesthesia. *ASA Newsletter*, **60**(6), 14–17.

Ekman, A., Lindholm, M.-L., Lennmarken, C. & Sandin, R. (2002). Reduction in the incidence of awareness using BIS monitoring. *Acta Anaesthesiologica Scandinavica*, **48**, 20–6.

Gravenstein, N. (1991). *Manual of Complications During Anaesthesia*. Philadelphia: Lippincott.

Hughs, S. & Griffiths, R. (2002). Anaesthesia monitoring techniques. *Anaesthesia and Intensive Care Medicine*. The Medicine Publishing Company Ltd, pp. 477–80.

Kenny, G. (2001). Techniques for measuring the depth of anaesthesia. *European Society of Anaesthesiologists*, Gothenburg.

Kumar, B. (2002). *Working in the Operating Department*, 2nd edn. London: Churchill Livingstone.

Leslie, K. & Myles, P. (2001). Awareness during general anaesthesia: is it worth worrying about? Bispectral index monitoring may be a solution to the problem (Editorial). *MJA*, **174**, 212–13.

McCarthy, G.J. (2000). *Awareness During Total Intravenous Anaesthesia and How to Avoid It*. Available at: http://www.sivauk.org/Belfast.McCarthy.htm (Accessed 16 January 2006).

Moerman, N., Bonke, B. & Oosting, J. (1993). Awareness and recall during general anesthesia. Facts and feeling. *Anesthesiology*, **79**, 454–64.

Morley, A., Derrick, J., Mainland, B., Lee, B. & Short, T.G. (2000). Closed loop control of anaesthesia: an assessment of the bispectral index as the target of control. *Anaesthesia*, **55**, 953–9.

Myles, P.S., Leslie, K., McNeil, J., Forbes, A. & Chan, M.T.V. (2004). Bispectral index monitoring during anaesthesia: the B-Aware randomised controlled trial. *The Lancet*, **363**(9423), 1757–63.

Myles, P.S., Symons, J.A. & Leslie, K. (2003). Anaesthetists' attitudes towards awareness and depth-of-anaesthesia monitoring. *Anaesthesia*, **58**, 11–16.

National Statistics. (2003). *Operative Procedure Statistics*. Available at: http://www.statistics.gov.uk/CCI/nscl.asp (Accessed 10 May 2006).

Nowak, R. (2004). *Monitor Detects Awareness During Anaesthesia*. Available at: http://www.newscientist.com/new/news.jsp?id=99994878 (Accessed 4 June 2004).

Osterman, J., Hopper, J., Heran, W., Keane, T. & Van Der Kolk, B. (2001). Awareness during anaesthesia and the development of traumatic stress disorder. *General Hospital Psychiatry*, **23**(4), 198–204.

Pain, L. (2002). Can we prevent recall during anaesthesia? *European Society of Anaesthesiologists*. Available at: http://www.euroanaesthesia.org/education/rc_nice/lrc3.html (Accessed 16 January 2006).

Plourde, G. (2002). BIS EEG monitoring: what it can and cannot do in regard to unintentional awareness. *Canadian Journal of Anaesthesia*, **49**, (Suppl 1), 12R.

Power, C., Crowe, C., Higgins, P. & Moriarty, D. C. (1998). Anaesthetic depth at induction. An evaluation using clinical eye signs and EEG polysomnography. *Anaesthesia*, **53**, 736–43.

Russell, I. F. (1993). Midazolam-Alfentanyl: an anaesthetic? An investigation using the isolated forearm technique. *British Journal of Anaesthesia*, **70**, 42–6.

Sandin, R. H. (2001). *Awareness 1960–2001; Incidence, Consequence, Prevention*. Available at: http://www.eurosiva.org/Archive/Goteborg/Abstracts/Sandin.htm (Accessed 21 November 2005).

Sandin, R. H., Enlund, G., Samuelsson, P. & Lennmarken, C. (2000). Awareness during anaesthesia: a prospective case study. *The Lancet*, **355**, 707–11.

Sice, P. J. A. (2005). *Depth of Anaesthesia. Update in Anaesthesia* Issue **19**(10). Available at: http://www.nda.ox.ac.uk/wfsa/html/u19/u1910_01.htm (Accessed 27 October 2005).

Simpson, P. J. & Popat, M. (2002). *Understanding Anaesthesia*, 4th edn. Edinburgh: Butterworth Heinemann.

Smith, A. F., Mort, M., Goodwin, D. & Pope, C. (2003). Making monitoring 'work': human-machine interaction and patient safety in anaesthesia. *Anaesthesia*, **58**, 1070–8.

Snow, J. (1847). On the inhalation of the vapour ether in surgical operations. London: Churchill. Cited in Power *et al.* (1998). Anaesthesia depth at induction an evaluation using clinical eye signs and EEG polysomnography. *Anaesthesia*, **53**, 736–43.

Tempe, D. K. & Siddiquie, R. A. (1999). Awareness during cardiac surgery. *Journal of Cardiothoracic and Vascular Anaesthesia*, **13**(2), 214–19.

The American Society of Anesthesiologists (ASA) House of Delegates. (2005). Practice advisory for intra-operative awareness and brain function monitoring. *American Society of Anesthesiologists*. Available at: http://www.asahq.org (Accessed 16 January 2006).

Yentis, S. M., Hirsch, N. P. & Smith, G. B. (2004). *Anaesthesia and Intensive Care A–Z; An Encyclopaedia of Principles and Practice*. Edinburgh: Butterworth Heinemann.

8

Aspects of perioperative neuroscience practice

Margaret Woods

Key Learning Points

- Understand neurological assessment
  - Coma scale measurement
  - Vital signs
  - Pupillary reaction
- Understand the principles of intracranial monitoring
- Understand the anaesthetic considerations for patients with head injury and subarachnoid haemorrhage
- Understand the anaesthetic assessment of the patient with a neurological illness

Introduction

Neuroscience is a rapidly evolving and dynamic speciality. Managing patients with neurological problems may be anxiety provoking and demanding, but rewarding when a successful outcome is achieved. Neuroscience includes various surgical and medical conditions ranging from acute conditions such as severe head injury and subarachnoid haemorrhage (SAH) to long-term conditions such as epilepsy or Parkinson's disease (PD). Patients with acute conditions may be managed at local hospitals in acute or critical care settings or may require referral for specialist intervention. Additionally, patients with long-term conditions may access acute services with problems, therefore an understanding of how their disorder impacts on their subsequent care is required by the

practitioner. The numbers of people with long-term neurological conditions are rising as a result of the increasing age of the population. Their care in the future will benefit from the implementation of the National Service Framework, which aims to create a more structured and integrated approach that is both supportive and appropriate at each stage of their lives (DH, 2005).

The aim of this chapter is to highlight the main points relating to the perioperative needs of neuroscience patients, with specific emphasis upon anaesthetic management. Even though care is mainly managed in specialist units, the outcome for such patients may be improved by expert knowledgeable care and attention in the preparation and safe transfer of these patients. In addition, neurological patients with long-term conditions may have both specialist anaesthetic needs relating to their neurological condition or more general anaesthetic needs which may be met in any acute setting.

Related anatomy and physiology

The brain, which comprises the cerebrum, cerebellum and brainstem, is protected by the skull and supported by three layers of coverings, the meninges. The three layers of meninges are the dura mater, the arachnoid mater and the pia mater. The cerebrum is partially separated into two hemispheres, which are in turn divided into lobes (Figure 8.1).

Core Topics in Operating Department Practice: Anaesthesia and Critical Care, eds. Brian Smith, Paul Rawling, Paul Wicker and Chris Jones. Published by Cambridge University Press. © Cambridge University Press 2007.

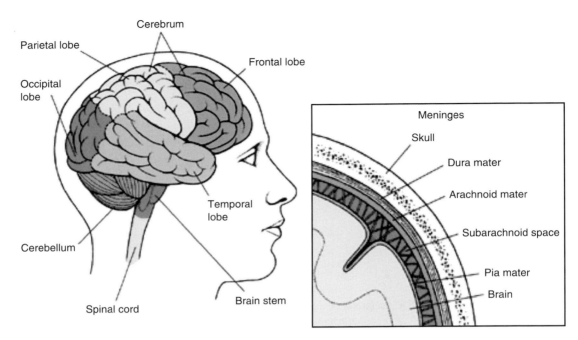

Figure 8.1 The brain has three main parts: the cerebrum, the brain stem, and the cerebellum. The meninges consists of three layers: the dura, arachnoids and pia mater. From The Merck Manual of Medical Information, Second Home Edition, (ed.) Mark H. Beers. Copyright 2003 by Merck & Co. Inc., Whitehouse Station, NJ.

Contained within the brain are four irregular-shaped cavities or ventricles, namely the right and left lateral ventricles, and the third and fourth ventricles. The ventricles are part of a closed system, the cerebrospinal fluid (CSF) pathway. CSF is formed by the choroid plexus, a collection of blood vessels in the ventricles and circulates in between the arachnoid and pia layers, known as the subarachnoid space around the brain and spinal cord. It is reabsorbed into the venous circulation through projections (arachnoid villi) in the arachnoid mater and returns to the venous circulation (Clancy & McVicar, 2002) (Figure 8.2).

and spinal cord and within the cerebral ventricles' (Hickey, 2003: 285). The brain, CSF and blood are contained within a rigid structure, the skull or cranium. The proportions of these contents are approximately brain 80%, blood 10% and CSF 10% (Hickey, 2003). These components are incompressible, that is, an increase in the volume of any one will result in an increase in ICP (Lindsay & Bone, 2004). In normal circumstances, ICP will remain relatively stable despite changes in the volume of blood or brain tissue due to reabsorption of CSF (Moss, 2001). Nevertheless there are a number of circumstances in which the ICP may rise (Table 8.1).

Intracranial pressure

The normal intracranial pressure (ICP) is approximately 0–15 mmHg and it is 'the pressure normally exerted by the CSF that circulates around the brain

Causes of raised ICP

The brain can accommodate increases in volume that occur over a lengthy period of time more easily than volume increases over a shorter period. This is

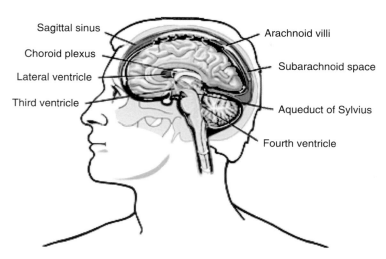

Sagittal sinus

Choroid plexus

Lateral ventricle

Third ventricle

Arachnoid villi

Subarachnoid space

Aqueduct of Sylvius

Fourth ventricle

Figure 8.2 Diagram of flow of cerebrospinal fluid. Reprinted with the permission of The Cleveland Clinic Foundation.

Table 8.1 Causes of raised intracranial pressure

Expanding mass	Tumour, haematoma, abscess
Increase in brain water content	Intracellular, extracellular oedema
Increase in cerebral blood volume	Vasodilation, e.g. hypercapnia, venous outflow obstruction, e.g. body position, prone
Increase in cerebrospinal fluid	Impaired absorption, e.g. subarachnoid haemorrhage, excessive secretion (rare)

Adapted from Lindsay & Bone, 2004.

because it has compensatory mechanisms, which can respond to rising pressure. If space is required because the ICP is rising, then CSF may be moved out of the skull and down around the spinal cord thus creating temporary space within the skull. This is an immediate compensatory mechanism. There are other mechanisms such as reduction of blood volume, decreased production of CSF and finally, compression of brain tissue. Compression of brain tissue will compound the original problem and cause a worsening of neurological symptoms by reducing the blood flow to the brain.

The brain, especially the cortex, which consists of grey matter because it is mainly composed of nerve cells (neurones), demands a constant blood supply to meet its high metabolic requirements. In an undamaged brain, cerebral blood flow is maintained by various regulatory mechanisms. One of the most important of these is autoregulation (Stanley & Hancox, 2001). The mean arterial blood pressure (MAP) is considered to be the pressure at which the brain is perfused. Cerebral perfusion pressure (CPP) is defined as the blood pressure gradient across the brain and is an estimate of the adequacy of the cerebral circulation (Hickey, 2003). Autoregulation allows fluctuations in the CPP without significantly altering cerebral blood flow (Stanley & Hancox, 2001; Lyndsay & Bone, 2004). Inadequate CCP will result in ischaemia or infarction depending on the severity of shortfall of cerebral blood flow.

Rising ICP eventually compresses the brain stem and forces parts of the cerebrum downwards through the tentorium cerebelli, a sheet

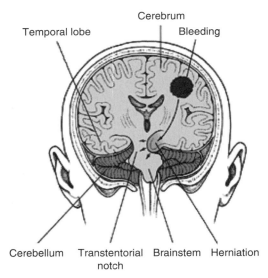

Figure 8.3 Transtentorial herniation of the brain. From The Merck Manual of Medical Information, Second Home Edition, edited by Mark H. Beers. Copyright 2003 by Merck & Co., Inc., Whitehouse Station, NJ.

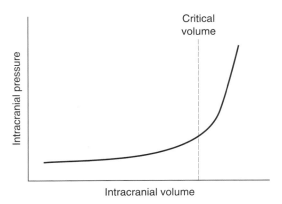

Figure 8.4 Pressure–volume curve. http://www.trauma.org/neuro/icp.html

of dura mater, which separates the cerebrum from the cerebellum (Figure 8.3). Displacement or herniation of the brain ensues and cerebral perfusion is severely compromised if ICP continues to rise unimpeded. Cerebral blood flow ceases when the ICP is equal to the MAP (Lyndsay & Bone, 2004) causing infarction of brain tissue.

Clinically, tentorial herniation commonly referred to as 'coning' is evidenced by a deepening of conscious level accompanied by worsening of neurological function. If pressure is unrelieved there may be dilation of the pupil on the same (ipsilateral) side, which fails to react to light or other pupillary abnormalities (Hickey, 2003). Small increases of volume are accommodated without a significant rise in ICP until compensatory mechanisms have been exhausted, at which point the ICP will rise rapidly (Figure 8.4). Alterations in vital signs such as a rising systolic blood pressure and bradycardia may also be evident and are indicative of brainstem dysfunction.

Assessment

Loss of consciousness is a sign of general dysfunction of the brain (Teasdale & Jennett, 1974) therefore monitoring a patient's conscious level will give an indication of improvement or deterioration in their condition. The purpose of undertaking neurological assessment is to compile a database of the patient's responses and general condition in order that the trend can be observed. Neurological assessment is a vital part of the patient's care and can incorporate a coma scale such as the Glasgow Coma Scale (GCS), vital signs such as blood pressure, heart rate, respiratory rate, temperature and pupillary responses. Motor function (limb movements and strength) and cranial nerve function (eye and facial movements) may also be assessed. Frequency of observations should be dictated by the patient's condition and the practitioner's professional judgement and should not be the subject of ritualistic practice (Edwards, 2001). Observation of head injuries in the accident and emergency department should at least consist of GCS; pupil size and reactivity; limb movements; respiratory rate; blood pressure; temperature; and blood oxygen saturation (pulse oximetry) (NICE, 2003).

The GCS is based upon evaluating behavioural responses, specifically eye opening, verbal

Table 8.2 The Glasgow Coma Scale

Glasgow Coma Scale		
Eye opening	spontaneously	4
	to speech	3
	to pain	2
	none	1
Verbal response	oriented	5
	confused	4
	inappropriate	3
	incomprehensible	2
	none	1
Motor response	obeys commands	6
	localises to pain	5
	withdraws from pain	4
	flexion to pain	3
	extension to pain	2
	nono	1
Maximum score		15

Source: Teasdale & Jennett, 1974.

response and motor response, to certain requests and stimuli (Jevon & Ewens, 2002). A numerical value is assigned to the level of response in each category, the minimum score achievable being 3, with a maximum score of 15 (Table 8.2). The GCS may be a 14-point scale or a 15-point scale. Both can be found in use in practice, which may cause some confusion for the practitioner (Wiese, 2003). Coma is estimated to be 8 or under and demands the early attention of an anaesthetist or intensivist to ensure that the airway is safely managed (NICE, 2003).

The GCS has long been the subject of debate with regard to its validity and reliability. Small studies showed that experienced practitioners used the tool more effectively (Rowley & Fielding, 1991; Ellis & Cavanagh, 1992), although it was originally intended that it should be a quick and easy to use tool, which various staff could use in different settings (Teasdale & Jennett, 1974).

Problems may be encountered when eliciting responses to pain, because there is a lack of clarity about the method, the frequency and the duration

of the testing (Price, 2002). Additionally, the GCS may not be the most appropriate tool for assessing the neurological status of ventilated and sedated patients (Price, 1996) and its use in the critical care environment has been superseded by continuous monitoring of physiological variables, in particular ICP and CPP (Price *et al.*, 2000). Despite the GCS's shortcomings, its international use suggests that it is a widely accepted tool for the assessment of coma (Price, 2002). Nevertheless, it is still subject to variability as are all observations (Teasdale *et al.*, 1978). Still, it remains a reliable way of objectively monitoring the clinical course of the patient with acute neurological dysfunction (Bateman, 2001).

Monitoring

Neurological assessment may be inadequate in the presence of neurological dysfunction, which is affecting the patient's conscious level to a significant degree. Raised ICP is the most common cause of death in neurosurgical patients, therefore monitoring the ICP will not only alert the practitioner to changes in the patient's condition but also provides a means of evaluating the effect of interventions which may have been deployed in an effort to reduce ICP (Gupta & Azami, 2002; Ravi & Morgan, 2003). Even though ICP monitoring may be used in a variety of disorders, monitoring is more commonly used in cerebral trauma (Springborg *et al.*, 2005).

Measurement of ICP may be established by means of a fluid-filled catheter similar to an arterial catheter, or solid catheters such as fibre-optic or strain gauge devices (Woodward, 2000). The common sites for ICP measurement are intraventricular and intraparenchymal (into the brain substance) although other sites are occasionally used (Gupta & Azami, 2002). Intracranial pressure may then be displayed numerically and as a waveform, which can be interpreted.

Intraventricular catheters allow both measurement of ICP and drainage of CSF, which may be a strategy used to relieve rising ICP (Citerio & Andrews, 2004; Ross & Eynon, 2005). Nevertheless, placement of the catheter may be difficult if the ventricle is distorted (Pattison *et al.*, 2005) and there is a higher risk of infection after 3 days of monitoring (Gupta & Azami, 2002).

Insertion of an intraparenchymal catheter may be undertaken safely in the critical care environment (Flint, 1999; Stanley & Hancox, 2001). Intraparenchymal catheters are accurate initially but may be less reliable 4–5 days after insertion (Citerio & Andrews, 2004). Nevertheless by that time their use may be less relevant in the management of the patient's condition.

The more widespread availability of ICP monitoring enables the patient to be monitored in a local hospital because transfer to a specialist centre may put the patient at further risk of deterioration (Macartney & Nightingale, 2001; Intensive Care Society, 2002). Even though ICP monitoring has been in use for a number of decades, there is no conclusive evidence of its value and more research is needed to clarify its role (Forsyth *et al.*, 2001). Nevertheless, it is a relatively inexpensive procedure with a low complication rate, which can inform the management of the seriously ill patient (Citerio & Andrews, 2004). Intracranial pressure monitoring can disclose raised ICP, which is not found on clinical evaluation alone (Stocchetti *et al.*, 2001). The National Institute of Clinical Excellence (NICE) will shortly consider the safety and efficacy of ICP monitoring and will issue guidance in the future (NICE, 2005).

Recent developments in monitoring have focused upon a multi-modal approach, that is, monitoring the ICP, cerebral perfusion and brain tissue oxygen (Gupta & Azami, 2002; Stevens, 2004). Nevertheless, the evidence of benefit from additional monitoring is poor and it may over-complicate management (Girling, 2004).

Monitoring can only be useful in guiding clinical practice if healthcare professionals are able to interpret the results. The use of ICP monitoring outside a neuro-critical care unit will necessitate that practitioners are suitably trained and supported in its use because results have to be interpreted and clinical decisions made based on these results (Ross & Eynon, 2005). Ultimately it is human skills and vigilance that determine either the success or failure of a monitoring system (Springborg *et al.*, 2005).

Head injury

Head injury is common, accounting for over 1 million people attending accident and emergency departments each year (DH, 2005). Damage can vary from slight to fatal injury. Patients sustaining injury severe enough to warrant admission to critical care or to undergo surgery are fortunately a small proportion of this group (NICE, 2003) although 5000 patients per year die in Britain as a result of their injuries (Lindsay & Bone, 2004). Deaths as a result of head injuries are falling through a combination of both preventative strategies and improved treatments. Preventative strategies have included the compulsory use of seat belts in vehicles and protective helmets for motorcyclists. Improved treatments include better resuscitation, transfer and early treatment at specialist centres when intervention is required.

Head injury may occur in isolation or as part of a multiple trauma presentation, particularly spinal injury (Morris *et al.*, 2004). Common causes for head injury are traffic accidents, falls, assaults, and sport injuries, to name but a few. Alcohol may also be a contributory factor (Christensen *et al.*, 2001). Road traffic accidents alone constitute 60% of the deaths from head injury (Lindsay & Bone, 2004). A person having a GCS of 8 or less is classed as having a severe head injury (Goh & Gupta, 2002). In adults, those most at risk of serious head injury are young males aged between 16 and 30 years. The loss of such a young person is a serious blow to both his family and society in general. There is also the consideration that many people may also be left with permanent disability requiring long-term care, which has both financial and service implications.

How brain damage occurs

Damage occurring as a result of head injury may be divided into two types: primary and secondary damage. Primary damage is that which is sustained at the time of the incident and as such there may be little that can be done to alter the effect of primary injury apart from preventative measures. Secondary damage is sustained in the aftermath or as a consequence of the primary damage (Girling, 2004). It may be caused by systemic factors such as hypoxia and hypotension or by compression of brain tissue. Compression may be caused by brain swelling (cerebral oedema) or by haematomas (intracranial haemorrhage) (Hickey, 2003).

Brain damage occurs predominantly when blunt forces are exerted on the skull. The brain may move inside the skull causing damage such as contusion, laceration and the formation of haematomas. The common types of haematoma are extradural, subdural or intracerebral, depending on the source of the bleed (Hickey, 2003) (Figure 8.5).

The brain may be subjected to acceleration, deceleration or rotational forces that may tear nerve fibres or axons resulting in widespread or diffuse microscopic damage known as diffuse axonal injury. Surgical intervention may not be necessary because there is no distinct mass, however, the patient may have significant injury depending on the amount of force that was exerted (Davis, 2000). This may be referred to as closed (non-penetrating) head injury.

Neurosurgical opinion must be sought with regard to the management of primary damage,

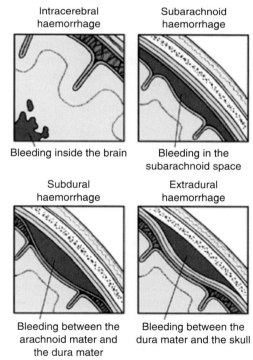

Figure 8.5 Sites of brain haemorrhage. From The Merck Manual of Medical Information, Second Home Edition, (ed.) Mark H. Beers. Copyright 2003 by Merck & Co., Inc., Whitehouse Station, NJ.

which may or may not be operable. Prompt intervention is advocated, within 4 hours or less (DH, 2005). Surgery will normally be undertaken at a specialist neuroscience centre, therefore rapid resuscitation and safe transfer will be needed to optimise outcome (improve patient's prognosis).

Secondary damage is incurred in the period following the original insult, often as a consequence of the primary injury, for example, raised ICP, ischaemia and oedema (Andrews, 2003; Cooper & Cramp, 2003). There are also alterations in the cerebral blood flow and an inflammatory response to brain tissue injury is initiated (Goh & Gupta, 2002; Jackson *et al.*, 2002). The effects of primary damage and subsequent alterations in cerebral function may be compounded by systemic problems of hypoxaemia, hypotension and pyrexia.

Autoregulation normally regulates cerebral blood flow, ensuring that the brain receives the exact amount required to carry out its metabolic functions. Autoregulation functions when the MAP is between 50 and 150 mmHg (Hickey, 2003). Unfortunately, cerebral autoregulation may be impaired after head injury and cerebral blood flow may fluctuate passively with changes in the MAP (Minassian *et al.*, 2002) thus potentially increasing the risk of cerebral ischaemia and infarction.

Management of head injury

The evidence base for the treatment of patients with severe head injury is very limited (Girling, 2004). The main aim of critical care management is to prevent secondary injury and to optimise cerebral oxygenation (Andrews, 2003). An important aspect of this aim may be achieved by the maintenance of adequate CPP. Targets for CPP may vary from 60 to 70 mmHg (Goh & Gupta, 2002; Hayes, 2002) to greater than 70 mmHg (Andrews, 2003; Lindsay & Bone, 2004). Calculation of the CPP is deduced by subtracting the ICP from the CPP, shown as: MAP (80 mmHg) − ICP (20 mmHg) = CPP (60 mmHg),

therefore it is necessary to have resources enabling the measurement of ICP.

Immediate management of the patient is focused on the prevention of secondary injury through proactive management of the airway and rapid resuscitation. Support of the airway may include intubation if conscious level is deteriorating. A GCS score of less than 8 is one of the indications for early intubation (NICE, 2003). Intubation should be as atraumatic as possible in order to prevent rises in ICP (Table 8.3). An IV induction agent and muscle relaxants should always be used in head-injured patients (Riley, 2001). Rapid sequence induction using succinylcholine may be necessary in emergency situations because protection of the airway against aspiration is a greater consideration. Muscle fasciculations (twitching) caused by succinylcholine may increase ICP (Moss, 2001), however its benefits far outweigh its risks (Simpson, 2001).

Anaesthetic agents may contribute to ICP; inhalational gases such as halothane and isoflurane cause cerebral vasodilation (Table 8.3). Furthermore both sedation and muscle relaxants may be used initially during the acute stage of head injury to suppress coughing and comply with ventilation, because both of these activities may increase ICP by increasing intrathoracic pressure (Moss, 2001). Relaxants are not however recommended for long-term use because they are associated with greater disability in survivors (Goh & Gupta, 2002).

The cardiovascular system should be stabilised through good venous access and fluid administration using both colloids (plasma expanders) and crystalloids as appropriate. Glucose solutions are to be avoided because hyperglycaemia can increase the risk of secondary brain injury (Riley, 2001). An elevated serum glucose level may be due to a stress response and may worsen neurological status by aggravating ischaemia (Hickey, 2003). Care is required in the general management and positioning of the patients in order not to inadvertently cause rises in ICP (Letvak & Hand, 2003) (Table 8.3).

Table 8.3 Factors known to increase intracranial pressure (ICP)

Respiratory	Hypercapnia (CO_2 potent vasodilator), hypoxaemia $pO_2 < 6.7$ Kpa (50 mmHg) cerebral vasodilation
	Respiratory procedures such as suctioning, intubation
	Anaesthetic agents such as halothane, isoflurane and enflurane cause vasodilation thus increasing cerebral blood flow and ICP
	Positive pressure ventilation with the addition of positive end expiratory pressure (PEEP), increases intrathoracic pressure, central venous pressure (CVP) and ICP
Body positioning	Trendelenburg, neck flexion, prone, extreme hip flexion, possible obstruction of venous return with increasesd intra-abdominal pressure and intrathoracic pressure
Activities	Valsalva's manoevre (straining at stool, moving in bed, sneezing) coughing, increased intra-abdominal pressure and intrathoracic pressure impeding venous return from the brain

Adapted from Hickey, 2003.

Neurological assessment is required in the perioperative environment although assessment may be complicated by the use of sedation and muscle relaxants. Therefore a level of consciousness cannot be determined. Nevertheless, pupils can be assessed for size, shape and reaction to light and vital signs must also be recorded. Increased systolic blood pressure and decreased heart rate are late signs of raised ICP and warrant immediate management (Letvak & Hand, 2003).

Drug therapy

Consideration must also be given to the patient's comfort and pain relief through the appropriate use of sedation and analgesia. Agitation and restlessness may also be a feature of head injury. Propofol is the most common choice for IV sedation. Propofol's sedative properties reduce the cerebral oxygen requirements by lowering the metabolic rate, however the systemic effect of this advantage is that there may be episodes of hypotension, which may compromise cerebral perfusion. Therefore cautious use is required. It is a short-acting drug and has the advantage that it can be weaned quickly allowing the conduction of a neurological assessment in approximately 5–10 minutes (Hickey, 2003).

Thiopentone, a long-acting barbiturate may be used for severe injury where the ICP is difficult to control, but there is no evidence that outcome is improved with its use (Roberts, 1999). Nevertheless, high doses of thiopentone should be used with caution because of the side-effect of cardiovascular depression and its use may be limited by slow clearance which may hinder early neurological assessment. Alfentanil is the analgesic of choice; it has a shorter elimination time, therefore it is useful if the patient requires short-term ventilation (Riley, 2001).

Mannitol, an osmotic diuretic, is an important therapy in the management of raised ICP. Through an osmotic gradient, fluid can be shifted from the extracellular space of the brain into the vascular system and excreted thereby reducing the volume of the brain. Roberts *et al.* (2004) concluded in their review that high-dose mannitol may be preferable in the preoperative management of patients with acute intracranial haematomas, however further research is required with regard to the optimal use of mannitol in this condition. Continued use of mannitol may result in dehydration therefore it is important that the patient has an indwelling catheter in place to monitor urinary output and that serum urea and electrolytes levels are also monitored (Hickey, 2003).

Ongoing research is in progress with little success to date into developing therapies to offset the effects of the inflammatory response seen in the subsequent days following injury (Hayes, 2002). Steroids, which were commonly used in the past decades, play no role in the management of head injury because it has been proved conclusively that they have a detrimental effect on outcome (CRASH Trial Collaborators, 2004).

Severe head injury can have a devastating effect on the patient and his family but specialist neuro-critical care results in improvements in recovery following severe head injury (Patel *et al.*, 2002).

Subarachnoid haemorrhage

Subarachnoid haemorrhage (SAH), bleeding into the subarachnoid space, is a type of stroke in which there is a sudden interruption to the blood supply to an area of the brain causing mild to severe ischaemia and possible infarction. Subarachnoid haemorrhage is less common than ischaemic stroke causing about 5% of all strokes but it can be devastating in its effects (Warlow *et al.*, 2003). Despite improvements in the management and treatment of SAH, the overall mortality from SAH remains high with 15% of patients dying before reaching hospital and a further 25% dying in hospital (Sutcliffe, 2002). Subarachnoid haemorrhage is the second commonest neurosurgical emergency (Gupta *et al.*, 1998).

There are a number of causes of SAH (which are beyond the scope of this chapter to discuss) but by far the most common is aneurysms, accounting for 70–75% of bleeds (Lindsay & Bone, 2004). An aneurysm is a weakness of the arterial wall which ruptures causing immediate onset of symptoms. The most common type of aneurysms is called a berry aneurysm because it has a distinct neck below a ballon-shaped bulge.

The extent of the haemorrhage will determine the severity of symptoms, which may range from mild, such as headache, to severe neurological deficit and coma. Aneurysms occur most commonly on the Circle of Willis, a small vascular structure at the base of the brain, which unites the two main blood supplies to the brain: the anterior and posterior circulations (Hickey, 2003) (Figure 8.6).

Subarachnoid haemorrhage is graded according to the severity of presentation. This has important implications for patients because those with minimal neurological deficit are suitable for intervention as soon as possible (Kopitnik *et al.*, 2003) or within 3–4 days of the initial bleed to minimise the risk of a devastating rebleed (Whitfield & Kirkpatrick, 2001). Delay in intervention may result in rebleeding, deterioration of neurological function and possible death.

Traditionally, treatment of SAH has been surgical intervention by craniotomy to secure the neck of the aneurysm and insertion of a surgical clip to occlude the neck of the aneurysm. Nevertheless, this method is becoming less common with the advent of less invasive methods. Alternative endovascular techniques, using a variety of methods, are also available for the management of SAH (Kirkpatrick, 2002).

One of the more common endovascular techniques is to use detachable platinum coils, which are inserted using radiological control to achieve thrombosis of ruptured and unruptured aneurysms. Endovascular coil treatment is significantly more likely to result in survival free of disability one year after SAH than neurosurgical intervention (ISAT, 2003) and the use of endovascular occlusion in the older patient (>65 years of age) appears to be promising (Sarkar *et al.*, 2001).

The implications for patients following endovascular procedure are first that it is a less invasive procedure and second, patients will require high dependency rather than intensive care post-procedure unless complications ensue. Nevertheless data are awaited from a five-year follow-up study to determine the long-term effects of coiling (Nicholls *et al.*, 2002). Both surgical and endovascular procedures are carried out at specialist neuroscience centres. Therefore all patients will

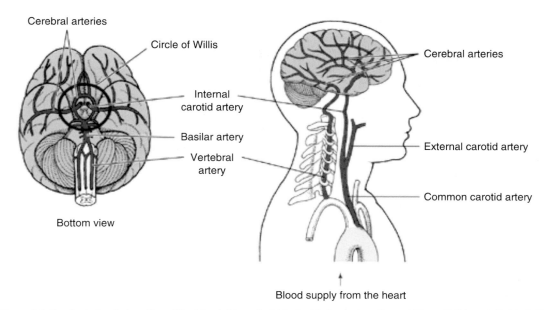

Figure 8.6 Cerebral circulation. From The Merck Manual of Medical Information, Second Home Edition, (ed.) Mark H. Beers. Copyright 2003 by Merck & Co., Inc., Whitehouse Station, NJ.

require expert skilled support during transfer to a specialist centre. Those patients in a poor neurological state are unlikely to be transferred until their condition improves sufficiently to justify the risks of transfer.

Anaesthetic requirements for patients with SAH are similar to patients with head injury. The main considerations are to maintain CPP, prevent rises in ICP and minimise metabolic demands (Quinn & Lindley, 2002). Anaesthetic practice is the same whether the aneurysm is secured by surgical or endovascular methods (Sutcliffe, 2002). Recent research has indicated that both propofol and sevoflurane agents compared satisfactorily when used with remifantanil in elective intracranial surgery (Sneyd *et al.*, 2005).

The patient with SAH is both at risk of re-bleeding and vasospasm (narrowing of cerebral blood vessels). The risk of re-bleeding is higher in the first 24–28 hours following the initial bleed, thereafter decreasing until the 7th–10th day (Hickey & Buckley, 2003). There is no specific

treatment to prevent re-bleeding apart from supportive therapy such as bed rest, maintaining optimal hydration and controlling headache although prophylactic measures to prevent deep vein thrombosis should include compression therapy rather than anticoagulation therapy.

The causes of vasospasm are not entirely clear but the effect is that the patient is at risk of further ischaemia through constriction of the blood vessels (Hickey & Buckley, 2003). Nimodipine, a calcium channel blocker which enhances blood flow, may be given either orally or intravenously for 21 days following SAH and has been shown to improve neurological outcome in patients with SAH (Rinkel *et al.*, 2005). Dehydration increases the risk of vasospasm and must be avoided by ensuring that the patient receives approximately 3 litres of fluid in 24 hours (Kirkpatrick, 2002; Sutcliffe, 2002). Good cerebral perfusion is also required to prevent further ischaemia although the use of hypertensive therapy should be avoided until the aneurysm has been secured. Management of electrolytes is also crucial because hyponatraemia (serum sodium less than 135 mEq/L) commonly occurs in patients with SAH and is complex in its causation, therefore careful monitoring of fluid balance is required. The incidence of hyponatraemia is increased in patients with a poor clinical grade of SAH with potentially detrimental effects if it is not promptly recognised and treated (Dooling & Winkelman, 2004).

Subarachnoid haemorrhage is a devastating condition with a high mortality rate (Pobereskin, 2001). Best outcomes for the patient are achieved where collaborative working is practised in a critical care environment within specialist centres (Gupta *et al.*, 1998).

Neurological conditions

An increasing proportion of patients presenting for surgery may suffer from a neurological disorder. Approximately 10 million people across the UK have a neurological condition, which may range from migraine to multiple sclerosis (DH, 2005). There are numerous neurological conditions, many of which are long-term and whose cause is unknown. It is beyond the scope of this chapter to be able to discuss neurological conditions in any degree of depth, consequently a selection is provided of the more common conditions.

There are some considerations, which will be common to most neurological illnesses and it is good practice for all patients scheduled to undergo surgery to be assessed in advance with a view to optimal perioperative management (Baxendale & Smith, 2001). In contrast to neurosurgical emergencies, the patient with a long-term condition may have the opportunity to prepare psychologically and physically for surgery. Through communication with the anaesthetist and surgical team they may have had the opportunity to discuss their needs and preferences.

Preoperative management must include careful assessment of respiratory and bulbar muscle (speech and swallowing) function (Thavasothy &

Hirsch, 2002). Consideration should be given to the possibility of respiratory impairment since some conditions such as motor neurone disease (Hickey, 2003), Guillain-Barré Syndrome (Richards & Cohen, 2003), myasthenia gravis (Thavasothy & Hirsch, 2002) and high spinal cord lesions (Cook, 2003) may produce respiratory inadequacy. Patients with such conditions are sensitive to anaesthetic agents, opioids and relaxants and a period of elective ventilation may be needed post-operatively. The airway may need to be protected if bulbar muscle function is compromised, because there is a risk of aspiration and the patient may require intubation or tracheostomy (Baxendale & Smith, 2001).

Epilepsy

In most patients with epilepsy, no identifiable cause can be found. When epilepsy presents later in life it may indicate neurological dysfunction and 40% of epilepsies occur as a result of injury or disease. There are many different types of epileptic episodes or seizures. Seizure activity may range from a brief loss of awareness to a major convulsion involving the whole body (Lindsay & Bone, 2004). Seizure activity may occur as a result of head injury, hypoglycaemia, drug overdose, alcoholism, or cerebral tumour. There is a higher level of incidence of epilepsy among older people (Brodie & Kwan, 2005). The majority of patients with epilepsy are managed in a community setting and are admitted to hospital for crises management (Lanfear, 2002).

It is important that patients that are prescribed anti-epileptic therapy who are undergoing anaesthesia should maintain their therapy throughout the perioperative period. Some anaesthetic agents, e.g. enflurane, have neuroexcitatory effects and should be avoided. Isoflurane or servoflurane are more advisable. Thiopentone is a potent anti-convulsant and is the intravenous induction agent of choice (Grant & Nimmo, 2001). Epilepsy surgery may be offered to some patients who are poorly controlled with anti-epileptic therapy (Gratrix & Enright, 2005).

Status epilepticus is a medical emergency that requires rapid intervention to prevent significant morbidity and mortality (Finney & Hirsch, 2005; Prasad *et al.*, 2005). Management is aimed at cessation of the seizure activity while maintaining tissue oxygenation. Lorazepam is recommended for immediate control of status epilepticus (Prasad *et al.*, 2005). Propofol is recommended for the management of status epilepticus that is unresponsive to benzodiazepines such as lorazepam or midazolam. Practitioners that practise in acute settings should familiarise themselves with the management of the patient having seizures.

Myasthenia gravis

Myasthenia gravis (MG) is a rare disorder characterised by painless muscle weakness (Haverson, 2004). It is a chronic autoimmune disease in which fluctuations in weakness and fatigue are clinical hallmarks (Mortenson Armstrong & Schumann, 2003). Facial, eye, swallowing and speech muscles may be affected to varying degrees. Whilst no specific cause can be identified in the majority of patients, however, a tumour of the thymus gland is one cause (Vincent *et al.*, 2001). There are a number of treatment options, which may help to improve the quality of life for patients with this condition. Anticholinesterase drugs, for example pyridostigmine, may be the first-line treatment option for the symptomatic management of MG, whilst not being a curative option (Hickey, 2003). A thymectomy or immunosuppressive therapy may also be considered.

Careful assessment is required prior to surgery particularly of respiratory and bulbar muscle function. Anaesthetic management depends on the severity of the disease, where possible local or regional anaesthesia should be considered. Caution should be exercised when using general anaesthesia, with the use of non-depolarising neuromuscular blocking drugs, such as atracurium, because patients with MG are extremely sensitive to these agents (Thavasothy & Hirsch, 2002).

Parkinson's disease

Parkinson's disease (PD) is a degenerative disease characterised by rigidity, tremor and bradykinesia (slowness of movement). Anaesthetic drugs may exacerbate the condition or interact with drug therapy used in its treatment. There is no ideal method of anaesthesia but in general it is preferable to stop PD treatment as late as possible preoperatively and to restart as soon as possible post-operatively (Errington *et al.*, 2002). In view of the fact that there is an ageing population in the UK, it is likely that PD patients will be encountered more commonly in the perioperative environment.

Conclusion

Neuroscience includes a variety of both acute and long-term conditions. Many patients will be encountered in general surgical and critical care settings; some patients will require management in specialist centres. Careful assessment and safe transfer is required if the patient is to achieve the best outcome. Neurological conditions may be degenerative and affect a wide age group. Patient-centred care will improve both quality of care and the patient experience.

REFERENCES

Andrews, P. J. D. (2003). Traumatic brain injury. In R. A. C. Hughes, ed., *Neurological Emergencies.* London: BMJ Books, pp. 34–66.

Bateman, D. E. (2001). Neurological assessment of coma. *Journal of Neurology, Neurosurgery and Psychiatry,* **71**(Suppl 1), 13–17.

Baxendale, B. & Smith, G. (2001). Preoperative assessment and premedication. In A. R. Aitkenhead, D. Rowbotham and G. Smith, eds., *Textbook of Anaesthesia*. Edinburgh: Churchill Livingstone, pp. 417–27.

Brodie, M. J. & Kwan, P. (2005). Epilepsy in elderly people. *British Medical Journal*, **3**(31), 1317–22.

Christensen, M. A., Janson, S. & Seago, J. A. (2001). Alcohol, head injury and pulmonary complications. *Journal of Neuroscience Nursing*, **33**(4), 184–9.

Citerio, G. & Andrews, P. J. D. (2004). Intracranial pressure Part two: Clinical application and technology. *Intensive Care Medicine*, **30**, 1882–5.

Clancy, J. & McVicar, A. J. (2002). *Physiology and Anatomy. A Homeostatic Approach*, 2nd edn. London: Arnold.

Cook, N. (2003). Respiratory care in spinal cord injury with associated brain injury: bridging the gap in critical care interventions. *Intensive and Critical Care Nursing*, **19**, 143–53.

Cooper, N. & Cramp, P. (2003). *Essential Guide to Acute Care*. London: BMJ Books.

CRASH (Corticosteroid Randomisation After Significant Head Injury) Trial Collaborators. (2004). Effect of intravenous corticosteroids on death within 14 days in 10008 adults with clinically significant head injury (MRC CRASH trial): randomised placebo-controlled trial. *The Lancet*, **364**, 1321–8.

Davis, A. E. (2000). Mechanisms of traumatic brain injury: biomechanical, structural and cellular considerations. *Critical Care Nursing Quarterly*, **23**(3), 1–13.

Department of Health. (2005). *The National Service Framework for Long-term Conditions*. London: Department of Health.

Dooling, E. & Winkelman, C. (2004). Hyponatraemia in the patient with subarachnoid haemorrhage. *Journal of Neuroscience Nursing*, **36**(3), 130–6.

Edwards, S. L. (2001). Using the Glasgow Coma Scale: analysis and limitations. *British Journal of Nursing*, **10**(2), 92–101.

Ellis, A. & Cavanagh, S. J. (1992). Aspects of neurosurgical assessment using the Glasgow Coma Scale. *Intensive and Critical Care Nursing*, **8**, 94–9.

Errington, D. R., Severn, A. M. & Meara, J. (2002). Parkinson's disease. *British Journal of Anaesthesia/ CEPD Reviews*, **2**(3), 69–73.

Finney, S. J. & Hirsch, N. P. (2005). Status epilepticus. *Current Anaesthesia and Critical Care*, **16**(3), 123–31.

Flint, G. (1999). Head injuries. *British Journal of Theatre Nursing*, **9**(1), 15–21.

Forsyth, R. J., Baxter, P. & Elliott, T. (2001). Routine intracranial monitoring in acute coma. *The Cochrane Database of Systematic Reviews* (issue 3). Available at: http://www.mrw.interscience.wiley.com (Accessed 24 August 2005).

Girling, K. (2004). Management of head injury in the intensive care unit. *Continuing Education in Anaesthesia, Critical Care and Pain*, **4**(2), 52–6.

Goh, J. & Gupta, A. K. (2002). The management of head injury and intracranial pressure. *Current Anaesthesia and Critical Care*, **13**, 129–37.

Grant, I. S. & Nimmo, G.R. (2001). Intercurrent disease and anaesthesia. In A. R. Aitkenhead, D. Rowbotham & G. Smith, eds., *Textbook of Anaesthesia*. Edinburgh: Churchill Livingstone, pp. 429–54.

Gratrix, A. P. & Enright, S. M. (2005). Epilepsy in anaesthesia and intensive care. *Continuing Education in Anaesthesia, Critical Care and Pain*, **5**(4), 118–21.

Gupta, A. K. & Azami, J. (2002). Update of neuromonitoring. *Current Anaesthesia and Critical Care*, **13**, 120–8.

Gupta, K. J., Finfer, S. R. & Morgan, M. K. (1998). Intensive care for subarachnoid haemorrhage: the state of the art. *Current Anaesthesia and Critical Care*, **9**, 202–8.

Haverson, R. F. (ed.) (2004). *Information Pack Medical Information (Medical Professionals)*. Derby: Myasthenia Gravis Association.

Hayes, M. (2002). Cerebral protection. *Current Anaesthesia and Critical Care*, **13**, 138–43.

Hickey, J. V. (2003). *The Clinical Practice of Neurological and Neurosurgical Nursing*, 5th edn. Philadelphia: Lippincott Williams and Wilkins.

Hickey, J. V. & Buckley, D. M. (2003). Cerebral aneurysms. In *The Clinical Practice of Neurological and Neurosurgical Nursing*. Philadelphia: Lippincott Williams and Wilkins, pp. 523–58.

Intensive Care Society. (2002). *Guidelines for the Transport of the Critically Ill Adult*. Available at: http://www. ics.ac.uk/updated June 2003 (Accessed 22 August 2005).

International Subarachnoid Aneurysm Trial (ISAT) Collaborators Group. (2003). International Subarachnoid Aneurysm Trial of Neurosurgical clipping versus endovascular coiling in 2143 patients with ruptured intracranial aneurysms: a randomised trial. *The Lancet*, **360**, 1267–74.

Jackson, R. G. M., Sales, K. M., McLaughlin, D. P. & Stamford, J. A. (2002). Traumatic brain injury: from model to man. *Current Anaesthesia & Critical Care*, **13**, 343–55.

Jevon, P. & Ewens, B. (2002). *Monitoring the Critically Ill Patient*. Oxford: Blackwell Science.

Kirkpatrick, P. J. (2002). Subarachnoid haemorrhage and intracranial aneurysms: what neurologists need to know. *Journal of Neurology, Neurosurgery and Psychiatry*, **73**(Suppl 1), 128–33.

Kopitnik, T. A., Croft, C., Moore, S. & White, J. A. (2003). Management of subarachnoid haemorrhage. In R. A. C. Hughes, ed., *Neurological Emergencies*. London: BMJ Books, pp. 247–95.

Lanfear, J. (2002). The individual with epilepsy. *Nursing Standard*, **16**(46), 43–53.

Letvak, S. & Hand, R. (2003). Postanesthesia care of the patient suffering from traumatic brain injury. *Journal of Perianesthesia Nursing*, **18**(6), 380–5.

Lindsay, K. W. & Bone, I. (2004). *Neurology and Neurosurgery Illustrated*, 4th edn. Edinburgh: Churchill Livingstone.

Macartney, I. & Nightingale, P. (2001). Transfer of the critically ill adult patient. *British Journal of Anaesthesia/CEPD Reviews*, **1**, 12–15.

Minassian, A. T., Dube, L., Guillaux, A. M. *et al.* (2002). Changes in intracranial pressure and cerebral autoregulation in patients with severe traumatic brain injury. *Critical Care Medicine*, **30**(7), 1616–21.

Morris, C. G., McCoy, E. P. & Lavery, G. G. (2004). Spinal immobilisation for unconscious patients with multiple injuries. *British Journal of Medicine*, **329**, 495–9.

Mortenson Armstrong, S. & Schumann, L. (2003). Myasthenia gravis: diagnosis and treatment. *Journal of American Academy of Nurse Practitioners*, **15**(2), 72–8.

Moss, E. (2001). The cerebral circulation. *British Journal of Anaesthesia/CEPD Reviews*, **1**(3), 67–71.

National Institute of Clinical Excellence. (2003). *Head Injury: Triage, Assessment, Investigation and Early Management of Head Injury in Infants, Children and Adults*. Available at: http://www.nice.org.uk/page.aspx?o=74657 (Accessed 23 August 2005).

National Institute of Clinical Excellence. (2005). *Intercranial Pressure Monitoring*. Available at: http://www.nice.org.uk/page.aspx?o=263496 (Accessed 23 August 2005).

Nicholls, D. A., Brown Jnr, R. D. & Meyer, F. B. (2002). Coils or clips in subarachnoid haemorrhage? *Journal of Stroke and Cerebrovascular Disease*, **11**(6), 295–7.

Patel, H. C., Menon, D. K., Tebbs, S. *et al.* (2002). Specialist neurocritical care and outcome from head injury. *Intensive Care Medicine*, **28**, 547–53.

Pattison, K., Wynne-Jones, G. & Imray, C. H. E. (2005). Monitoring intracranial pressure, perfusion and metabolism. *Continuing Education in Anaesthesia, Critical Care and Pain*, **5**(4), 130–3.

Pobereskin, L. H. (2001). Incidence and outcome of subarachnoid haemorrhage: a retrospective population based study. *Journal of Neurology, Neurosurgery and Psychiatry*, **70**, 340–3.

Prasad, K., Al-Roomi, K., Krishnan, P. R. & Sequeira, R. (2005). Anticonvulsant therapy for status epilepticus. *The Cochrane Database of Systematic Reviews*, Issue 4. Art. No.: CD003723. DOI: 10.1002/14651858. CD003723.pub2.

Price, T. (1996). An evaluation of neuro-assesment tools in the intensive care unit. *Nursing in Critical Care*, **1**(2), 72–7.

Price, T. (2002). Painful stimuli and the Glasgow Coma Scale. *Nursing in Critical Care*, **7**(1), 19–23.

Price, T., Miller, L. & de Scossa, M. (2000). The Glasgow Coma Scale in intensive care: a study. *Nursing in Critical Care*, **5**(4), 170–3.

Quinn, A. C. & Lindley, A. (2002). Subarachnoid haemorrhage. *Current Anaesthesia and Critical Care*, **13**, 144–52.

Ravi, R. & Morgan, R. J. (2003). Intracranial pressure monitoring. *Current Anaesthesia & Critical Care*, **14**, 229–35.

Richards, K. J. C. & Cohen, A. T. (2003). Guillain-Barré syndrome. *British Journal of Anaesthesia*, **3**(2), 46–9.

Riley, B. (2001). The intensive care unit. In A. R. Aitkenhead, D. Rowbotham and G. Smith, eds., *Textbook of Anaesthesia*. Edinburgh: Churchill Livingstone, pp. 722–37.

Rinkel, G. J. E., Feigin, V. L., Algra, A. *et al.* (2005). Calcium antagonists for aneurysmal subarachnoid haemorrhage. *The Cochrane Database of Systematic Reviews*, Issue 1. Art. No.: CD000277. DOI: 10.1002/14651858. CD000277.pub2.

Roberts, I. (1999). Barbiturates for acute traumatic brain injury. *The Cochrane Database of Systematic Reviews*, Issue 3. Available at: http://www.mrw.interscience. wiley.com (Accessed 23 August 2005).

Roberts, I., Scheerhout, G. & Wakai, A. (2004). Mannitol for acute traumatic brain injury (Cochrane Review). In *The Cochrane Library*, Issue 3. Chichester, UK: John Wiley & Sons Ltd.

Ross, N. & Eynon, C. A. (2005). Intracranial pressure monitoring. *Current Anaesthesia and Critical Care*, **16**, 255–61.

Rowley, G. & Fielding, K. (1991). Reliability and accuracy of the Glasgow Coma Scale with experienced and inexperienced users. *The Lancet*, **337**, 535–8.

Sarkar, P. K., D'Souza, C. & Ballantyne, S. (2001). Treatment of aneurysmal subarachnoid haemorrhage in elderly patients. *Journal of Clinical Pharmacy and Therapeutics*, **26**, 247–56.

Simpson, P. J. (2001). Neurosurgical anaesthesia. In A. R. Aitkenhead, D. Rowbotham & G. Smith, eds., *Textbook of Anaesthesia*. Edinburgh: Churchill Livingstone, pp. 688–98.

Sneyd, J. R., Andrews, C. J. H. & Tsubokawa, T. (2005). Comparison of propofol/remifentanil and sevflurane/remifentanil for maintenance of anaesthesia for elective intracranial surgery. *British Journal of Anaesthesia*, **94**(6), 778–83.

Springborg, J. B., Frederiksen, H. J., Eskesen, V. & Olsen, N. V. (2005). Trends in monitoring patients with aneurysmal subarachnoid haemorrhage. *British Journal of Anaesthesia*, **94**, 259–70.

Stanley, I. R. & Hancox, D. (2001). Initial management of severe head injury: is cerebral perfusion pressure maintained? *Care of the Critically Ill*, **17**(5), 166–8.

Stevens, W. J. (2004). Multimodal monitoring: head injury management using Sjv O2 and LICVOX. *Journal of Neuroscience Nursing*, **36**(6), 332–9.

Stocchetti, N., Penny, K. I., Dearden, M. *et al.* (2001). Intensive care management of head-injured patients in Europe: a survey from the European Brain Injury Consortium. *Intensive Care Medicine*, **27**, 200–406.

Sutcliffe, A. J. (2002). Subarachnoid haemorrhage due to cerebral aneurysm, I. *British Journal of Anaesthesia/CEPD Reviews*, **2**(2), 45–8.

Teasdale, G. & Jennett, B. (1974). Assessment of coma and impaired consciousness. *The Lancet*, **2**(7872), 81–4.

Teasdale, G., Knill-Jones, R. & Van Der Sande, J. (1978). Observer variability in assessing impaired consciousness and coma. *Journal of Neurology, Neurosurgery and Psychiatry*, **41**, 603–10.

Thavasothy, M. & Hirsch, N. (2002). Myasthenia gravis. *British Journal of Anaesthesia*, **2**(3), 88–90.

Vincent, A., Palace, J. & Hilton-Jones, D. (2001). Myasthenia gravis. *The Lancet*, **357**, 2122–8.

Warlow, C., Sudlow, C., Dennis, M., Wardlaw, J. & Sandercock, P. (2003). Stroke. *The Lancet*, **362**, 1211–24.

Whitfield, P. C. & Kirkpatrick, P. J. (2001). Timing of surgery for aneurysmal subarachnoid haemorrhage. *The Cochrane Database of Systematic Reviews*, Issue 1. Art. No.: CD001697. DOI: 10.1002/14651858.CD001697. www.mrw.interscience.wiley.com/cochrane/clsysrev/articles/CD01697/frame.html (Accessed 23 August 2005).

Wiese, M. F. (2003). British hospitals and different versions of the Glasgow coma scale: telephone survey. *British Journal of Medicine*, **327**, 782–3.

Woodward, P. (2000). *Intensive Care Nursing. A Framework for Practice*. London: Routledge.

9

Resuscitation

Rob Campbell

Key Learning Points

- Understand resuscitation for acute management of cardio-respiratory arrest and periarrest
- Recognise the historic movements in resuscitation
- Identify and discuss the patient treatment options using the resuscitation algorithms

Many methods of resuscitation that we now take for granted were developed in the 1950s, including for example, Dr Peter Safar's work with mouth-to-mouth ventilation and oxygen saturation.

One of the earliest and most possible accounts of resuscitation comes in the Old Testament in the second book of Kings: '. . . And he went up, and lay upon the child, and put his mouth upon his mouth, and his eyes upon his eyes, and his hands upon his hands; and he stretched himself upon the child; and the flesh of the child waxed warm' (Bible, 2 Kings, iv, 34). This passage is a potential description of the biblical figure Elijah performing mouth-to-mouth resuscitation.

The ancient Egyptians over 3500 years ago recorded resuscitation attempts that involved hanging the victim by their legs and applying intermittent pressure to their chest to aid inspiration and expiration.

In 1767 the first life-saving society was founded in Holland, closely followed in Britain in 1774. These early societies focused on near-drowning incidents. This emphasis continued up to the 1960s with the Holgar Neilson method of moving the arms through 180 degrees in a pumping action with the victim lying flat on their back, being the preferred means of removing water from the lungs thus aiding oxygenation.

The Russian method of resuscitation used in the early nineteenth century can be compared with recent research into induced mild cerebral hypothermia; the Russians buried the patient in snow up to their neck making any form of resuscitation attempt difficult. By not covering the head they missed a potential benefit of this technique.

Modern resuscitation began in 1960. Dr William Kouwenhoven, an electrical engineer at Johns Hopkins University, was working on developing an external defibrillator. During the trials of this device, when the electrodes were firmly applied to the thorax a palpable cardiac output (carotid pulse) was noticed. This breakthrough became closed cardiac compression which is now commonly referred to as cardio pulmonary resuscitation (CPR). The ratios between ventilations and compressions were not fixed for many years but slowly changed overtime to what we currently employ as our ratio, 30 compressions to 2 ventilations.

In the late 1980s there was recognition that treating cardio-respiratory arrests was not

Core Topics in Operating Department Practice: Anaesthesia and Critical Care, eds. Brian Smith, Paul Rawling, Paul Wicker and Chris Jones. Published by Cambridge University Press. © Cambridge University Press 2007.

standardised irrespective of whether the guidelines were known. Consequently, the Advanced Life-Support (ALS) course arose. This course seeks to bring a common approach to dealing with the arrested patient. Over its short life span it has evolved and been influenced by evidence-based medicine. Currently, the course uses an approach that focuses on the periarrest patient as well as the arrested patient.

Whatever culture and whatever period in humankind's history there have been attempts to revive patients from clear death (Bible Gateway, 2005). Some of these activities have succeeded encouraging the patient's life to continue, but on balance most were unsuccessful. Yet that has not deterred mankind from trying and to this day resuscitation is a multibillion dollar industry (Skyaid, 2006).

Pathways leading to the need for resuscitation

The anaesthetic practitioner may be involved in resuscitation that might range from perioperative incidents, those that occur during a procedure, the recovery phase or in another area within the hospital and indeed occasionally outside hospital.

The anaesthetic practitioner should be equipped and have an understanding of how and why these events occur and how to aid in managing them.

In years gone by resuscitation was regarded as a reactive process where the patient would arrest and then attempts were made to revive them. This did not always prove to be successful causing a large degree of cynicism to develop among healthcare professionals, to the value of resuscitation. That cynicism still exists in some form, however, in the last few years, the emphasis has been to be proactive, that is, to recognise there is a problem and to take corrective action.

To that end, there has been the emergence of various courses such as acute life threatening events-recognition and treatment (A.L.E.R.T.™). These courses dovetail with objective scoring that are designed to assess how ill the patient is. The current ALS course philosophy also goes in this direction. The main adjunct to these courses has been the necessary arrival of outreach teams. These are invariably intensive therapy unit (ITU) nurses whose role it is to assess and identify patients who are compromised and need corrective therapy. That may mean treatment on the ward or transfer to a critical care area.

Broadly, three common pathways lead to eventual circulatory failure. Those being respiratory, cardiovascular and trauma.

If we follow these four the purpose of this section is to apply this view to the areas that anaesthetic practitioners may find themselves coming up against.

Respiratory causes

The core of anaesthesia apart from making someone unconscious or making them pain-free revolves around managing the airway and the control of respiration.

The pathways to respiratory compromise can be pathological, mechanical/trauma related or the inability of the individual to control a patient's airway.

Pathologies

One of the commonest one is asthma which can affect both the young and elderly in equal measure and if not recognised can and does lead to death. Also, outlined below are some other respiratory-related diseases that if unchecked carry a risk of morbidity.

Asthma

Asthma

On observation/examination

Tachypnoea – obtain respiratory rate

Tachycardia

Initially blood pressure will rise then fall as the severity
   increases towards cardiovascular collapse

Accessorary muscle usage. The patient will assume a
   posture that helps them to breath. This is the so
   called "tripod position"

Altered blood gases. Initially an alkolotic picture
   followed by an acidotic picture

Sternal notch recession

Cyanosis

Fatigue

Expiratory wheeze

Peripheral cyanosis

Central cyanosis (bad)

Tension pneumothorax

Hyper expanded chest

Treatment

100% Oxygenate

Assist ventilation as necessary

5mg Salbutamol nebuliser (may be repeated)

200mg Hydrocortisone

Ipratropium 250 – 500mg where high dose B_2 agonist &
   hydrocortisone therapy has been ineffective

Attach SpO^2 & ECG monitoring

IV access with blood taken for appropriate analysis.

Reassess A. B. Cs

Consider aminophyline

Consider elective ventilation

**CONTACT HELP, ESPECIALLY
   ANAESTHETIC HELP**

Chronic obstructive pulmonary disease

Chronic obstructive pulmonary disease

Symptoms/features	Treatment
On observation	**CONTACT HELP, ESPECIALLY ANAESTHETIC HELP**
Chronic cough	Give high flow oxygen and reduce with effective titration
Increased **sputum** (mucus coughed from the airways)	SpO^2 monitoring
Shortness of breath	Bronchodilators
Limitation of physical activity	IV access with bloods for bioanalysis
	Corticosteriods
	Expectorants in chronic cases of emphysema

Pneumonia

Pneumonia

Symptoms/features	Treatment
On observation	Oxygen
Tachypnoea bronchial breathing	Assist ventilation if necessary
Tachycardia	SpO^2 monitor
Dysphagia	IV access with bloods for bioanalysis
Antibiotics	Fluids
Chest pains	ECG monitor
Sweating	
Shaking chills	
Offensive coloured sputum	
Cyanosis and altered blood pressure readings as the severity increases	

Mechanical/trauma

One of the most significant causes of anaesthetic deaths relates to difficulty of airway management. Out of 750 cases of death reported to the medical defence Union in the UK over a 12-year period. The causes leading to these deaths were attributed to poor technique in 326 cases, with a 100 because of intubation errors.

Taylor *et al.* (1976) conducted a study of 41 cardiac arrests in patients who were otherwise healthy but were undergoing elective surgery. The principal cause of these deaths was due to hypoxic, anoxic arrest. Of these 41 arrests, three were successfully resuscitated.

Simple airway obstruction

Simple airway obstruction

Symptoms/features

On observation

Tachpnoea & tachycardia. As the severity increases and no treatment is applied then the tachpnoea and tachycardia will give way to a slowing of breathing and circulation

Initially blood pressure will rise then fall as the severity increases towards cardiovascular collapse

Altered blood gases – initially an alkolotic picture followed by an acidotic picture

Posture – leaning forward and trying to draw breath

Cyanosis SpO^2 ↓

Recessed mandible – no muscle tone

Visible foreign objects, whether inhaled or regurgitated

Stridor – snoring type noise heard on inspiration

Cardiorespiratory collapse

Treatment

Remove the obstruction by:

Opening the airway with head tilt chin lift;

Suctioning out the obstruction;

Removing the object with a forceps (Magill's);

Manually with one's own fingers(s)

Then assess your patient's breathing, circulation and consciousness and administer oxygen and actively ventilate as required

---

Ventilatory failure

The lungs are responsible for transporting inhaled air into the bloodstream by means of diffusion at the alveoli as well as carrying CO_2 out of the bloodstream and into the lungs to be exhaled. Respiratory failure is when there is insufficient oxygen being drawn in or insufficient CO_2 being exhaled. This is described as type 1 respiratory failure and is hypoxaemia.

In ventilatory failure, it is more the retention of CO_2 and its build-up that causes ventilatory failure. The causes can range from restrictive chest disorders, brain stem respiratory drive malfunction and chronic obstructive pulmonary disease.

Ventilatory failure

Symptoms/features	Treatment
On observation	Oxygen
Tachypnoea in acute circumstances	In severe cases ventilatory support
Tachycardia	IV access with bloods for bioanalysis
Altered blood pressure	Cardiovascular support > fluids,
Cyanosis	bronchodilators > B₂ agonists, anticholengergics and
Hypercapnea (Co² monitor)	theophyline
Fever (pneumonia)	Corticosteroids to reduce inflammation. Takes time to work
Coughing foul sputum	in the acute setting
Inability to expand and contract their thorax. This may	
be because of trauma or another pathology such as	
motor neurone disease	

Tension pneumothorax

This can be because of asthma or in the case of young, fit and male adults occur spontaneously.

Whatever the cause it can be a life-threatening event and requires rapid recognition and treatment.

Tension pneumothorax

Symptoms/features	Treatment
On observation	Oxygen and ventilatory support as required
Dyspnoea	Insert large bore cannula into the second intercostal
Tachypnoea	space in the midclavicular line on the affected side.
Unilateral breath sounds (absent on the affected side)	Remember to remove the trocar portion of the cannula
Hyper-resonant pitch on the affected side	and survey the position as retensioning occurs because
Deviated trachea (deviates a way from the affected side;	of the cannula shifting position. This is only a temporising
not always obvious – late sign)	measure until a chest drain is inserted
Raised jugular venous pressure	IV access with bloods for bioanalysis
Accessory muscle usage	In severe cases, ALS procedures may be required
Cardio respiratory arrest	

Burns

A patient presenting to theatre following severe burns, i.e. third-degree with full thoracic circumferential burns may have restrictive chest movements because of tightening skin and muscle due to excessive heat. To allow breathing an escharotomy is performed to allow chest movement. With third-degree burns, there is no involvement of pain as the nerve endings have been destroyed.

Caution is needed with suxamethonium chloride in burns patients. Burns patients have an increase in serum potassium. This can be worsened by suxamethonium chloride.

Burns

Symptoms/features	Treatment
On observation	Oxygen
Tachypnoea in acute circumstances	In severe cases ventilatory support
Tachycardia	IV access with bloods taken for bioanalysis
Altered blood pressure	Cardiovascular support > fluids
Cyanosis	
Hypercapnea (CO_2 monitor)	
Altered blood gases	

Haemothorax (penetrating/blunt trauma)

Haemothorax is when there is a significant build-up of blood in the pleural cavity. This collection is caused by either trauma, clotting disorders, vascular disorders or pulmonary emboli.

From the perspective of the anaesthetic practitioner they will come across this in the emergency department (ED) or in severe cases where the patient has bypassed the ED and gone straight to

---

Haemothorax (penetrating/blunt trauma)

Symptoms/features	Treatment
On observation	Oxygenation
Dyspnoea and reduction of breath sounds	In severe cases active ventilation
Tachypnoea	Aspiration/drainage of fluid from the chest*
Occlusive dressing taped down three sides.	Open chest wound.
Tachycardia	IV access with bloods for bioanalysis
Pale and clammy	Fluid replacement (warmed)
Dull to percussion	Pain relief – for flail segment this is painful and to aid
Falling blood pressure and symptoms associated with shock	respiration and to help the patient an epidural may be
Lung tissue damage leading to hypoxia	required or local anaesthesia to the intercostal muscles
Mediastinal shift (deviation away from the affected side)	If the patient has a thoracotomy then an endobronchial
Radiological changes	tube is required
Visible trauma to the chest wall (anterior, posterior and bilateral midaxillary lines)	

---

*A thoractomy may be indicated if the fluid loss from any drain eexceeds 200 ml per hour or there is estimated to be 1500 ml in the thoracic cavity.

theatre. If there is anaesthetic involvement it is safe to say that serious cardiovascular collapse is likely, and consequently surgery would be considered.

A pneumothorax can occur with a haemothorax (haemopnuemothorax) but it is rare and is associated with such injuries as flail chest. Flail chest is where sufficient force has been applied to cause more than one rib to fracture and for the fracture to have a proximal and distal break to the sternum. As the patient breathes in, the ribcage rises, the flail segment will fall and when the patient breathes out the ribcage falls, but the segment will rise. This contralateral movement is painful and has a severe impact on the efficiency of respiration.

Pulmonary emboli

This is where a blood clot forms and occludes a pulmonary arteriole thus affecting respiratory efficiency. The clot may be formed by fat, air, amniotic fluid or blood.

Pulmonary emboli

Symptoms/features	Treatment
On observation	Oxygen
Invariably a history of lower extremity venous thrombosis	Cannulate if not already
Tachypnoea	Thrombolytic therapy
Dyspnoea/nasal flaring	Pain relief
Splinting of ribs when breathing. The patient is bent over holding their ribs	In severe cases, the patient will suffer a cardiac arrest
May produce bloody sputum	Other than good basic life-support with vigorous CPR to break the emboli up, the prognosis is poor
Light-headed, fainting and dizzy	Cardiac bypass with thoracic surgery may be an option
Low blood pressure	
Tachycardia leading to absent or slow pulse rate	
Chest pain	
Skin – pale clammy and cold	
Abdominal cramps	

Cardiovascular causes

Like respiratory problems this to can be divided between pathological and mechanical in origin.
- Pathological
  - Hypertensive crisis
  - Myocardial infarction
  - Heart failure.
- Systemic problems
  - Kidney malfunction.
- Cardiac arrest

Hypertensive crisis

Hypertension is a disease that is common in the industrialised world and is caused by inactivity as much as by having a genetic tendency to cardiovascular disease. A small minority go on to have hypertensive crises (Vidt, 2006). This is where, because of the elevation of pressure, end organ dysfunction occurs, thus compromising tissue oxygenation.

Hypertensive crisis

Symptoms/features	Treatment
On observation	Oxygen
Blood pressure in excess of 220/140	Cannulate if not already
Cardiac enlargement	Antihypertensive therapy and early intensive care admission
Congestive heart failure	Care should be taken in reducing the blood pressure as the end
Focal neurological deficits	organs compensate to tolerate a higher pressure
Torpor	Therefore, any rapid drop to blood pressure can have
Headache	significant perfusion effects
Nausea / vomiting	The operating practitioner should be aware of some of the drugs used
Renal failure	in antihypertensive therapy
Coma	These range from ACE inhibitors to alpha- and beta-adrenergic blocking
	drugs that can be taken in tablet form. For more serious cases
	IV drugs are required
	Sodium nitroprusside
	Nitroglycerin, Labetalol
	Phentolamine

Myocardial infarction

A myocardial infarction is more commonly referred to as a heart attack. Either way both terms are frightening. From a pathophysiological point of view a coronary vessel becomes blocked thus impeding the supply of oxygenated blood and nutrients to that portion of the heart. What occurs next is the myocardium dies and becomes necrotic and subsequently leads to fibrosis.

Myocardial infarction

Symptoms/features	Treatment
On observation	Oxygen with SpO_2 monitoring.
Chest pain	Cannulate (if not already)
Pain radiating down the left arm, around the left side of the neck, back, epigastrium and jaw	Thrombolytic therapy
Breathing ↓ or ↑ Cough	Aspirin 300mg to be chewed
Sweating / pallor	Pain relief and antiemetics
Tachycardia	Take bloods for troponins* and other standard bloods
Nausea and/or abdominal pain often are present in infarcts involving the inferior wall	ECG – this may or may not show anything. Changes do not take place for anything up to 6 hours
Anxiety	In the event of cardiac arrest follow the correct ALS protocols
Light-headedness and syncope	
Arrhythmias/dysrrhythmias	
Cardiac arrest	
Some of these features may be masked due to anaesthesia	

---

*Troponin levels manifest 12 hours after the event.

If the patient can be thrombolysed then the section of muscle may be salvaged. This event can occur while the patient is on the table undergoing surgery or waiting in the anaesthetic room or any time anywhere. The anaesthetic practitioner needs to be aware of the clinical features and the possible therapies for the patient.

For a patient undergoing surgery and who suffers a myocardial infarction can present many problems in diagnosing the event. For example, pallor and sweating may be mistaken for pain due to inadequate analgesia for the surgical procedure.

Trauma

The purpose of this chapter is not to discuss the aetiology or kinematics of trauma, but to look at what the theatre practitioner needs to be aware of in the acute management of trauma. Nevertheless, it should be acknowledged that the kinematics of trauma are important and can point the way to the types of injury the patient may have suffered.

By trauma, we think of the polytrauma events that are depicted on television. This level of trauma is described as a disease process of the young and usually the commonest disease process of people in the first 40 years of life. Having said that, we should never forget the single trauma events that befall the elderly and infirm.

In a sense, trauma can be categorised as a mechanical event that can lead to cardio-respiratory arrest if it goes unchecked or is so severe that cardiac arrest is certain.

Hypovolaemia or fluid depletion is a common affair in trauma and can directly or indirectly lead to death.

Trauma

Symptoms/features	Treatment
On observation	A
On a spinal board	Clear, secure and oxygenate the patient; ensure the oxygen supply
The patient will present on a spinal board with their	is on a high flow rate setting
head and neck immobilised between two foam	Suction present
blocks with 2 straps – 1 across the chin and the other	If the patient needs intubating then the patient's head and
across the forehead	neck will have to be released from the spinal board's
There are additional straps across the thorax, pelvis	head blocks as well the cervical collar. As the blocks
and knees	are removed, the head and neck must be immobilised
Lastly the patient should have cervical collar	manually even when intubation is taking place
Obvious signs of fluid loss	Intubation should be undertaken by someone who is
Obvious injuries	skilled in this procedure
Difficulty of breathing with either rapid respiratory rate,	
or slow and erratic or stopped altogether	B
Sweaty with pallor. This can be because of pain or	Assess breathing and ventilate the patient as necessary
blood loss	Attach SpO_2
As blood loss increases, the patient becomes more	Examine, palpate, percuss and auscultate the thorax
white / grey and anaemic in appearance	(anteriorly, laterally and posteriorly)
Cold to touch	Chest drains may be required, as may other
In burns cases the patient may have red and painful	specialist items
skin to full thickness burns that are dry and not	
painful to the touch	

C
Measure pulse rate
Measure BP or capillary refill
Insert 2 large cannulae into the veins in the patient's
    antecubital fossa
Before connecting infusion bags take blood samples for:
Crossmatch
Full blood count
Toxicolgy
Any other warranted biochemical analysis
In hypovolaemic loss, BP to be kept between 90–100mmHg.
    Any greater pressure may "blow" off clots and promote
    further bleeding
The fluid used depends on Trust Hospital policy. However,
    the large molecular volume expanders may be used,
    but can interfere with the clotting cascade or any future
    attempts at crossmatching. They may even induce
    anaphylaxis. Therefore crystalloids tend to be used
    Physiologic NaCl being the safest

D
Neurological assessment. If a Glasgow coma scale can be
    taken, then do so, However, the AVPU scoring will be
    enough in a primary survey. The patient is categorised by
    ascribing them a letter:
A = Alert
V = Respond to voice
P = Respond to pain
U = Unresponsive
The letters P & U equate to 8 or less on the Glasgow coma
    score. Therefore, the patient will require active ventilatory
    support i.e. intubation
If the patient is showing obvious signs of distress and is
    trying to get off the spinal board then to prevent any
    further injury the patient may have to be released.
    This is a last resort and reasoning with the patient should
    be the first line to be taken

E
Expose the patient. Look for any observable signs on
    the patient's body. Also, palpate as necessary.
    This is so other injuries or any other pathology
    may be detected
There is also an element of environmental control
    to be managed. Keep the patient warm. Measure
    temperature

As mentioned this is not a trauma textbook so therefore the reader should note there are many types of trauma that range from thoracic to special circumstances on how to deal with a pregnant patient. For a more in-depth study, the readers should avail themselves of a specific trauma textbook or undertake a trauma course.

Nevertheless, the anaesthetic practitioner must be able to recognise and be ready to help with the care of a trauma victim. It is well documented that the first hour is critical if the patient is going to survive.

Life-support algorithms

If a patient suffers a cardio-respiratory arrest the anaesthetic practitioner should be able to perform Basic Life-Support as well as having knowledge of the universal algorithm. The latter algorithm relates to treating a shockable or non-shockable cardio-respiratory arrest.

Basic Life-Support or CPR (Cardio Pulmonary Resuscitation) is a time-buying manoeuvre with a prime function to oxygenate the brain while waiting for help to arrive or during the application of the universal algorithm.

The 2005 guidelines draw between layperson and In-Hospital Resuscitation (Figure 9.1). With In-Hospital Resuscitation, some actions can occur simultaneously. For example, someone can be sent to summon help, another sent to bring the resuscitation equipment trolley while another individual assesses the patient.

If the patient is responsive to a gentle shake and being loudly asked if they are alright, then depending on local protocols further medical help may be called on. Nevertheless, the patient should receive a full assessment of their ABCDE (airway, breathing, circulation, disability and exposure) with oxygenation and IV cannulation may be required.

Outlined in the previous box are the major observable features plus the symptoms the patient may display in an A.B.C. manner. The early management of the patient should be to conduct a primary survey. This is not so much a diagnostic activity as so much of a resuscitation exercise. The idea is to identify the life-threatening injuries in their order of magnitude and to deal with them. Once the patient has been stabilised, can a diagnostic approach be taken? Please note that diagnoses are made in the primary survey because what has happened is blatantly obvious.

If the patient does not respond to any audio tactile stimulation then they should be turned onto their back, if not done so already.

- Airway opened using a head tilt chin lift.
- Inspect the mouth for any visible foreign body or debris. This should be removed using a finger sweep, forceps or suction as appropriate.
- In the event of trauma, the patient should receive manual in-line stabilisation with either a jaw thrust or chin lift in combination. If this does not help then the head should be tilted into extension in small increments until the airway is acquired and maintained. An open airway has precedence over any potential cervical fractures.
- Assess breathing by keeping the airway open, look, listen and feel for a full 10 seconds.

Those who have clinical experience may wish to palpate the carotid artery but for no more than 10 seconds. This may be performed simultaneously while checking for breathing or after the breathing check.

Once cardiac arrest has been determined, one person should start CPR, another sent to call the resuscitation team if not already done so and to then bring the resuscitation trolley to the patient (Resuscitation Council (UK), 2005).

The anaesthetic practitioner, as part of the resuscitation team responding to the call should,

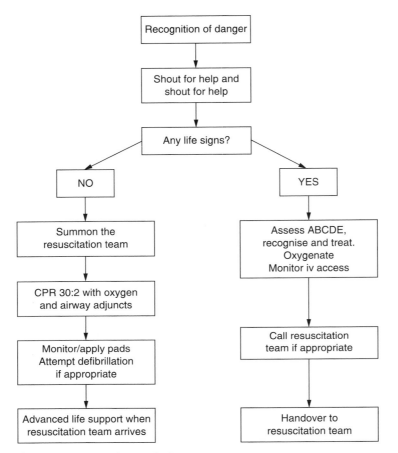

Figure 9.1 In-Hospital Resuscitation.
Source: By kind permission of the Resuscitation Council (UK).

when he or she arrives, make themselves known to the person running the resuscitation attempt and then as appropriate check and use the airway management equipment they have selected. Please note that when ventilating the patient, before inserting an laryngeal mask (LMA) or endotrachael tube, the ventilations should be delivered with a 1-second inspiratory time. Once an LMA or an endotrachael tube has been inserted then compressions and ventilations can be independent of each other.

Once the team arrive or the defibrillator monitor arrives, then the cardiac-arrest rhythm can be assessed and the appropriate treatment instituted.

The sequence of events is going to depend on the location within the hospital, the availability of staff and distance for the resuscitation team to travel as well as many other variables. Therefore, any success will be influenced by these factors.

In the event of performing Basic Life-Support on a pregnant patient who is in her third trimester the gravid uterus will put pressure on the inferior vena cava. Therefore, the patient should have a wedge inserted under her right lumbar region to relieve the compression.

Impeding the patient's blood flow can result in the patient losing consciousness with hypoperfusion.

Respiratory arrest

This is where the patient is unconscious, not breathing but has palpable cardiac output. Under this circumstance, the patient will be ventilated with 100% oxygen and have administered 10 ventilations for approximately 1 minute, and then circulation will be re-evaluated. If the patient has not recommenced breathing then another 1 minute of ventilation will be performed with a further re-evaluation. This will continue until the patient starts breathing, help arrives or the patient succumbs to a cardio-respiratory arrest, in which case chest compressions are started and the 30:2 ratio is applied. The form that help takes will depend on local protocols covering this eventuality.

This algorithm (Figure 9.2) acknowledges an A.B.C. assessment has been performed and where appropriate Basic Life-Support has been instituted. The emphasis under these circumstances is towards fast and safe treatment, especially in the patient with a shockable arrest where the use of a defibrillator is necessary.

In cardio-respiratory arrest the defibrillator is used to deliver a non-synchronised shock to a patient in ventricular fibrillation (VF) although a patient in pulseless ventricular tachycardia (VT) will be treated in the same way.

Ventricular fibrillation (Figure 9.3) occurs secondary to ischaemic damage to the heart muscle with contributing factors such as catecholamine release, hypoxaemia, fluid/electrolyte imbalances and the use of drugs.

The fibrillating heart is able to propel little or no blood into the systemic or pulmonary circulatory systems. Thus, the patient will be rendered unconscious with no respiratory or cardiac effort.

Ventricular fibrillation occurs in 70% of pre-hospital cardio-respiratory arrests (Kazzi, 2004).

Treatment for this condition is defibrillation. The anaesthetic practitioner should at least be able to use an automated external defibrillator (AED). This device determines if the cardiac condition is shockable, selects the required energy and then charges up to the desired energy setting. These devices have been around since the 1980s and with economies of scale are cheaper than manual devices and can be used safely by individuals with little or no medical training other than in the use of this device and basic life support. Ideally, the anaesthetic practitioner should be able to use a manual defibrillator, but for various reasons this is not always possible.

Ventricular tachycardia (VT) (Figure 9.4) is a rapid and sustained beat that originates in either the right or left ventricle. The cause may be because of myocardial infarction or valvular disorders. If the VT is unstable, it will deteriorate into VF, which if left untreated will lead to death.

The patient will have an electrical rate on the electrocardiogram monitor that is more than 100 beats per minute, thus classifying it as a tachycardia. The complexes in VT are easily recognisable by an electrocardiogram.

Physiologically, the ventricles are opening and closing at such a rate that they get little opportunity to fill with blood. This results in systemic hypoperfusion. Because of no palpable output, it is treated in the same manner as VF. If the patient has palpable output then the anaesthetic practitioner will need to distinguish between symptomatic or asymptomatic VT.

Non-shockable cardio-respiratory arrest

This will be either asystole or pulseless electrical activity. These two conditions carry a high degree of mortality/morbidity and despite having clear guidelines for treatment they are still difficult to reverse.

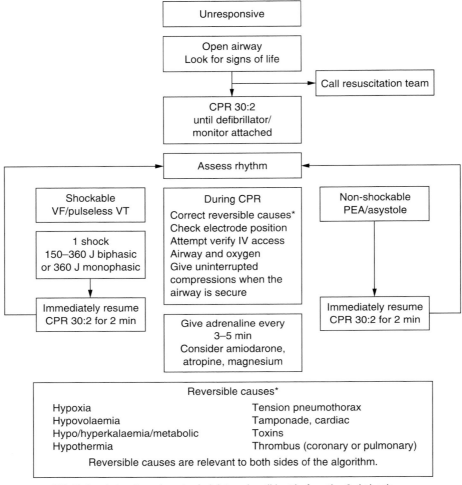

Figure 9.2 Universal Algorithm 4 (Adult).
Source: By kind permission of the Resuscitation Council (UK).

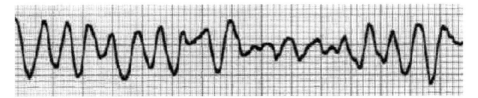

Figure 9.3 Ventricular fibrillation.

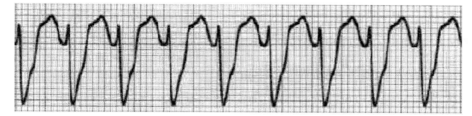

Figure 9.4 Ventricular tachycardia.

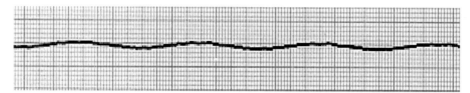

Figure 9.5 Asystole.

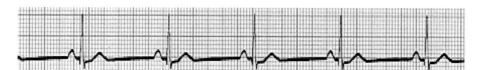

Figure 9.6 Pulseless electrical activity.

Asystole

This is characterised on the electrocardiogram as a wandering baseline with no visible P, Q, R, S, T waves. Sometimes, wide slurred complexes may be seen which are indicative of agonal rhythm. The cause of this condition can be as a result of primary or secondary insult.

Primary

Damage to the conductive pathway of the heart, such as sclerosing of the sino-atrial node which leads to heart block and ultimately to asystole.

Secondary

The conductive pathway fails because of such problems as the patient becoming hyperkalaemic, sustaining a pulmonary embolus, blocked airway, hypothermia or sustaining overdoses of narcotics or sedatives (Caggiano, 2006).

Whether the cause is primary or secondary, resuscitation has to begin almost immediately if there is to be any chance of success.

Pulseless electrical activity

During non-shockable cardio-respiratory arrest, there is recognisable electrical activity on the electrocardiogram but no palpable or recordable output.

This type of cardio-respiratory arrest is commonly seen within hospitals and is difficult to treat. To treat this condition the anaesthetic practitioner must have a clear idea about why the patient has arrested. Once that is known then the correct treatment may be applied.

In order to achieve this, effective documentation with patient notes and communication between healthcare professionals is needed. In the author's experience of having attended many arrests between 1988 and the present there is never a clear idea as to why the patient has suffered a pulseless electrical activity arrest. Therefore, any treatment that is applied is more supportive than definitive.

In treating pulseless electrical activity the reversible causes have been codified into the 4 Hs and the 4 Ts. It should be noted that these reversible causes are not exclusive to this condition but can also be applied to the reversal of asystole and VF. If the patient is successfully resuscitated then really this is the most important phase. At this point, the patient is still vulnerable to relapsing into cardio-respiratory arrest. Therefore, all further care should be directed towards preventing this from happening.

If the anaesthetic practitioner is involved in a successful resuscitation attempt outside of theatre, then the patient will have to be moved to a high dependency care setting whether that is coronary, (CCU) intensive therarapy unit or high dependency unit (ITU/HDU).

Moving a critically ill patient requires much forethought and each hospital should have clear guidelines as part of its CPR policy on moving critically ill patients within the organisation.

Once the patient has been successfully moved to a definitive care setting they may well require ventilatory support, cardiovascular support as well as supportive drug therapy.

If the cardio-respiratory arrest occurred within theatre, the anaesthetic practitioner still has a critical role to play in assisting the anaesthetist in the management of the airway. The perioperative staff should all be basic-life-support competent at the very least, preferably trained to first responder level (NHS Plan, 2000).

Whichever organisation the anaesthetic practitioner belongs to it should have clear and explicit guidelines about the management of emergencies within the theatre department.

Nevertheless, the issue of transportation is still an important one and should be conducted in the same way as if it were occurring from elsewhere within the hospital. The advantage however is the distance between theatre to critical care should be short.

4 Hs	Treatment
Hypovolaemia	Fluid challenge
Hypoxia	Isolate, secure and control the airway and ventilate with 100% oxygen
Hypo/hyperkalaemia and hypocalcaemia	Correct electrolyte imbalance
Hypothermia	Warm the patient
4 Ts	
Tension pneumothorax	Release the tension
Tamponade	Aspirate any fluid from the pericardium
Toxic/therapeutic overdose	Apply reversal agent/supportive therapy
Thromboembolic	Vigorous basic life support to fragmentise the clot or place the patient on cardiac bypass

Please note that this is relevant to shockable cases as well as non-shockable.

Modified circumstances

Under certain circumstances, the anaesthetic practitioner will need to know when to modify the treatment protocols to consider special circumstances.

Pregnancy

As mentioned above in the basic life support section the patient requires a wedge under their right-hand side to relieve caval compression. From the advanced life-support perspective the following is required.

Airway management

The patient is at increased risk of aspiration due to an incompetent cardiac sphincter valve and reduced gut emptying. Airway management is exacerbated by the patient having full dentition, breast engorgement which reduces the room for the laryngoscope handle and glottic oedema.

The fundus of the uterus mobilising high into the abdomen displacing the viscera upwards causing reduced chest compliance, which means a rise in respiratory rate with a reduction in tidal volume.

Circulatory volume increases from 63 ml/kg to 82 ml/kg. There is a rise in red cells but this is more than offset by an increase in plasma volume. The plasma volume increases by a greater proportion to prevent the circulatory volume from becoming too concentrated. The red cell component increases to allow for foetal circulation as well as the potential loss of fluid at childbirth.

Due to this increase, the patient can 'mask' fluid loss if becoming hypovolaemic. This means in effect the patient can mask their symptoms much in the same way as children do until it is too late.

Hypothermia

The anaesthetic practitioner may come across this problem either in theatre or in the accident and emergency (A&E) department. In the former case, it is usually down to inadequate preparation for keeping the patient warm during a prolonged surgical procedure.

From the surgical perspective, it is better to prepare for this eventuality by having a warming mattress or other device and having a means of delivering warm humidified gases. Nevertheless, if the unexpected occurs it is difficult to remedy during surgery unless there is an overriding priority to do so. The only measures that can be undertaken short of this are to attach a humidifier, attach adequate temperature measurement, infuse warm fluids up to 40°C in temperature, or to turn up the heat and humidification in theatre. The

probability of the patient going into cardiac arrest in theatre is unlikely. The anaesthetic practitioner is more likely to see cardiac arrest because of hypothermia in the A&E department rather than in theatre.

Hypothermia is split into three categories:
mild 32–35°C
moderate 30–32°C
severe >30°C.

In the event of cardiac arrest coupled with severe hypothermia, the patient can be rewarmed at the same speed at which they became hypothermic. If the patient is in VF then it will usually be refractory. Nevertheless, three shocks may be administered. If this does not stop the problem then the practitioner should know that it now becomes continual basic life support with 500 mcg of adrenaline every 6 minutes until the patient reaches the minimal optimal defibrillation temperature of 31°C. Once this has been reached, then treatment can revert to the conventional pattern.

In moderate and mild hypothermia the treatment measure of rewarming may be applied.

Immersion

This is defined as the victim being in water but not submerged. Therefore, in the UK's climate the patient is likely to be hypothermic if having been exposed for a lengthy period of time.

Submersion, as the term implies, is where the victim goes underwater with the chance of ingesting liquid. Drowning is classified as death within 24 hours of having been submerged.

For patients who have been immersed for a significant period of time, irrespective of the temperature, the rescuer should extract the patient horizontally. The pressure of water surrounding the patient has a 'squeeze' effect that causes a relative hypotension. Therefore, when the patient is lifted out they will 'faint' due to this relative hypotension. The faint is caused by fluid redistributing from the body's core back to the peripheries.

To manage the hypothermia remove the patient's clothes and rewarm the patient in the manner described earlier.

Poisoning

The anaesthetic practitioner will usually come across this problem while supporting the anaesthetist in the A&E department. The initial phase is a rapid A.B.C.D.E. evaluation with supportive therapy. If it is known what the patient has ingested and the antidote is known then that may be administered. In cases where the antidote is not known then a member of the team can go 'on-line' to Toxbase™ and seek advice or alternatively phone one of the poisons centres.

If the patient is treated successfully then they should be transferred to intensive care or to a specialised centre. Any transportation should be carefully considered prior to its undertaking.

The commonest drug overdoses are shown below.

Drug/agent	Antidote
Alcohol	Glucose
Paracetamol	N–Acetylesistine
Benzodiazepines	Flumanizil
Tranquillizers	Depends on drug category
Opiates/narcotics	Narcan
Beta-blockers	Glucagon
Bleach/caustic agents	

Unless the patient has presented in hospital within an hour of taking the substance then it is unusual to do a gastric lavage.

Periarrest algorithms

There are some specific conditions that precede full-blown cardio-respiratory arrest. These conditions are referred to as the periarrest algorithms.

As the term implies the patient has the potential to deteriorate and therefore the anaesthetic practitioner should know what the algorithms are. The algorithms are designed to be of use for non-experts and are a consensus throughout Europe on how to manage these conditions. The main point to stress is the anaesthetic practitioner should be able to recognise the condition at the start and assist with basic treatment while waiting for more expert help to arrive.

Whatever the periarrest condition, the anaesthetic practitioner must keep in their mind uppermost at all times the rule of evaluating and treating A., B., C., D. and E. (Under stable conditions take a 12-lead ECG to aid diagnosis and correct treatment.)

If the patient is treated in this way then they can be safe in the knowledge that they will be providing the right treatment pattern (Resuscitation Council (UK), 2005).

Broad complex tachycardia

This condition tends to predominate from middle-age onwards and comes about because of problems within the heart. As mentioned above the beat arises out of the ventricles and is going at such a rate to define it as a tachycardia, however, in the periarrest stage the patient has palpable cardiac output. The anaesthetic practitioner needs to know whether the patient is symptomatic or not. The factors in the box below are the significant symptoms.

Symptoms/adverse signs
BP <90 mmHg chest pain
Heart failure heart rate > 150 min^{-1}
Loss of consciousness

Apart from determining the display of symptoms the anaesthetic practitioner must still apply an A.B.C. approach with assessment and treatment.

As can be seen from the protocol if the patient is symptomatic then the patient is to be cardioverted with 120–150 J biphasic or 200 J monophasic. Increase the energy settings incrementally if the initial shocks prove ineffective.

If cardioversion is ineffective then drug therapy is the next treatment option. Administer 300 mg of amiodarone IV over 10–20 minutes followed by 900 mg of amiodarone over 24 hours.

In unstable broad complex tachycardia cardioversion is more reliable in terminating the tachyarrhythmia while drugs act more slowly and have a reduced efficacy in comparison to electricity. Drugs are preferred for the more stable patients.

If the patient presents as asymptomatic then there has to be a determination about whether the broad QRS is regular or irregular.

If it is regular then the patient is given 300 mg IV amiodarone over 20–60 minutes then followed by 900 mg over 24 hours.

If it is irregular then expert help must be sought at the earliest opportunity as the possibilities include:

- atrial bundle branch block (treat as for narrow complex tachycardia)
- pre-excited AF (consider amiodarone)
- polymorphic VT (Torades des Pointes. Give 2 g of magnesium over 10 minutes) (Resuscitation Council (UK), 2005).

Narrow complex tachycardia

This condition is atrial in origin and tends to have a faster cardiac rate than VT. Whereas VT predominates in the older population, supraventricular tachycardia (SVT) predominates in the younger population. Like VT the anaesthetic practitioner has to determine whether the patient is symptomatic or not.

Narrow tachycardia can be subdivided into four subgroups:

Sinus tachycardia. This condition comes about as a stress-related problem, anaemia, fluid loss and heart failure to name a few.

Treatment revolves around assessing and treating the underlying condition. Trying to slow the rate and rhythm usually makes matters worse.

AVRNT (AV nodal re-entry tachycardia). This is the commonest type of paroxysmal SVT that is benign in nature unless the patient has any underlying structural heart defects. With this condition the cardiac rate is well in excess of normal (80–100 bpm) and with any atrial activity difficult to observe.

AVRT (AV re-entry tachycardia). Like AVRNT this is usually benign unless there is any structural cardiac defect with a narrow complex tachycardia being the commonest presenting type.

Atrial flutter with regular AV conduction (often 2:1). By its presentation it can be difficult to distinguish it between AVRNT and AVRT. This is because of the difficulty of observing flutter waves or indeed atrial activity.

This condition with a 2:1 block almost has an atrial rate of 30, i.e. 300 bpm which results in a tachycardia of 150 bpm.

Treatment for regular narrow complex tachycardia whether stable or otherwise must always begin with assessment and treatment of the patient's A., B., C., D. and E.s.

If the patient's condition is unstable then they will require synchronised cardioversion. Nevertheless, it is permissible to administer 6 mg of adenosine while waiting for equipment and personnel to be assembled (Resuscitation Council (UK), 2005).

Stable narrow complex tachycardia

Start with carotid sinus massage or the Valsalva manoeuvre. This will normally terminate up to 25% of paroxysmal SVT. Ensure the patient is monitored and observe for any flutter waves.

These manoeuvres include the following.

Unilateral massaging of the carotid sinus

Occulo cardiac reflex

Valsalva manoeuvre. This may often mean asking the patient to blow into a 20-ml syringe with the objective of blowing the plunger up the barrel of the syringe.

If this does not work use adenosine 6 mg via a rapid bolus with the patient still monitored. If the ventricular rate slows, observe for any flutter waves. If any are observed then treat accordingly.

If the 6 mg dose fails then repeat with 12 mg and then after 1–2 minutes, assuming failure, give a further 12 mg.

If adenosine fails to terminate the condition or there is a contraindication to adenosine use 2.5–5 mg of Verapamil IV over 2 minutes (Resuscitation Council (UK), 2005).

Irregular narrow complex tachycardia

The first step is to summon expert help as soon as possible.

The most likely cause of the irregularity is atrial fibrillation with uncontrolled ventricular response or rarely atrial flutter with a variable atrioventricular block. If the patient is symptomatic then deliver synchronised cardioversion with 70–100 J, if using a biphasic defibrillator (100 J, monophasic).

If the patient is stable then the treatment options are as follows.

• Antiarrhythmics that facilitate chemical defibrillation
• Drugs that control cardiac rate
• Synchronised cardioversion
• Anticoagulant therapy to prevent thrombus.

Patients who have been in atrial fibrillation for more than 48 hours will require 3 weeks of anticoagulant therapy before synchronised cardioversion. If however transoesophageal echo cardiography shows there is no atrial thrombus, then synchronised cardioversion can be performed sooner than 3 weeks.

In patients who present earlier than 48 hours then rhythm-controlling drugs can be used. Amiodarone should be administered 300 mg over 20–60 minutes followed by 900 mg over 24 hours. Another option is to use synchronised cardioversion as it carries a greater likelihood of being successful than chemical cardioversion (Resuscitation Council (UK), 2005).

Bradycardia

Technically a heart rate below 60 beats per minute constitutes bradycardia. Nevertheless, it is better from a clinical perspective to assess it as being 40 beats per minute or less with or without haemodynamic compromise.

As with the tachydysrhythmias, bradycardia is divided between being symptomatic or asymptomatic. If the patient has no adverse signs, it is unlikely to degenerate into anything more sinister, and if not compromised, the patient is observed for any untoward changes. If adverse signs are observed then the appropriate part of the algorithm below is followed.

It should be noted that the administration of 2–10 mcg/min[1] of adrenaline IV is something that should be done by an experienced anaesthetist or intensive care physician and not by a medical practitioner who does not routinely use adrenaline IV. The anaesthetic practitioner and emergency medical staff should have a good working knowledge of external pacing. External pacing is an effective method of temporising until the patient can be moved to a place where a pacing wire may be inserted.

Setting up external pacemakers is straightforward but the practitioner needs to be familiar with the system employed by their hospital. Whilst the defibrillator element of the machine has the standard 1.2.3. approach, the setting up of external pacemakers differs from one manufacturer to another. Nevertheless, all machines will have a control for setting the required heart rate and another for increasing/decreasing the current, which is measured in milliamps.

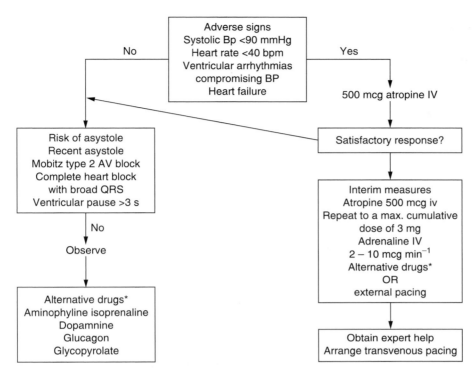

Figure 9.7 Bradycardia algorithm.
Source: By kind permission of the Resuscitation Council (UK).

It is quite common for some machines to have electrodes that can be capable of acting as defibrillation electrodes as well as pacing electrodes.

Pacing terms are listed below.

Pacing terms

Threshold. The current at which artificial QRS complexes are propagated.

Capture. This is when artificial QRS complexes have been propagated.

Demand. Artificial complexes are induced where the machine senses 'dropped' QRS complexes.

Fixed. The pacing system will propagate artificial QRS complexes irrespective of whether there is a dropped beat or not. The rate will remain fixed.

When using one of these systems the anaesthetic practitioner must always remember to keep the patient monitored for their vital signs, especially whilst being transported.

The anaesthetic practitioner should be aware that percussion pacing this technique may be used as a temporising measure. The person undertaking this should deliver gentle blows in the precordium lateral to the lower left margin to the sternal edge. In terms of positioning it may be necessary to move marginally in other directions until electrical capture occurs. (Resuscitation Council (UK), 2005).

Paediatric emergencies

The anaesthetic practitioner may be involved with neonatal and paediatric emergencies that either arise within theatre or elsewhere within the hospital.

Therefore, the anaesthetic practitioner needs to have an understanding of the pathways that lead to cardio-respiratory collapse in the paediatric population.

In childhood, the greatest degree of mortality occurs in the first year of life. Until recently, the greatest cause of mortality was due to sudden infant death syndrome or cot death. Because of effective healthcare promotion, cot death rates have been reduced from just under 396 in 1995 to just under 183 in 2003 (Corbin, 2003).

When the child becomes of school-age the principal cause of death is related to neoplasms with trauma coming second and infectious diseases coming behind congenital abnormalities (PHPLS Manual). This sequence follows into early adulthood.

Given these pathways, the treatment of paediatric patients emphasises the early recognition of a problem and taking action to prevent matters from getting any worse, in other words being proactive as opposed to reactive.

The anaesthetic practitioner needs to be aware of any 'Do Not Attempt Resuscitation' (DNAR) order.

In managing the acute circumstance, the same A.B.C.D.E. approach still applies.

Compromised patients will go into cardio-respiratory arrest either by decreasing respiratory drive or through circulatory collapse.

Therefore, the anaesthetic practitioner is required to know the paediatric basic and advanced life-support algorithms. Not only should they be aware of this they should also understand that they need to obtain as soon as possible an idea of what caused the patient to arrest. They may then be able to help in supplying the appropriate treatment pattern.

Paediatric age definitions are listed below.

Infant.   Birth to first birthday

Child.   From first birthday to puberty.

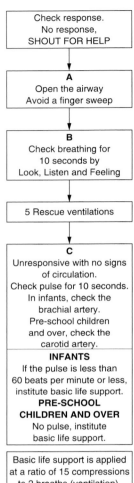

Figure 9.8 Algorithm for Health Care Professionals with a duty to respond and with two or more rescuers. *Source:* By kind permission of the Resuscitation Council (UK).

Notable anatomical and physiological differences

Infants	The head should be placed in the neutral position to open the airway. This is because of the shortness of the larynx, its elastic nature combined with disproportionately larger occipital bone which forces the head into a flexed position
	Instead of mouth-to-mouth, the rescuer should cover the patient's mouth and nose and blow gently over 1–1.5 seconds using the air volume within their cheeks. This is to prevent any lung damage or gastric insufflation
	Checking of pulse. In infants the neck is short and while they do have carotid arteries they are difficult to palpate. Therefore, it is easier to palpate the brachial artery. Other central arteries may also be palpated, i.e. femoral. Indeed a pulse can be found in the fontanella. (An infant's skull bones have not yet fused therefore a pulse may be felt at this point)
	Cardiac arrest is defined as having 60 beats per minute or less
	Chest compressions are applied by first locating the appropriate position, 1 finger's breadth inferior from the internipple line with 2 fingers applied to the sternum. Pressure applied is one third of the resting diameter of the thorax
	There is an initial shout or summons for help at the start of the protocol. However, if no one has responded to this cry for help then basic life support (BLS) is performed for 1 minute and then seeking help is actively undertaken. In the case of an infant, BLS can be performed 'on the move'
Children	The head can be extended to open the airway. Mouth to mouth can be performed as well as drawing air from the rescuer's own lungs in order to expand the patient's chest
	For checking a pulse, the carotids or other central arteries may be palpated. The patient should have an absent pulse before starting BLS. However, if the patient has a pulse rate less than 60 beats per minute and is unconscious with respiratory compromise then treat as cardiac arrest
	To landmark for chest compressions it is 1 finger's breadth from the distal tip of the xiphiod process placing the heal of the rescuer's other hand adjacent to the finger. Depending on the age and size of the patient one hand may be used to exert compression pressure or two hands as in the same fashion used for adult patients

Advanced life support

The arrested paediatric patient is more likely to be in a non-shockable rhythm than a shockable one. This reflects the nature of paediatric arrests. They tend to be the final consequence of some other form of organ or system failure.

This loop is followed until the patient is resuscitated or the attempt is terminated.

AEDs can be used in children over the age of 8 using the same energy settings as used in adults. If the AED can attenuate its energy settings and paediatric pads are available then it may be used in children from 1 year to 8 years of age.

Adrenaline on the non-shockable side is given as soon as IV or IO access has been established and then repeated doses are made every other cycle. The anaesthetic practitioner should be aware of the reversible causes and assist the nursing and medical staff in eliminating the possible reversible causes. In the case of VF or pulseless VT adrenaline is first given just before the third shock and then every other cycle.

If the patient is successfully resuscitated then the anaesthetic practitioner should be aware

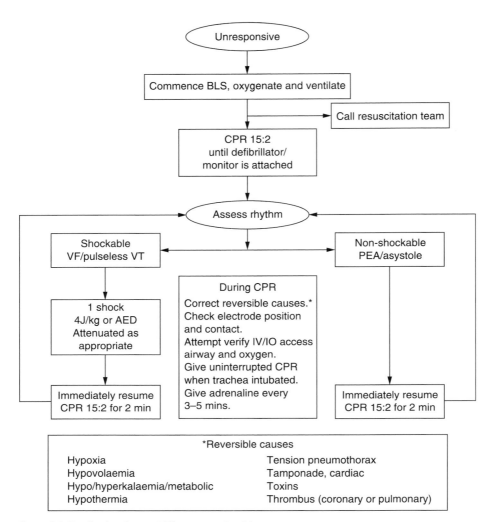

Figure 9.9 Paediatric advanced life support algorithm.
Source: By kind permission of the Resuscitation Council (UK).

of their organisation's intra-hospital transport policy.

It is not always the case that the anaesthetic practitioner is involved in breaking bad news to a patient's relatives. Nevertheless, if they do find themselves in this position then it should be in a supportive role to the registered medical practitioner or the ward nursing staff who will have had greater degree of contact with the patient's relatives.

REFERENCES

ALS Manual, reprinted edn. February 2002, Chapter 13.

BibleGateway. (2005). Available at: www.biblegateway. com/passage/?search=2Ki%204:18-37&version=9 (Accessed 10 May 2006).

Caggiano, R. (2006). *Asystole*. Available at: www. emedicine.com/EMERG/topic44.htm (Accessed 6 May 2006).

Corbin, T. (2003). *Sudden Infant Deaths and Unascertained Deaths in England & Wales 1995–2003.* Available at http://www.gnn.gov.uk/content/detail.asp?ReleaseID=167884&NewsAreaID=2&NavigatedFromSearch=True (Accessed 8 May 2006).

Kazzi, A.A. (2004). *Ventricular Fibrillation.* Available at: www.emedicine.com/emerg/topic633.htm (Accessed 6 May 2006).

NHS Plan. (2000). Chief Nursing Officer's 10 key objectives. Objective No 7.

PHPLS Manual, 2nd edn. P4 table 1.2, Blackwell BMJ Books.

Resuscitation Council (UK). (2005). Guidelines.

Skyaid. (2006). *History of CPR.* Available at: www.skyaid.org/Skyaid%20Org/Medical/history_of_resuscitation.htm (Accessed 10 May 2006).

Taylor, G., Larson, P. & Prestrich, R. (1976). Unexpected cardiac arrest during anaesthesia and surgery. *JAMA,* **236,** 2758.

Vidt, D. (2006). *Hypertensive Crises, Emergencies & Urgencies. Cleveland Clinic.* Available at: www.clevelandclinicmeded.com/diseasemanagement/nephrology/crises/crises.htm (Accessed 9 May 2006).

10

Intravenous induction versus inhalation induction for general anaesthesia in paediatrics

Teresa Hardcastle

Key Learning Points
- Preferred techniques
- The use of premedication
- Intravenous induction techniques
- Induction agents used
- Inhalational induction techniques
- Inhalational agents used in anaesthesia of paediatric patients

The two methods for induction of general anaesthesia are intravenous and inhalational. Intravenous is more frequently used than inhalational induction in adults whereas in paediatric anaesthesia both intravenous and inhalational induction techniques are widely used.

Paediatric anaesthesia is a challenging speciality in itself. Children are not small adults. The spectrum of diseases they suffer from is different from adults and their responses to disease and injury may differ both physically and psychologically. The differences in the anatomy and physiology of neonates, infants and children have important consequences in many aspects of anaesthesia (Aitkenhead *et al.*, 2003). According to Mellor (2004) the technical difficulties that are associated with small size together with the child's psychological and developmental understanding may prove more challenging for induction of anaesthesia in the child compared with the adult. The special demands of inducing anaesthesia in children necessitate the unique skills of the anaesthesia team. One of the many challenges for the anaesthesia team is to minimise distress for the child at induction of anaesthesia (Holm-Knudsen *et al.*, 1998).

According to Messeri *et al.* (2004) the induction of anaesthesia for surgery is a stressful time for both child and family. Donnelly (2005) argues that a young child's emotional development is immature and that the presence of a parent or carer will provide reassurance to maintain the child's sense of security. It is suggested by Palermo *et al.* (2000) that the presence of parents is not always effective as they are emotionally involved in the event and are therefore vulnerable in supporting the child themselves and thus can cause greater distress for the child. A smooth and perfect induction is rewarding for the anaesthesia team and helps allay parental anxiety (Christiansen & Chambers, 2005). Nevertheless, it is important not only to prepare the child but also to support the family for what is to be expected in the perioperative environment to ensure smooth induction of anaesthesia.

Induction of anaesthesia in children is broadly achieved with the same agents and techniques that are used in adults (Mellor, 2004). Many would argue in paediatrics as to which is the least traumatic method of anaesthetic induction. In the United States inhalation induction is the most common technique used whereas in the United Kingdom and other parts of the world intravenous induction appears to be used more commonly (Aguilera *et al.*, 2003).

Core Topics in Operating Department Practice: Anaesthesia and Critical Care, eds. Brian Smith, Paul Rawling, Paul Wicker and Chris Jones. Published by Cambridge University Press. © Cambridge University Press 2007.

According to Aitkenhead *et al.* (2003) children possess great insight and during the preoperative visit by the anaesthetist a child may ask the anaesthetist questions and request a preferred mode of induction. Evidently the technique for induction will depend on the status and the health of the child as to whether a rapid sequence induction of anaesthesia is indicated. In the case of a rapid sequence induction the clinical status of the child will overshadow the child's wishes.

It is not always routine to administer a premedication to children undergoing surgery. Many paediatric surgical procedures are performed on a day-case basis, to avoid an overnight hospital stay, resulting in minimal disruption to the child and family. According to Holm-Knudsen *et al.* (1998) many anaesthetists have a policy of selective premedication based on their assessment of the child and the circumstances of the surgery and anaesthesia. Children who have behavioural problems or who have had traumatic experiences with previous anaesthetics and have preoperative anxiety are more likely to have a premedication prior to coming to theatre. The usual drug of choice is midazolam 0.5 mg per kg orally 30 minutes preoperatively. The timing of administration is crucial to facilitate the full sedative effect. Disruption to the theatre list can have catastrophic implications on the desired effect of the premedication, subsequently the child arrives in the anaesthetic room frightened and emotionally distressed. The decision not to use premedication is commonly influenced by the perceived adverse effects such as delayed recovery from anaesthesia, disorientation during recovery and paradoxical reactions such as anxiety and behavioural changes (Holm-Knudsen *et al.*, 1998). A study carried out by Messeri *et al.* (2004) examined the effect of both premedication and parental presence on preoperative anxiety during induction of anaesthesia and concluded that there was no significant difference in the presence of stress between children who did and did not receive premedication with midazolam. They observed that parental presence, low anxiety level of the parent and the age of the child actually determined a reaction of less stress in children during induction of anaesthesia.

Intravenous induction has become less traumatic for children since the introduction of topical anaesthetics such as EMLA® (Eutectic Mixture of Local Anaesthetic) and Ametop® (Amethocain Topical). Pain endured during intravenous cannulation can cause psychological trauma to a child and lead to the development of needle phobia (Smalley, 1999). Topical anaesthetics are used to numb the skin and reduce pain for procedures such as venepuncture and venous cannulation. The topical anaesthetic is usually applied to the skin over the anticipated site for venous cannulation on the dorsum of the hands or feet and is covered with an adhesive plastic dressing and sometimes bandaged. The cream or gel needs to be covered to allow for the anaesthetic to be absorbed and effectively numb the skin. Two sites are normally chosen if there is a doubt about the efficacy of the vein.

Ametop® is a topical anaesthetic gel that contains amethocaine and it should not be used on the preterm neonate or infant under the age of 1 month. It is put in place 30–40 minutes prior to induction of anaesthesia and should not be left in place for more than an hour. The site will remain numb for 4–6 hours. The area where the gel has been applied may appear red and swollen and it may itch as the effect of the gel increases the size of the blood vessels (BNF for Children, 2005a).

EMLA® is a topical anaesthetic cream which contains lidocaine and prilocaine. It can be used on children over the age of 1 year but its use is contraindicated in neonates. It should be applied at least an hour before the procedure and may be left on for 4–5 hours. The site will remain numb for up to 6 hours (BNF for Children, 2005b). EMLA® can have the effect of causing temporary paleness to skin and also causing vasoconstriction which in turn may cause difficulty cannulating the identified vein.

Children are informed by the anaesthetist and nursing staff on the ward that when they go to theatre for their operation they will have a small scratch on the back of their hand before they go to sleep. The anaesthesia and nursing staff refer to the topical anaesthetic as the 'magic cream' and children commonly use this term.

Many children fear the idea of a needle as evidently they associate this with experiencing pain. Much has been written over the years concerning the use of distraction techniques to reduce anxiety and distress in children undergoing painful procedures (Collins, 1999; Kleiber & Harper, 1999). Distraction according to McCaffrey and Beebe (1989) is re-focusing the attention away from pain or the anticipation of pain onto something else. Distraction techniques used in the anaesthetic room vary and can involve the use of the child's favourite toy, discussion regarding favourite television programme, music, reading a story or playing with a toy. A study aimed at assessing, preparing and distracting children during procedures such as intravenous cannulation carried out by Wood (2002) acknowledged the need for effective distraction and the importance of parental involvement. Consequently a parent can play a significant role in the use of distraction techniques, since the child will trust and relate to their parent. At the same time as the parent distracts their child, the anaesthetist inserts the intravenous cannula concealing the needle from the child. Most children are inquisitive and like to look where the cannula has been positioned and comprehend where the special medicine will go to send them to sleep, to have their operation.

Many children become distressed when they are placed onto the theatre trolley on arrival into the anaesthetic room. The anaesthetist who encounters a very distressed child in these circumstances may ask the parent to sit on a stool with their child on their lap. This avoids the separation anxiety that a child experiences by being placed on an unfamiliar, overwhelming trolley in a strange room. The anaesthetist asks the parent to cuddle their child, placing one of the child's arms around the parent's back out of the child's sight distracting them at the same time as the intravenous cannula is inserted by the anaesthetist. Anaesthesia is induced with the child cuddling the parent. Nevertheless as soon as the induction agent has taken effect the child is immediately and safely taken from the parent by the anaesthesia team and placed on the theatre trolley. However, the use of this technique for induction would depend on the status and the health of the child and would not be suitable if a rapid sequence induction of anaesthesia was indicated.

Propofol is a short-acting, non-barbiturate intravenous anaesthetic agent that is used for both induction and maintenance of anaesthesia in adults and children (Aitkenhead et al., 2003). It is presented in an aqueous solution in soya oil and egg phosphatide (Mellor, 2004). According to Moore (1998) propofol produces a rapid smooth induction of anaesthesia. One main advantage of using propofol in paediatrics is the rapid recovery facilitating a speedy discharge especially in day surgery. The use of propofol is associated with a significant reduction in post-operative nausea and vomiting (Moore et al., 2003; Gwinutt, 2004). Nevertheless, the main disadvantage of propofol is pain upon injection; this can be lessened with the addition of lidocaine 0.2 mg/kg (Aitkenhead et al., 2003).

Sodium thiopentone is a widely used intravenous induction agent. According to Mellor (2004) it was first introduced in the 1930s and has been the basis of intravenous induction for many years. It is a water-soluble barbiturate and is supplied as a yellow powder to be dissolved in water before use. Its main use in paediatrics is for rapid sequence induction. According to Aitkenhead et al. (2003) a dose of 5–6 mg/kg of a 2.5% solution is required in a healthy child. Induction of anaesthesia is smooth and rapid with minimal excitatory effects such as involuntary movement or hiccuping (Gwinutt, 2004). One of its main advantages is that it is pain-free on injection but recovery tends to be slow. Sodium thiopentone, because of its alkalinity, if injected extravascularly, will cause tissue necrosis (Mellor, 2004).

Anaesthesia is commonly induced in children and infants by means of a gaseous induction via a facemask with a volatile agent. Inhalational induction is preferred by some children who fear the insertion of an intravenous cannula, are needle phobic, have had a psychologically traumatic experience in the past with intravenous induction or prefer this method of induction. An inhalational induction is often used in babies and small infants because of difficulties obtaining venous access (Bagshaw & Stack, 1999). Occasionally the insertion of an intravenous cannula may be difficult if the veins are not obvious. Mellor (2004) argues that it is harder when the child has a large amount of subcutaneous fat, which is common in toddlers, and that veins become smaller in cold, dehydrated and frightened children.

Other indications for inhalational induction of anaesthesia are the perceived difficult intubation or removal of inhaled foreign body from the airway, a common occurrence especially in young children. With a perceived difficult intubation or removal of foreign body from the airway, the use of intravenous induction could give rise to a sudden loss of airway control, apnoea that in turn would lead to hypoxia. With inhalational induction the child's airway is tested with the gradual onset of anaesthesia whilst spontaneous breathing is sustained. Inhalational induction can be smooth and fast but can trigger problems such as breath holding and laryngospasm particularly if the airway is stimulated in the light planes of anaesthesia (Kandasamy & Sivalingam, 2000).

The type of facemask used for inhalational induction has changed considerably over the years. The black rubber facemask was used for many years and came in different shapes and sizes. Many children were frightened of these facemasks and were sometimes left with disturbed memories of a black facemask with the unforgettable odour of rubber being placed over their face. Today the facemasks used for inhalational induction are manufactured in clear lightly coloured plastic and come in many sizes ranging from neonatal size to large adult size and come with a variety of scents including cherry, vanilla, strawberry and bubblegum. The concept behind the different scents is influential to the child's acceptance of the facemask. The child is thus able to choose the scent they prefer for their gaseous induction. According to Aitkenhead et al. (2003) the clear plastic scented facemasks are not only more acceptable to children but they have the added advantage of allowing respiration and the presence of vomitus to be observed.

Many games can be played with children as part of the inhalational induction technique using the scented facemasks but the success of this technique relies on how receptive the child is. Games whereby the child holds the facemask close to their face pretending to be a pilot or an astronaut can be encouraged or the child is persuaded to see how big they can blow the balloon which is at the end of the Ayre's T-piece anaesthetic circuit also known as a Mapleson E (or F if an open-ended rebreathing bag is included which is a Jackson Rees modification) which in turn influences the child to breathe the gas. Some children prefer their parent to hold the mask for them rather than holding it themselves. Occasionally there is a child who has an excessive fear of the anaesthetic facemask. Przybylo et al. (2005) suggest that it is common for a co-operative child to refuse having the facemask placed on their face during the induction of anaesthesia. Przybylo et al. (2005) conducted a study into mask fear in children and found that some children complained that they did not like the experience of wanting to fight the mask, of feeling dizzy, claustrophobic and not being able to breathe. One other technique that may be used by the anaesthetist is the anaesthetist cups one hand around the angle mount connector without the facemask and places their hand near to the child's face but not completely covering it. The child then breathes the gas in a purposeful calm and peaceful environment at the same time as listening to the reassuring voice of a parent or the anaesthetist. Nevertheless, it is essential for the anaesthetist to direct the fresh gas flow away from the child's eyes as the anaesthetic gases can cause eye irritation (Aitkenhead *et al.*, 2003).

The child who is to have an inhalation induction may possibly refuse to sit on the theatre trolley or table. To avoid separation anxiety the child may sit on a parent's lap and be cuddled whilst having a gas induction. Nevertheless, the use of this technique for induction would depend on the status and the health of the child and the preference of the anaesthetist. The child is immediately and safely taken from the parent by the anaesthesia team and positioned on the theatre trolley once the child is asleep. The anaesthetist holds the facemask maintaining a clear airway with good ventilation until a deeply anaesthetised state is reached (Mellor, 2004). It is vital, once a deep anaesthesia state is reached, to insert an intravenous cannula to establish vascular access for the use of drugs and administration of fluids should laryngospasm or hypotension occur (Schwartz *et al.*, 2004). It may be necessary for two anaesthetists to be present as part of the anaesthesia team which will facilitate the maintenance of the child's airway whilst at the same time establishing venous access.

Inhalational induction agents are otherwise known as volatile agents. Volatile anaesthetic agents are liquids that have a high-saturated vapour pressure and low boiling point that are administered via inhalation through the lungs, entering the circulation through the alveolar capillaries. These agents can be used for induction but are chiefly used for the maintenance of anaesthesia. Volatile agents are supplied via calibrated vaporisers using carrier gases such as air, oxygen or oxygen nitrous oxide mixes (Torrance & Serginson, 1997).

Halothane was introduced in the 1950s and was the gold standard volatile agent that was used for inhalational induction of anaesthesia that dominated paediatric anaesthesia for more than half a century without any serious opposition from other volatile anaesthetic agents (Bagshaw & Stack, 1999; Aitkenhead *et al.*, 2003; Lerman, 2004). The smell is non-irritant and not unpleasant and usually tolerated well by children. Nevertheless, Lien *et al.* (1996) argue that although it is tolerated well the inhalation induction is relatively slow because of its higher blood gas partition coefficient. Emergence from anaesthesia using halothane is longer compared with some of the newer volatile agents (Aitkenhead *et al.*, 2003) and therefore its use in paediatric day case surgery is virtually non-existent. Nevertheless, one disadvantage of its use is that it can effect the myocardium causing depression of myocardial contractility, reducing cardiac output and vascular resistance thus lowering arterial blood pressure. With repeated halothane anaesthesia the liver may be affected and thus develop an inflammatory response. Consequently as a precautionary measure halothane is not administered within 3 months of a previous administration (Oakley & Van Limborgh, 2005).

Sevoflurane is a volatile anaesthetic agent with a low blood gas partition coefficient and a pleasant non-pungent odour (Viitanen *et al.*, 2000). It has taken over and replaced halothane in many hospitals especially in the paediatric setting. It has been used in Japan since the 1970s (Mellor, 2004), was introduced in the United States and the United Kingdom during the mid 1990s (Schwartz *et al.*, 2004) and owing to its low pungency is well accepted by children. When first introduced in the UK sevoflurane was selectively used due to its high cost.

It has several advantages compared with halothane including a quicker smoother anaesthetic induction causing few arrhythmias, minimal cardiac depression and hepatic and renal toxicities (Lerman, 2004). In paediatrics a rapid induction of anaesthesia is less emotionally distressing for both parent and child. Even though sevoflurane produces a swifter onset of anaesthesia where a child rapidly loses their eyelash reflex, excitement is not uncommon during induction of anaesthesia (Dubois *et al.*, 1999; Mellor, 2004; Schwartz *et al.*, 2004). Schwartz *et al.* (2004) argue that eye closure and loss of lid reflex do not guarantee a deep enough state of anaesthesia. Anaesthetists administering a gaseous induction are acutely aware that it is necessary to insert an intravenous cannula as soon as it is possible to provide a means of administering drugs and fluids should a difficulty arise. Nevertheless, a response to painful stimuli increasing the chance of laryngospasm may be observed on intravenous cannulation whilst the child is in the light stages of anaesthesia. This requires the skill of the anaesthetist to know when the child has reached a deep enough level of anaesthesia to attempt intravenous cannulation. Schwartz *et al.* (2004) conducted a study into early intravenous cannulation in children during inhalational anaesthesia and concluded that it is better to wait 2 minutes after the child loses the eyelash reflex before attempting intravenous cannulation, thus reducing the chance of laryngospasm. One other possible disadvantage of this agent for inhalational induction is respiratory depression resulting in breath holding before a level of deep anaesthesia is achieved (Mellor, 2004).

Isoflurane, another anaesthetic volatile agent, lies between halothane and enflurane in its potency (Gwinutt, 2004). Its advantage over halothane is that it does not depress myocardial contractility, cause renal or hepatic toxicity, and can be repeated at short intervals. It is ideal to use in surgery that requires hypotension as its effect is by vasodilatation rather than depressing the contractility of the myocardium.

Isoflurane when it was first introduced in the 1980s offered a new agent that had lower blood solubility with a faster onset of anaesthetic induction (Bagshaw & Stack, 1999). Nevertheless isoflurane has an unpleasant smell and pungent odour and is not tolerated by children and therefore its use for inhalational induction is ineffective. One other disadvantage in using this volatile agent for inhalational induction is the possible incidence of airway complications (Bagshaw & Stack, 1999; Gwinutt, 2004).

Desflurane was introduced into clinical practice in the 1990s and because of its low blood-gas and blood-tissue solubility provides a rapid emergence even after prolonged anaesthesia. Nevertheless, it soon became apparent that this volatile agent was inappropriate for inhalational induction because of its strong pungency (Bagshaw & Stack, 1999). Murat (2002) argues that in four published clinical trials on the use of desflurane for inhalational induction in paediatrics there were airway complications such as breath holding, laryngospasm, coughing, and hypoxaemia reported in more than 50% of children. The BNF (2005) states that desflurane is contraindicated for inhalation induction in children because coughing, breath holding, apnoea, laryngospasm and increased secretions can occur.

Nitrous oxide is a sweet-smelling, non-irritant gas used as a carrier for most inhalational anaesthetic agents (Aitkenhead *et al.*, 2003). When administering an inhalational induction to a child some anaesthetists prefer to administer nitrous oxide and oxygen alone to begin with which allows the child to become familiar with the smell whilst reducing their awarenes before introducing sevoflurane. Other anaesthetists prefer to induce sevoflurane at 8% with oxygen alone resulting in a faster induction where the child loses consciousness which is less stressful for both child and parent. Nevertheless, Dubois *et al.* (1999) compared techniques used for sevoflurane induction and found that by adding nitrous oxide at induction the loss of consciousness was much faster and resulted in a reduced phase of excitement. Bortone *et al.* (2002) argue that previous studies have found that there is a higher incidence in PONV (Post Operative Nausea and Vomiting) with the combination of nitrous oxide and inhalational anaesthetic agents. Nevertheless, in their study they concluded that the use of nitrous oxide was not associated with an increased incidence of PONV in children who had undergone testicle and inguinal hernia surgical procedures. They supported the use of nitrous oxide with sevoflurane to reduce anxiety with inhalational induction.

Intravenous and inhalational methods of inducing anaesthesia are both widely used techniques in paediatrics. Intravenous induction has become less traumatic for a child since the introduction of the topical local anaesthetic creams, however timing and theatre scheduling can disrupt the desired effect of the creams. It is obvious that distraction techniques play an important role in intravenous induction. A child who does not visibly see a needle will not anticipate the fear of pain. There will of course be children who have had a distressing experience in the past with needles and will always fear the pain, however even in these cases distraction can be effective. The parent plays an important role with the child in minimalising anxiety and fear. The parents themselves need to be fully prepared for what will happen in the anaesthetic room, communication via the ward staff and anaesthetic team being vital to success.

Inhalational techniques have changed over the last 10 years since the introduction of sevoflurane which has taken over from halothane as the gold standard for gaseous induction. Induction and emergence from anaesthesia is much faster. Children often request this method of induction as sevoflurane has the added advantage of having a pleasant smell and less pungent odour. The facemasks used to induce anaesthesia are far removed from the old black rubber that many children found frightening to the more pleasant clear plastic, scented facemasks that are much more acceptable to a child.

Children suffer from separation anxiety and the anaesthetic team are acutely aware of this and depending on the health and status of the child where possible will induce anaesthesia with a young child sat on the parent's knee. For the anaesthetic team minimising the anxiety of the child and parent, together with the demands of inducing anaesthesia is a challenge and requires great skill especially if the lack of co-operation of the child is predictable and requires a management plan in advance.

REFERENCES

Aguilera, I. M., Patel, D., Meakin, G. H. & Masterson, J. (2003). Perioperative anxiety and postoperative behavioural disturbances in children undergoing intravenous or inhalation induction of anaesthesia. *Paediatric Anaesthesia*, **13**, 501−7.

Aitkenhead, A. R., Rowbotham, D. J. & Smith, G. (2003). *Textbook of Anaesthesia*, 4th edn. London: Churchill Livingstone.

Bagshaw, O. N. T. & Stack, C. G. (1999). A comparison of halothane and isoflurane for gaseous induction of anaesthesia in infants. *Paediatric Anaesthesia*, **9**, 25−9.

BNF. (2005). *Volatile Liquid Anaesthetics. Desflurane*. Available at: http://bnf.org/bnf/bnf/50/noframes/6573. htm (Accessed 21 November 2005).

BNF for Children. (2005a). *Ametop*®. Available at: http://www.bnfc.nhs.uk/bnfc/bnfc/current/40704.htm (Accessed 17 November 2005).

BNF for Children. (2005b). *EMLA*®. Available at: http://www.bnfc.nhs.uk/bnfc/bnfc/current/6693.htm? q=%22emla%22#_hit (Accessed 17 November 2005).

Bortone, L., Picetti, E. & Mergoni, M. (2002). Anaesthesia with sevoflurane in children: nitrous oxide does not increase postoperative nausea and vomiting. *Paediatric Anaesthesia*, **12**, 775−9.

Christiansen, E. & Chambers, N. (2005). Case report. Induction of anaesthesia in a combative child; management and issues. *Paediatric Anaesthesia*, **15**, 421−5.

Collins, P. (1999). Restraining children for painful procedures. *Paediatric Nursing*, **11**(3), 15−16.

Donnelly, J. (2005). Care of children and adolescents. In K. Woodhead & P. Wicker, eds., *A Textbook of Perioperative Care*. London: Elsevier Churchill Livingstone, pp. 267−83.

Dubois, M. C., Piat, V., Constant, I., Lamblin, O. & Murat, I. (1999). Comparison of three techniques for induction of anaesthesia with sevoflurane in children. *Paediatric Anaesthesia*, **9**, 19−23.

Gwinutt, C. (2004). *Lecture Notes On Clinical Anaesthesia*, 2nd edn. London: Blackwell.

Holm-Knudsen, R., Carlin, P. & McKenzie, F. (1998). Distress at induction of anaesthesia in children. A survey of incidence, associated factors and recovery characteristics. *Paediatric Anaesthesia*, **8**(5), 383−92.

Kandasamy, R. & Sivalingam, P. (2000). Use of sevoflurane in difficult airways. *Acta Anaesthesiologica Scandinavica*, **44**, 627−9.

Kleiber, C. & Harper, D. C. (1999). Effects of distraction on children's pain and distress during medical procedures: a meta-analysis. *Nursing Research*, **48**(1), 44−9.

Lerman, J. (2004). Inhalational anaesthetics. *Paediatric Anaesthesia*, **14**, 380–3.

Lien, C.A., Hemmings, H.C., Belomont, M.R. *et al.* (1996). A comparison: the efficacy of sevoflurane-nitrous oxide or propofol-nitrous oxide for induction and maintenance of general anaesthesia. *Journal of Clinical Anaesthesia*, **8**, 639–43.

McCaffrey, M. & Beebe, A. (1989). *Pain: Clinical Manual for Nursing Practice.* St Louis: Mosby.

Mellor, J. (2004). Induction of anaesthesia in paediatric patients. *Update in Anaesthesia*, **18**(8), 1. Available at: http://www.nda.ox.ac.uk/wfsa/html/u18/u1808_01.htm#pharm (Accessed 21 November 2005).

Messeri, A., Caprilli, S. & Busoni, P. (2004). Anaesthesia induction in children: a psychological evaluation of the efficiency of parents' presence. *Paediatric Anaesthesia*, **14**, 551–6.

Moore, J.K., Moore, E.W., Elliott, R.A. *et al.* (2003). Propofol and halothane versus sevoflurane in paediatric day-case surgery: induction and recovery characteristics. *British Journal of Anaesthesia*, **90**(4), 461–6.

Moore, N. (1998). Total Intravenous Anaesthesia (TIVA) in paediatrics: advantages and disadvantages. *Paediatric Anaesthesia*, **8**(3), 189–94.

Murat, I. (2002). Editorial. Is there a place for desflurane in paediatric anaesthesia? *Paediatric Anaesthesia*, **12**, 663–4.

Oakley, M. & Van Limborgh, M. (2005). Care of the patient undergoing anaesthesia. In K. Woodhead & P. Wicker, eds., *A Textbook of Perioperative Care.* London: Elsevier Churchill Livingstone, pp. 147–60.

Palermo, T.M., Tripi, P.A. & Burgess, E. (2000). Parental presence during anaesthesia induction for outpatient surgery of the infant. *Paediatric Anaesthesia*, **10**, 487–91.

Przybylo, H.J., Tarbell, S.E. & Stevenson, G.W. (2005). Mask fear in children presenting for anaesthesia: aversion, phobia or both? *Paediatric Anaesthesia*, **15**(5), 336–70.

Schwartz, D., Connelly, N.R., Gutta, S., Freeman, K. & Gibson, C. (2004). Early intravenous cannulation in children during sevoflurane induction. *Paediatric Anaesthesia*, **14**: 820–4.

Smalley, A. (1999). Needle phobia. *Paediatric Nursing*, **11**(2), 17–20.

Torrance, C. & Serginson, E. (1997). *Surgical Nursing.* London: Elsevier Science.

Viitanen, H., Baer, G. & Annila, P. (2000). Recovery characteristics of sevoflurane or halothane for day-case anesthesia in children aged 1–3 years. *Acta Anaesthesiologica Scandinavica*, **44**, 101–6.

Wood, C. (2002). Introducing a protocol for procedural pain. *Paediatric Nursing*, **14**(8), 30–3.

11

Managing difficult intubations

Michael A. Sewell

Key Learning Points
- Available aids and techniques for both predicted and unexpected failed or difficult intubations
- The importance of preoperative airway assessment and its impact on induction

Introduction

As the anaesthetic assistant's role develops, with opportunities arising for some to become non-medical anaesthetists (anaesthesia practitioner), preoperative assessments are already being carried out by anaesthetic assistants in a number of hospitals. This chapter aims to outline the prediction and management of difficult intubations for the participant, be it junior anaesthetist, non-medical anaesthetist or anaesthetic assistant. For those who will not be assessing or managing difficult airways, this chapter will provide valuable insight and enable the anaesthetic assistant to anticipate the needs of the anaesthetist.

A preoperative visit from the anaesthetist is appreciated by patients and has been shown to be more effective in reducing anxiety than premedication. The aim of the preoperative assessment is to ensure the patient's health is optimal and any potential difficulties during anaesthesia are anticipated. In the United Kingdom, it has traditionally been the role of the anaesthetist to perform the assessment of the airway and subsequent

procedure of intubation for elective surgery, although no test is 100% reliable in predicting difficult intubation.

A history of previous difficult intubation is important, but a history of straightforward intubation some years earlier may be falsely reassuring. Whether we like it or not, we all change physically with age; increasing weight, reduced spinal flexion or changing disease processes means possible implications for airway management. The overweight patient with a poorly defined neck will often cause the anaesthetic assistant to prepare for a difficult intubation without necessarily being conscious of the reason for their actions. A poorly defined neck will certainly hinder the anaesthetist in creating an effective seal whilst using a mask, a problem seen frequently by the anaesthetic assistant and readily recognised. This is a rather simplistic example, but nonetheless indicative of a conditioned response on the part of the anaesthetic assistant.

Failed intubation may be the result of an anticipated degree of difficulty with the airway or a totally unexpected event. Prediction and management of difficult intubations requires investigative examination and attention to detail. Clinical examination of the patient and assessment of the airway are useful in identifying patients posing the risk of a potentially difficult intubation. Nevertheless, it is not unusual to be confronted with a patient of normal appearance in whom the glottis cannot

Core Topics in Operating Department Practice: Anaesthesia and Critical Care, eds. Brian Smith, Paul Rawling, Paul Wicker and Chris Jones. Published by Cambridge University Press. © Cambridge University Press 2007.

be visualised on direct laryngoscopy. Visualisation of the glottis is only possible under direct laryngoscopy when the patient is anaesthetised. Sometimes visualisation of the vocal cords is restricted, for example due to a large tongue and/or epiglottis.

It is essential to define '*difficult airway*' and '*difficult intubation*' precisely, as this is important in the evaluation of an incident. Using an anaesthetic aid such as a bougie or cricoid pressure when the cords are not visible, may not be difficult for some practitioners. Pearce (1998) recognised that the skill of the person intubating has an impact on the success and quality of the intubation.

Samsoon and Young (1987) defined difficult intubation as '*inadequate visualisation of the glottis*' and failed orotracheal intubation as '*inability to insert a tracheal tube from the oropharynx into the trachea*'. The interpretation of Feldman *et al.* (1989) is that '*difficult intubation lies somewhere between an easy intubation and an impossible one*'.

Assessment

The initial stage of the preoperative visit should deal with basic airway questions such as:
- Do you wear dentures, crowns, partial plate or a bridge? Are any of your teeth loose, cracked, chipped or capped?
- Has any blood relative ever had any problems during an anaesthetic?
- Can you open your mouth fully?
- Have you ever been treated for a problem of the jaw joint?
- Do you have neck stiffness or problems moving your head?
- Do you snore, or do others say you snore?

This would then be followed by a physical examination. There is a fundamental link between assessing the airway and the prediction of a difficult intubation, formally identified by Mallampati (1983). It is possible to anticipate

difficult intubation in nearly all cases by evaluating the three critical anatomical areas of the airway which include a) relative tongue/pharyngeal size; b) the mandibular space; and finally, c) the movement of the atlanto-occipital and mandibular joints.

Area A: relative tongue/pharyngeal size

Significant correlation was found between airway class and degree of ease or difficulty of exposure of the glottis by direct laryngoscopy in a study by Mallampati. The Mallampati test (1983) devised three classifications of airway:

  Class I: uvula, faucial pillars, soft palate visible
  Class II: faucial pillars, soft palate visible
  Class III: only soft palate visible.

This classification was further modified by Samsoon and Young (1987) to include a fourth classification which represents an extreme version of the original third classification in which the soft palate is completely masked by the tongue and only the hard palate is visible.

The revised Mallampati classification

To evoke the Mallampati classification (Figure 11.1), the patient remains seated with their head in a neutral position and opens his or her mouth as widely as possible and protrudes their tongue to the maximum extent. Patients are encouraged not to talk during this assessment to avoid providing a false result.

Area B: the mandibular space

The distance from the inner surface of the mandible to the thyroid cartilage during neck extension should be at least three large finger breadths (50 mm) in adults. Also, an inability to bring the lower incisors edge to edge with the upper incisors, i.e. impaired mandibular protrusion, is an important warning that laryngoscopy may be difficult.

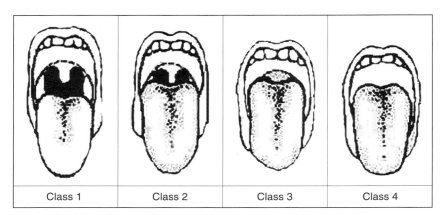

| Class 1 | Class 2 | Class 3 | Class 4 |

Figure 11.1 The revised Mallampati classification.

Area C: mobility of the atlanto-axial and TM joints

The neck is examined for masses with particular attention to the possible influence of these on the position and mobility of the trachea. The optimal position for intubation is the so called '*sniffing the morning air*' position and neck position should be assessed with this in mind. With the lower neck flexed, as is inclined to happen with a standard pillow under the head, the normal angle of head extension is 80° with lesser degree representing greater limitation and increased potential for difficult laryngoscopy. In this regard, patients with diabetes mellitus are often difficult to intubate and one of the reasons for this is the stiffness of the mentioned joints.

Throughout the anaesthetic literature it is well established that patients with rheumatoid arthritis (hypoplastic mandible), obstructive sleep apnoea, presence of neoplasm extending into the airway, swelling, infections (quinsy, epiglottitis, infectious mononucleosis) or haematoma of the mouth, tongue, pharynx, larynx, trachea or neck would be associated with difficult intubation (Illingworth & Simpson, 1998).

Endocrine disorders, for example acromegaly, can produce abnormalities to the upper airway, e.g. macroglossia, thickening of the pharyngeal or laryngeal tissues, or hypertrophy of the aryepiglottic folds. In addition to this, large nose, lips and overhanging teeth can make ventilation difficult (Rushman *et al.*, 1999). Small mandible size, an inability to protrude the jaw, short, thick neck and overweight patients can also be of concern for intubation (Morgan & Mikhail, 1996).

Management

When confronting a potentially difficult airway, it is important to remain calm. Assess the degree of difficulty and seek senior assistance if available. Pay particular attention to ventilation, ensuring the patient is adequately oxygenated and anaesthetised at all times, and it may be necessary to consider waking the patient. The drama of a difficult intubation can easily escalate when there are multiple attempts at laryngoscopy in a hypoxic patient with a mouth full of blood and secretions. The use of rapidly redistributed intravenous induction agents such as propofol will allow rapid return of consciousness unless the patient receives adequate amounts of a volatile agent or further incremental doses of the induction agent.

If ventilation can be maintained using a mask without too much difficulty and gas exchange can be maintained, there are a number of manoeuvres and aids available to improve the chances of correct endotracheal placement.

Patient positioning

As mentioned earlier, the '*sniffing the morning air*' position is the single most important manoeuvre that can improve intubation conditions. This position is sometimes 'exaggerated' by placing a pillow under the shoulders, allowing the head to fall back, which actually places the larynx forward and out of alignment. The neck is flexed onto the chest with the aid of a pillow before the head is extended so that the face is tilted back. In this position, the oral, pharyngeal and tracheal axes are aligned.

The frequently seen practice of placing one hand on the chin and the other on the back of the head to force the head into severe extension produces a very poor alignment, pushing the larynx into an anterior position. In patients with osteoporosis or rheumatoid arthritis, this technique runs the risk of fracturing the odontoid peg against the body of C1. In very obese patients, it may be necessary to place pillows under the shoulders and neck as well as the head to allow the head to be extended on the neck.

Laryngoscopy technique

- Check to verify effect of induction and paralytic agent.
- Optimise patient position, if needed (see above).
- With suction available at hand, hold the laryngoscope in the left hand and the endotracheal tube (ETT) in the right hand.
- Open the patient's mouth with a right-handed scissor technique.
- Insert the laryngoscope blade on the right side of the mouth and use it to sweep the tongue to the left.
- Advance the blade until landmarks are recognised, usually the tip of the epiglottis or the arytenoid cartilages.

- Lift (do not lever) the laryngoscope in the direction of the handle to lift the tongue and posterial pharyngeal structures out of the line of sight, bringing the glottis into view.
- When the vocal cords or the arytenoid cartilages are clearly seen, advance the tube down the right side of the mouth, keeping the vocal cords in view until the last possible moment, then advance the tube through the vocal cords.
- Insert the tube to 23 cm (at incisors) in men and 21 cm in women, then inflate the cuff.
- Attach the bag ventilator to the tube and verify tube position immediately.
  1. Listen for breath sounds over epigastrium (one breath), then to each hemithorax in the midaxillary line (one breath on each side).
  2. Attach CO_2 detector to tube or use end-tidal CO_2 monitor to verify return of CO_2 with each breath.
  3. Use oesophageal syringe or bulb syringe to verify tube is in noncollapsing trachea (caution: this technique may be falsely negative if tube is in oesophagus and stomach is full of air).
- Secure tube in position and consider requesting chest X-ray to confirm position if appropriate.
- Ensure proper attachment to mechanical ventilator and review ventilator settings.
- Consider ongoing sedation, particularly if induction agent may wear off before paralytic agent.

Gum elastic bougie

Also known as an Eschmann Tracheal Introducer (ETI) (Eschmann Health Care, Kent, UK), the bougie is a straight, semi-rigid stylette-like device with a bent tip that can be used when intubation is (or is predicted to be) difficult – often helpful when the tracheal opening is anterior to the visual field. During laryngoscopy, the bougie is carefully advanced into the larynx and through the cords until the tip enters a mainstem bronchus. While maintaining the laryngoscope and bougie in position, an assistant threads an ETT over the end of the bougie, into the larynx. Once the ETT is in place, the bougie is removed.

Stylet

If you are going to use a stylet, it should be inserted into the ETT and bent to resemble a hockey stick to facilitate intubation of an anteriorly positioned larynx. Even if you do not plan on using a stylet, one should be within easy access in case the intubation proves to be more difficult than anticipated. A pre-curved malleable stylet when placed within an ETT will enable the tube to be curved and thus aid the placement of the tube, especially when the larynx is anteriorly situated. The stylet on no account should be allowed to protrude beyond the tip of the ETT, as this may cause trauma to the larynx.

Lightwand

Lightwands, when inserted into an ETT, may be useful for blind intubations of the trachea (when the laryngeal opening cannot be visualised). The end of the ETT is at the entrance of the trachea when light is well transilluminated through the neck (the jack o'lantern effect). In this situation a distinct glow can be seen below the thyroid cartilage which is not apparent when the light is placed in the oesophagus. The lightwand is usually advanced without the aid of a laryngoscope and once into the trachea the internal stylet that gives the wand its stiffness can be retracted to allow the pliable wand to be advanced into the trachea and used as a guide for the placement of the ETT.

Alternative laryngoscope blades

The standard Macintosh laryngoscope was introduced in 1943. It has a relatively short curved blade designed to rest in the vallecula and lift the epiglottis. Several laryngoscope blades are available, some of which are described below.

Miller

Straight-bladed laryngoscope with a slight curve at the tip. This blade is longer, narrower and smaller at the tip and is designed to trap and lift the epiglottis.

McCoy

The McCoy levering laryngoscope (McCoy, 1993) has a 25-mm hinged blade tip controlled by a spring-loaded lever that is aligned along the handle of the laryngoscope which allows elevation of the epiglottis without the use of excess forces on the pharyngeal tissue.

Bullard

The Bullard laryngoscope is a rigid-bladed indirect fibre-optic laryngoscope with a shape designed to match the airway. The fibre-optic bundle passes along the posterior aspect of the blade and ends 26 mm from the distal tip of the blade, allowing excellent visualisation of the larynx. Intubation can be achieved using an attached intubating stylet with preloaded ETT. Even though this device requires a considerable amount of practice it is particularly useful in those patients with upper airway pathology, limited mouth opening or an immobile or unstable cervical spine. Bullard™ Elite Laryngoscope (Circon, ACMI, Stamford, CT) is the most recent version of the Bullard laryngoscope and is the only indirect fibre-optic laryngoscope which incorporates attachable metal stylets for use and can be utilised with a conventional laryngoscope handle. It also has a working channel for oxygen insufflation, suction, and instillation of local anaesthetics and it is available in both adult and paediatric sizes (newborn infant and child).

Prism

The Huffman prism is an example of a laryngoscope using refraction to aid visualisation of the larynx. It employs a modification of the Macintosh blade whereby a block of transparent plastic in a prism shape is attached to the proximal end of the blade. The ends of the prism are polished to provide optically flat surfaces, the nearest to the eye being cut at 90 degrees to the line of vision and the distal surface at 30 degrees. The net result to the view obtained is a refraction of approximately 30 degrees.

Polio

The polio blade was originally designed to enable patients in an iron lung to be ventilated. In the UK, the polio blade is a 90-degree adaptor located between the handle and the blade of the standard Macintosh laryngoscope. It allows the easier introduction of the blade in situations where the chest gets in the way of the handle.

Laryngeal mask airway

The laryngeal mask airway (LMA) is a useful means of airway control in difficult and failed intubations, invented by Dr Archie Brain at the London Hospital Whitechapel in 1981. Note that the LMA has been shown to be life-saving in cases of failed intubation in obstetric anaesthesia (Gataure & Hughes, 1995). A number of insertion methods have been advocated and in the case of difficulty, it seems wise to use a familiar technique. Since its introduction into clinical practice, the LMA has been used in more than 100 million patients worldwide without fatality. Even though it was originally developed for airway management of routine cases with spontaneous ventilation, in America it is now listed in the ASA Difficult Airway Algorithm in five different places as either an airway (ventilatory device) or a conduit for endotracheal intubation. It can be used in both paediatric and adult patients in whom ventilation with a facemask or intubation is difficult or impossible. Also, it can be used as a 'bridge to extubation' and with pressure support or positive pressure ventilation. There have been several new variants of the LMA including the LMA Classic (standard LMA), LMA Flexible™ (wire reinforced flexible LMA), LMA Unique™ (disposable LMA), LMA Fastrach™ (intubating LMA) and most recently, the LMA Proseal™ (gastric LMA). The Proseal™ was designed with a modified posterior cuff to improve the laryngeal seal and incorporates a second tube to provide a channel for gastric tube placement or passage of regurgitated fluid. It is postulated that the Proseal™ will replace the LMA Classic, as it is designed to provide a better seal, as well as protect the airway against aspiration.

If intubation is difficult and the airway can be secured with a laryngeal mask there are several choices available:

- Use the LMA to oxygenate the patient whilst allowing to wake up. Consider regional anaesthesia or securing the airway by alternative means.
- Use the LMA to maintain anaesthesia. The laryngeal mask can be used for both spontaneous and controlled ventilation. The laryngeal mask is in popular use in gynaecological surgery (such as laparoscopy) and there have been reports of its use in patients normally requiring intubation (such as coronary artery bypass grafting). Although quite widely used in this manner, Sidaras and Hunter concluded in 2001 '...we suggest that the time has not yet come to pass when we can appreciate fully the risks of artificially ventilating a patient through a LMA'.
- Use the LMA to intubate the trachea. In adults a well-lubricated uncut cuffed 6-mm internal diameter ETT can be passed through the lumen of a size 3 or 4 laryngeal mask. The patient needs to be correctly positioned 'sniffing the morning air' and the laryngeal mask needs to be correctly sited with no downfolding of the epiglottis. The patient should be deeply anaesthetised with or without muscle relaxation to prevent coughing or laryngospasm. Rotation of the tube through 90 degrees will prevent the bevel of the tube catching on the bars of the laryngeal mask

aperture, and the tube can then be passed into the trachea. If cricoid pressure has been applied, this tends to be compromised by the presence of the laryngeal mask and should be continued at least until the moment of intubation when it may need to be momentarily released. If difficulty is encountered the position of the head and neck may be altered, firstly by extension of the atlanto-occipital joint and then with varying degrees of flexion of the neck. If an ETT larger than a size 6.0 is required, a gum elastic bougie can be passed through the laryngeal mask into the trachea, the LMA removed, and then the ETT railroaded over the bougie into place.

Blind nasal intubation

Nasal intubation is similar to oral intubation except that the ETT is advanced through the nose into the oropharynx before laryngoscopy. If the patient is awake, local anaesthetic drops and nerve blocks can be used. A lubricated ETT is introduced along the floor of the nose, below the inferior nasal turbinate, perpendicular to the face. Often, a nasopharyngeal airway can be used. The tube is advanced until it can be visualised in the oropharynx. If the tube is not in the midline it will tend to lodge in the pyriform fossa and this usually exhibits as a bulge on the anterior aspect of the neck. If the tube enters the oesophagus, it can often be relocated in the trachea by first withdrawing and then advancing again. This technique requires a great deal of practice and is not recommended for the novice. A topical vasoconstrictor solution (such as xylometazoline spray) should be used to mini-mise the risk of bleeding from the nasal mucosa.

Retrograde intubation

Retrograde intubation is an excellent technique for securing a difficult airway either alone or in conjunction with other alternative airway techniques. The technique is simple, straightforward, and should be a skill of every anaesthesia care provider. It is especially useful in patients with limited neck mobility (cervical spine pathology) or who have suffered airway trauma. Recent advancements in the technique include the introduction of the Arndt Airway Exchange Catheter™ and needle holder to the pre-existing retrograde intubation set. The Arndt catheter will allow patient oxygenation if necessary during the procedure, and is recommended for use with endotracheal tubes of 5.0 mm or larger.

Retrograde intubation involves the passage of a catheter through a cricothyroid incision upwards so as to protrude at the mouth. It is then possible to use the catheter to railroad an ETT into the larynx. The technique may be carried out under local or general anaesthesia but it has complications and is not recommended for the inexperienced. Complications include:

- bleeding
- perforation of the posterior wall of the trachea with the needle
- subcutaneous emphysema of the neck
- pneumothorax
- infection at the puncture site.

Jet ventilation

Transtracheal jet ventilation is a well-accepted method for securing ventilation in rigid and interventional bronchoscopy. It is applied in rigid bronchoscopy with a specially designed jet valve and in fibrescopes in which the jet injector is attached to the suction channel without intervening tubing. It may also be used to prophylactically secure a difficult airway by placing a cricothyrotomy catheter, or an airway exchange catheter into the trachea in order to establish effective ventilation prior to induction of anesthesia.

Flexible fibreoptic bronchoscopic intubation (FBI)

Using a flexible bronchoscope to intubate the trachea. The endotracheal tube is passed directly over the bronchoscope prior to use, and then threaded down the scope and into the trachea.

This technique allows direct visualisation of the airway, with confirmation of the position of the ETT by direct vision. Oxygen may be insufflated through the suction port of the bronchoscope.

Fibreoptic bronchoscopic intubation requires expensive, fragile equipment and special care must be taken during cleaning and storage of the equipment. There is a significant learning curve for FBI, requiring repeated practice in normal patients to allow mastery. There may be difficulty if blood or heavy secretions are present in the upper airway.

The technique is easier to learn and master in elective cases, but can be used to great effect by skilled practitioners in cases of unexpected difficult intubation. Fibreoptic bronchoscopic intubation can be used in awake/sedated patients, asleep/breathing patients and asleep/paralysed patients. A retrograde wire guide may be passed up the suction port of the bronchoscope to guide the scope into the trachea. In young patients, a smaller bronchoscope may be used, or a wire guide may be passed into the trachea from the suction port of the bronchoscope. The scope is withdrawn and repositioned to ensure proper placement of the wire, which is used as a guide for placement of the endotracheal tube either directly or after placement of a catheter to provide a stiffer guide for intubation. Fibreoptic bronchoscopic intubation is also useful for preoperative evaluation and diagnosis of patients with suspected difficult airways.

A dedicated fibreoptic flexible laryngoscope is also available, and used in a similar manner.

Management of the unexpected failed intubation

A suitable failed intubation drill is mandatory. Generally patients do not come to harm because they cannot be intubated; they come to harm because of inadequate oxygenation, inadequate anaesthesia, trauma to the airway and aspiration. Persistent and prolonged attempts at intubation using conventional laryngoscopy cause oedema and bleeding in the airway with progressive difficulty in ventilation. Over-vigorous mask ventilation fills the stomach with gas, leading to an increase in the likelihood of regurgitation, adding further to the problems.

A major problem relating to the use of a failed intubation drill is the timing of the decision as to when it should be implemented. Even though there must be an early acceptance of failure, it is probably reasonable to have three or four attempts at endotracheal intubation using some of the aids or techniques described earlier. The use of unfamiliar equipment such as alternative laryngoscope blades is likely to compound the problem.

Awake intubation is indicated in the following patients: those with congenital airway anomalies; those with trauma to the face, airway or cervical spine; and those with a history of previous difficult intubation. The practical technique of awake intubation is described below. Even though awake intubation is an unpleasant experience for the patient, it provides a number of advantages:
- The airway is preserved.
- There is no loss of muscle tone.
- Consciousness and respiration are unaffected.

Awake intubation technique

Use sedative premedication cautiously and not at all in the presence of severe airway compromise. Anticholinergic premedication may be given to reduce secretions. Prescribe aspiration prophylaxis (such as ranitidine and sodium citrate) preoperatively. Check ALL equipment in the anaesthetic room, attach monitoring and secure intravenous access. Prepare the airway by achieving local anaesthesia. Spray the nasal mucosa with a vasoconstrictor if this is the chosen route. Having loaded the chosen endotracheal tube onto the fibreoptic scope, proceed via the mouth or nose until the larynx is visualised. Pass the tube off the scope into the trachea and check for correct placement.

The equipment and procedures mentioned above are not the sought-after 'get out of jail free' card, and without experience and confidence, are unlikely to render a difficult situation any better. Confidence can only be gained through familiarity with the equipment and technique. Observing an anticipated difficult intubation, prior to undertaking the same under the mentorship of an experienced practitioner, will pay dividends when the unexpected occurs.

REFERENCES

Feldman, S., Harrop-Griffiths, W. & Hirsch, N. (1989). *Problems in Anaesthesia Analysis and Management.* Oxford: Heinemann Medical Books.

Gataure, P. S. & Hughes, J. A. (1995). The laryngeal mask airway in obstetric anaesthesia. *Canadian Journal of Anaesthesia*, **42**, 130–3.

Illingworth, K. A. & Simpson, K. H. (1998). *Anaesthesia and Analgesia in Emergency Medicine*, 2nd edn. Oxford: Oxford University Press.

Mallampati, S. R. (1983). Clinical sign to predict difficult tracheal intubation. *Canadian Anaesthetists' Society Journal*, **30**, 316–17.

McCoy, E. P. & Mirakhur, R. K. (1993). The levering laryngoscope. *Anaesthesia*, **48**, 516–19.

Morgan, E. G. & Mikhail, M. S. (1996). *Clinical Anesthesiology*, 2nd edn. Stamford Connecticut: Appleton & Lange.

Pearce, A. (1998). *Evaluation of the Airway*. London: The Difficult Airway Society.

Rushman, G. B., Davies, N. J. & Cashman, J. N. (1999). *Lee's Synopsis of Anaesthesia*, 12th edn. Oxford: Butterworth Heinemann.

Samsoon, G. I. & Young, J. R. (1987). Difficult tracheal intubations: a retrospective study. *Anaesthesia*, **83**, 1129–35.

Sidaras, G. & Hunter, J. M. (2001). *British Journal of Anaesthesia*, **86**, 749–53.

12

Obstetric anaesthesia

Tom Williams

Key Learning Points

The approach of this chapter is to be 'about' obstetric anaesthesia rather than a commentary on anaesthetic techniques. The intention is to provide the anaesthetic practitioner (AP) with a suitable level of knowledge to support practice by enabling a link to related surgical procedures, patient conditions, altered anatomy and physiology and adjusted biochemistry that creates the potentially hazardous situations unique to this speciality. In tandem with this will be the incorporation of the contribution of the AP and how their role and responsibilities impact upon procedures and outcomes.

- Altered anatomy, physiology and biochemistry
- Related conditions
- Treatment modalities
- Surgical interventions
- Anaesthetic techniques
- Scope of practice

Introduction

Obstetric anaesthesia is now recognised as an anaesthetic sub-speciality and acceptance is confirmed by the establishment in the UK of the Obstetric Anaesthetists Association (OAA). This acceptance as a stand-alone speciality is due in part to the inherent risk factors and potential hazards presented by the obstetric patient combined with the objective to establish a consistent anaesthetic approach to the speciality. Accordingly, the position of the attending anaesthetic practitioner (AP) becomes one of specialist, suitably knowledgeable and armed with an understanding of anaesthetic needs and interventions required in this particular setting.

When discussing obstetric anaesthesia there is an inclination to limit discussion to caesarean section (C/S) or consider it as the benchmark. Nevertheless, related procedures such as evacuation of retained products of conception (ERPC) at the minor end of the scale and placental abruption at the other, warrant equal attention while procedures such as ectopic pregnancy should be included as they are by nature, obstetric orientated, in spite of the latter often being viewed as a general gynaecology emergency. In taking this view then, it could be argued that all obstetric anaesthesia procedures are by definition 'emergencies'.

In conjunction with the anticipated concerns and considerations of anaesthesia generally, obstetric anaesthetists also have to be mindful of an extending catalogue of inherent factors and related conditions, although theoretically being presented with a healthy patient, or in many instances, two patients, the 'two lives' situation, being just one anomaly unique to this speciality. The normal 'pregnant condition' in itself, even in the absence of additional disease states, presents a physical, physiological and biochemical challenge due to the myriad number of bodily changes that

Core Topics in Operating Department Practice: Anaesthesia and Critical Care, eds. Brian Smith, Paul Rawling, Paul Wicker and Chris Jones. Published by Cambridge University Press. © Cambridge University Press 2007.

develop throughout pregnancy and for the most part, accumulate during the third trimester, the most common time for anaesthetic intervention. At full term or during this stage, the cardiovascular changes the anaesthetist has to compensate for, include a 30–40% increase in cardiac output with an accompanying rise in heart rate and stroke volume as well as the potential for supine hypotension and pregnancy-induced hypertension.

Body-size increase is in part due to fluid retention and accompanying oedema but in addition, blood volume rises by up to 50% while the plasma volume increase is not proportional to the increase in red blood cells and so produces haemo-dilution leading to a 'physiological anaemia'. The increase in retained body water can also have a bearing on intubation in the form of pharyngeal and laryngeal oedema, making visualisation and recognition of the intubating landmarks more difficult. Crucial alterations to the respiratory system include a 40% rise in tidal volume and 15% increase in respiratory rate, both compensatory mechanisms intended to meet the increased oxygen demand and elimination of carbon dioxide. Additionally there is a decreased reserve due to a reduced functional residual capacity (FRC). Physical adjustments that have a bearing on respiratory physiology include the ribs becoming lifted and splayed making the mother more reliant on diaphragmatic breathing while upward displacement of the diaphragm by the enlarging uterus can cause the heart to shift anteriorly and to the left (Ciliberto & Marx, 1998). Pain, especially during labour, also has a bearing on pregnancy-adjusted physiology. It can cause hyperventilation leading to maternal hypocarbia and respiratory alkalosis. These have the effect of reducing tissue oxygen transport which is already compromised by the increased oxygen consumption at this stage (Rudra, 2004).

Several of these cardiac and respiratory changes become more pronounced by the naturally nervous state when the mother requires surgical intervention, so besides the physiological implications of this combination, there is a requirement to be alert to the psychological needs of the patient. Comforting, reassurance and the establishment of an environment as conducive to normality as possible is important and the AP can play their part in this as advocate to the patient as feelings of vulnerability can further heighten anxiety, especially during anaesthetic preparation activity.

Additional factors include a temperature increase of approximately 1°C, the possibility of gestational diabetes and the creation of a hyper-coaguable state due to elevated hormone levels. In late pregnancy fibrinogen levels can double that of a non-pregnant woman and the platelet count also rises (Ciliberto & Marx, 1998). Nevertheless, during pregnancy neither clotting nor bleeding times are unduly abnormal and there is a decrease in fibrinolytic activity which actually helps to prevent bleeding during delivery.

Hormonal activity in the form of progesterone is a factor in relation to vomiting and regurgitation as it delays stomach emptying during labour and at term. Incompetence of the oesophageal sphincter during this period is also thought to be due to hormonal influence. This situation is further exacerbated if pethidine is the analgesic of choice (Morgan, 1987). Gastric stasis and fasting, both lower pH causing increased acidity and the need to inhibit hydrochloric acid (H_2SO_4) production by neutralising with antacid therapy, orally or via intramuscular (IM) or intravenous (IV) routes. Ranitidine is a popular H_2 blocker (antacid) used for injection and sodium citrate as an oral measure prior to anaesthetic induction.

Along with nausea and vomiting associated with labour, both anaesthesia and surgery potentiate the situation through various mechanisms. Nausea and vomiting in early pregnancy or first trimester (morning sickness), correctly termed hyperemesis gravidarum is due to different factors. Various methods of anti-emetic therapy are employed during the perioperative phase with a prophylactic regime involving ondansetron, or supplementing a patient controlled analgesia (PCA) regime with a drug such as droperidol. Alternatives include stemetil and metoclopramide, with the latter greatly assisting gastric emptying

(Ciliberto & Marx, 1998). It is worth noting that Yuill & Gwinnutt (2003) consider anti-emetic use in pregnancy controversial because of the risk of teratogenicity, meaning that it may cause malformation of the foetus. In the event of general anaesthesia, these pharmaceutical measures are utilised in conjunction with rapid sequence induction. Overall this has the aim of reducing lung damage should aspiration occur and lead to chemical pneumonitis, also referred to as Mendelson's syndrome and aspiration pneumonitis. A pH of approximately 2.5 is recognised as sufficient to initiate serious lung injury. If gastric contents are aspirated the patient may develop hypoxia, hypotension, bronchospasm and pulmonary oedema, with a mortality rate in the region of 5%. Debate over the volume of aspirate needed to produce such effects continues as it is accepted that leakage of gastric contents on a minor scale occurs generally during anaesthetics but without noticeable effects, however it seems to be agreed that between 25 ml and 50 ml in adults would be sufficient to initiate more serious complications (Wenstone, 2000). Even in situations when vaginal delivery under light analgesia or sedation is in progress, there remains the possibility of complications that may instigate surgical intervention and aspiration remains a consideration as upper airway competence is well maintained under light anaesthesia but lost with mild sedation using barbiturates and benzodiazepines (Rudra, 2004).

In anatomical or physical terms, body-size increase is an obvious change and there are many consequences of this size and shape adjustment. The woman's centre of gravity changes and the development of a spinal 'lordosis' can increase the need for lumbar support, both of paramount importance when the mother is placed in the supine position on the narrow and tilted operating table. According to Owen (2002) hormonal influence softens pelvic cartilage allowing extra bone movement and this heightens the potential for injury and pain especially during placement into the lithotomy position if hip rotation and over

abduction occur. Intubation difficulties can be increased due to shortening and thickening of the neck and breast enlargement may hinder normal laryngoscope insertion, requiring the AP to be familiar with difficult and failed intubation procedure. Faura (2004) considers awake intubation a possibility when difficult intubation is anticipated. Intubation adjuncts differ little from standard except for a variety of laryngoscopes with the Mackintosh 'Polio' blade being popular. Its wide 135-degree angle is of great value when small or inadequate mouth opening combines with short neck and enlarged breasts. During the last few weeks of pregnancy most mothers feel faint while lying on their backs. Carrie *et al.* (2000) state that this is due to compression of the vena cava between the gravid uterus and vertebral column hindering venous return, to such an extent, that compensatory mechanisms and collateral circulation come in to play as the heart is deprived and cannot maintain an adequate output. Renal hypertension due to compression of the renal artery by the gravid uterus is another hazard (Tortora & Grabowski, 2003).

This overview of pregnancy-related changes should be sufficient to give an appreciation of the complication potential that can develop but combine these with the reason(s) for anaesthesia and surgery and the anaesthetic team are presented with a crisis situation equal to any emergency event, irrespective of speciality.

As already suggested most obstetric anaesthetic cases can be classified as emergencies and a significant feature with most is haemorrhage, which can in any setting progress to hypovolaemic shock. The uterus receives approximately 10–15% of maternal cardiac output at term (Brighouse, 2002) clarifying the need to appreciate the hypovolaemic potential. Nevertheless, almost by way of good fortune, the increase in blood volume associated with late pregnancy can go some way to providing protection from the effects of haemorrhage but blood loss combined with additional factors such as prolonged labour, electrolyte imbalance and maternal exhaustion can progress and lead to cardiogenic and distributive shock. Obstetric shock has become a recognised term but treatment regimes are more or less the same as for other forms but with possibly more control on the use of vasopressors as the rise in blood pressure can also bring about a potentially damaging hypertension in this particular setting. Venous return can also be hindered and combined; these actions can have catastrophic effects on the placenta and foetus.

Large blood and fluid replacement due to severe haemorrhage introduces its own complications. Transfusion involving four or more units of blood is not uncommon in many of the related conditions in obstetrics. The term 'massive transfusion' is often used and indicates the replacement of half the circulating volume within 1 hour. The loss of blood in itself leads to heat reduction followed by replacement with cold fluids which compounds this further. This tendency to hypothermia extends clotting times and the transfusion of large blood and fluid volumes can produce a dilutional coagulopathy (Ducloy & de Flandre, 2002). Cold stored blood is more viscous and therefore harder to infuse, has higher levels of free potassium, can instigate metabolic acidosis due to its lowered pH while there are reduced clotting factors and functional platelets. Hypothermia also impairs the release of oxygen from haemoglobin, depresses liver function and so the rate at which drugs are metabolised, renal function slows and insulin production is suppressed leading to higher blood glucose levels. Post-operatively, shivering triggered by hypothermia can lead to an elevation in metabolic rate and an increase in oxygen consumption.

It is not normal practice to cross-match obstetric patients although grouping and saving serum is standard practice in most obstetric units, however, it is usual to have a ready supply of O-negative blood available. Fresh frozen plasma (FFP) and plasma expanders may also be required so consistent core temperature reading is mandatory as major haemorrhage and fluid replacement greatly increase the potential for inadvertent hypothermia (IH) to occur. Therefore patient and fluid-warming

systems in combination with rapid infusion techniques may be required.

According to Carrie *et al.* (2000) haemorrhage is an ever-present risk with parturition and there are a number of conditions and complications of late pregnancy which involve excessive blood loss and so bring about the need for anaesthetic and surgical intervention. This surgical intervention is usually in the form of C/S with the aim of preserving the foetus and controlling haemorrhage.

Placental abruption usually occurs after the 28th week of gestation. In this condition, a portion of the placenta separates from its uterine attachment allowing the escape of maternal blood. Ducloy and de Flandre (2002) state that haemorrhage is often underestimated as occult blood collects in the uterus around the placenta and foetus and can remain concealed within the uterine cavity or track down and escape at the cervix. Causation is usually associated with hypertension and often accompanies pre-eclampsia and pregnancy-induced hypertension.

Placenta previa can occur in the ante- or intra-partum phase. It involves the implantation of the placenta into the lower segment of the uterus at the opening from the uterus into the vagina so preventing vaginal delivery. As the uterus dilates in late pregnancy it causes the placenta to separate by tearing. In the related condition of *placenta percreta*, the placenta grows through the uterus while with *placenta accreta* the placenta invades the myometrium (Harvey, 2004). This is more likely in those who have had previous uterine surgery.

Uterine rupture occurs either during labour or the later weeks of pregnancy, the cause is usually due to separation of a weakened scar after previous uterine surgery (Eldridge, 2000, cited by Harvey, 2005). Delayed delivery following administration of an oxytocic can also be a cause. Treatment will involve either laparotomy for repair and/or combined with C/S if necessary.

Post-partum haemorrhage is described by Chamberlain (1995) as excessive bleeding of more than 500 ml from the genital tract after the birth of the child. It may be immediate or if it occurs between 24 hours and 6 weeks is classified as primary and beyond this period is termed secondary haemorrhage. This can be following placenta previa and abruption or when products are retained in the uterus preventing sufficient retraction to stem bleeding or ineffective uterine contraction.

Further conditions which fit into the description of foetal distress and determine C/S are described below. *Prolapsed (umbilical) cord* involves the downward displacement of the cord before the foetus presents. With *vasa previa* a foetal blood vessel lies over the os and is in danger of rupture and *shoulder dystocia* is failure of the foetal shoulders to traverse the pelvis after delivery of the head. This is more likely to progress to episiotomy and application of external pelvic pressure with the mother in the lithotomy or left lateral position than open surgery. All of the above conditions can threaten the viability of the foetus and lead to C/S. In fact anything that interferes with foetal oxygenation will cause foetal distress (Chamberlain, 1995). Approximately 30% of *breech* births also result in emergency C/S (Dobson, 2004).

Even though obstetric anaesthesia is specialised and to some extent standardised in procedure, it does not conform or adhere to a universal model or algorithm but in general will involve the avoidance of drugs and agents that cross the placental barrier, depress foetal vital signs, cause myocardial or respiratory depression and initiate untimely uterine contractions. Preoperative preparation, whether elective or emergency would have involved establishing an IV line and measures to control and neutralise gastric acid with oral antacids given as close to theatre time as possible. Fasting would only be an issue in the case of an elective procedure. Premedication is not standard or indeed desirable, especially narcotics and drugs used for sedation due to the depressant effect on the foetus (Carrie *et al.*, 2000). Nevertheless, pethidine remains standard with midwives and delivery room staff during expected normal birth

and this must be kept in mind if such a scenario converts to one requiring anaesthesia and surgery.

The potential for aortocaval compression in patients at this stage determines that they should never be allowed to lay flat. During transfer to theatre this may require the mother to assume the left lateral position and once on the operating table should be positioned supine with a 15-degree left-sided tilt (Nelson, 1999). This may involve the use of a wedge or actual lateral rotation of the table itself (Harvey, 2004).

In order to maintain adequate oxygen saturation levels, pre-oxygenation is mandatory. Besides the immediate benefits to mother and baby it provides an oxygen reserve which may be required during intubation. There is no definitive duration for pre-oxygenation but to be fully effective it should be a minimum of 3 minutes. This is thought to be sufficient time to not only saturate the red cells but provide extra reserves by displacing a degree of pulmonary nitrogen and being taken up by the plasma.

The potential for vomiting and regurgitation has already been referred to and therefore employment of a rapid sequence induction is mandatory. Following pre-oxygenation and ongoing explanation to the patient, the anaesthetist will begin induction. Carrie *et al.* (2000) state that with the exception of the frequently used muscle relaxants, most drugs used in anaesthesia readily cross the placental barrier in significant quantities. Ryan (2000) states that as regurgitation can start once induction and neuromuscular blocking agents have been given, cricoid pressure (Sellick's manoeuvre), must be applied by the AP who should be suitably trained and familiar with this crucial procedure. If applied correctly, it prevents stomach contents reaching the patient's airway and entails applying pressure with the thumb and first two fingers downward upon the cricoid cartilage (Ryan, 2000). This acts to compress the oesophagus between the trachea and cervical spine, closing off the oesophagus. Classical Sellick's manoeuvre actually involves counter pressure with the assistant's other hand cupped behind the patient's neck.

A number of variations are in common practice, namely using one hand while the other is free to pass intubation equipment which should be prepared and to hand. The pressure should be maintained until the endotracheal tube (ETT) is in place and the cuff inflated and only released upon the instruction of the anaesthetist. Immediate fixation of the ETT is essential in order to prevent inadvertent displacement. Besides the aspiration hazards associated with incorrectly applied cricoid pressure, there is the possibility that it could also hinder visualisation of intubation landmarks. Anaesthesia is kept deliberately light due to the depressant effects on the foetus but a consequence of this is maternal awareness. Therefore any narcotic agents and inhalational supplementation are held back until the foetus is delivered and only then is anaesthesia deepened. It is at this point that the tilted table will need levelling out. Suxamethonium remains the drug of choice for intubation followed by a non-depolarising muscle relaxant as part of the maintenance regime. Nevertheless, suxamethonium is not without undesirable properties. Even though it allows intubation within approximately 30 seconds, there is a period when no spontaneous breathing can take place and any attempt to apply positive ventilation via the facemask could force gases into the stomach and so exacerbate the tendency to regurgitation. It is here that the value of pre-oxygenation may be realised. The longer acting non-depolarising muscle relaxant is given when the effects of the depolarising agent have abated. The muscle fasiculation produced increases intragastric pressure and the paralysis produced increases the potential for regurgitation. In the event of aspiration the AP needs to be familiar with treatment protocols which could involve head-down tilt of the operating table, lateral positioning, suction, ventilation with 100% oxygen followed by drug therapy including bronchodilators, steroids, antibiotics and depending on severity, pulmonary lavage, chest physiotherapy and the possibility of mechanical ventilation combined with positive end expiratory pressure (PEEP) in the most severely affected.

The signs of aspiration may include laryngospasm, bronchospasm, airway obstruction, tachypnoea, tachycardia and a fall in oxygen saturation with the possibility of hypotension and cyanosis (Wenstone, 2000). Signs may be immediate or manifest at a later stage leading to misdiagnosis. If the situation happened during induction for an emergency procedure, the anaesthetist would be responsible for prioritising and synchronising actions between treatment of the aspiration and continuing surgery.

All of the commonly used inhalational agents readily cross the placental barrier and the concentration in the foetal blood quickly approaches the levels in the mother. An additional contraindication is that in general they hinder uterine contraction and so increase the potential for post-partum haemorrhage. Nevertheless, many have been reported to have benefits in labour using sub-anaesthetic concentrations in conjunction with oxygen + nitrous oxide, when they have minimal effect on the foetus and uterine contraction (Rudra, 2004). Respiratory changes during pregnancy enhance anaesthetic uptake as the increase in resting ventilation delivers more agent into the alveoli (Ciliberto, 1998).

Alongside analgesics, anti-emetics and antibiotics, oxytocics are the only other drugs commonly used. Even though they are not anaesthetic related, they are standard in the obstetric anaesthetist's pharmacology armamentarium. They are administered via a single shot, intended to bring about uterine contraction as the foetus is being delivered, or as an infusion if the surgeon indicates that the uterus is flaccid and lacking tone.

Oxytocics are also referred to as uterotonics. There are three in common use: syntocinon, ergometrine and syntometrine, which is a combined preparation of the other two. They have the action of contracting the myometrium, although in differing manners and for varying durations. This action can actually compromise placental blood flow and lead to foetal hypoxia. Ergometrine especially has the additional unwanted side effects of causing nausea and vomiting and can induce a general vasoconstriction leading to a rise in blood pressure, an effect unwanted if the mother is already hypertensive.

Interestingly, according to Ciliberto and Marx (1998) the auto transfusion of blood from the contracting uterus reduces the impact of maternal blood loss at birth.

Besides the high profile C/S and emergencies involving severe blood loss, there are a number of procedures common to obstetric anaesthesia which are viewed as less serious, however many of the inherent risks are still present.

Forceps delivery and *vacuum extraction*, or *vontouse*, usually take the form of a trial and if unsuccessful, progresses to C/S and so accordingly involve an anaesthetic pre-planned with this in mind. Nevertheless, as some form of analgesia is usual for these procedures, pudendal block, caudal or epidural should be anticipated. Although *ectopic* pregnancy is increasingly preceded by laparoscopic investigation, the anaesthetic approach will be as for an emergency utilising rapid sequence induction and being prepared for major haemorrhage and shock. ERPC involves post-partum bleeding because of debris, which prevents effective retraction of the uterus. General anaesthesia is the norm for these patients, with time since delivery and eating determining technique.

The potential for embolism, particularly thromboembolism, is ever present with any speciality, indeed with any patient undergoing a lengthy hospital stay but there are increased factors with obstetric patients, especially those requiring surgery. Amniotic embolism is unique to the obstetric situation and occurs usually during or just after delivery when amniotic fluid gains access to the circulation, possibly due to placental abruption, leading to shock and obstruction of pulmonary blood flow and triggering an anaphylactoid response. Effects are devastating, immediate and usually fatal, not least because of the unfamiliar and uncommon nature of the condition in delivery suites. Immediate signs would include hypocarbia, hypoxia and hypotension. Thrombo prophylactic

measures to prevent deep venous thrombosis (DVT), which is a precursor to pulmonary embolism, tend to centre on physical measures such as thrombo-embolism deterrent (TED) stockings or flowtron devices intended to maintain venous blood flow by external massaging.

Monitoring for obstetric anaesthesia differs little if at all from standard anaesthetic monitoring and adheres to the recommendations of the Association of Anaesthetists of Great Britain and Ireland (AAGBI, 2000) and OAA. The AAGBI regard it as essential that core standards of monitoring apply whenever a patient is anaesthetised, irrespective of duration or location. Whether involving general anaesthetic or regional analgesia, minimum monitoring will include, pulse oximetry, non-invasive blood pressure and electrocardiography, with the addition of inspired oxygen and end-tidal carbon dioxide monitoring in the case of general anaesthesia. Despite the view that nothing replaces personal vigilance, there is substantial evidence that monitoring reduces risks of incidents. The Australian Incident Monitoring Study (1993) reported that 52% of incidents were detected first by a monitor with the pulse oximeter and capnograph being predominant in this detection. Even though they are not standard, methods of monitoring potential awareness, as with all branches of anaesthesia, are finding their way into the speciality.

Eclampsia is an associated condition, although not necessarily anaesthesia related and can involve the anaesthetic team antenatally. The condition may occur before, during or shortly after delivery (Chamberlain, 1995) and is characterised by convulsions which may develop if pre-eclampsia is left untreated. Actual causation is unknown but insufficient blood flow to the uterus is suspected. Placental abruption often accompanies the condition. It is during the pre-eclamptic stage at which the anaesthetist and AP might become involved when the patient will require intensive care management prior to possible delivery of the foetus by C/S. If pre-eclampsia progresses it may become necessary to sedate the patient and introduce positive pressure ventilation along with invasive blood pressure and central venous pressure monitoring. Pre-eclampsia usually occurs after the 20th week of gestation and involves hypertension, proteinuria, oedema and oliguria and is classified as mild, moderate or severe (Torr & James, 1998). Depending on the degree of effect, the patient may also suffer cerebral irritability, visual disturbance, pulmonary oedema and hypoxia. Management will involve reducing the blood pressure, controlling the convulsions, correcting the fluid balance and any coagulation abnormalities. Hydralazine is commonly used to treat the hypotension and magnesium sulphate is regularly the drug of choice in the treatment of convulsions and works by producing cerebral vasodilatation. Sedation is essential and benzodiazepines are often considered but due to the possible detrimental effects on the maternal airway and foetus, must be used with care and in conjunction with suitable monitoring. Pethidine is also contraindicated as the metabolites produced during its breakdown can actually cause convulsions (Rudra, 2004). Fruesemide remains the standard diuretic in the treatment of the oedema. Convulsions can be triggered by noise, bright lights and activity that can invoke anxiety so if the patient does have to be taken to theatre the AP will be a prime mover in controlling anything that may have a detrimental effect, i.e. bright theatre lighting, increased staff activity and any accompanying noise normally generated when setting up theatre.

The value of regional analgesia is well established (within obstetric anaesthesia), especially epidural and spinal techniques. The regular use of the former became popular as an epidural service on delivery suites providing a pain-free, awake birth. If vaginal birth became difficult and proceeded to forceps or C/S, the facility for analgesia was already in place, avoiding the need for general anaesthesia with all its inherent problems of airway and aspiration management. The indwelling epidural catheter could be used to supplement necessary analgesia for surgery and post-operative pain management. The realisation

of the benefits of regional analgesia then led to the spinal approach becoming popular for both elective and emergency C/S. The single-shot technique however can be unsuitable should surgery duration outlast analgesic effect, while the need for post-operative pain control has to be provided by additional means. Almost as a natural next step, the combined spinal/epidural (CSE) or combined spinal/epidural analgesia (CSEA) has gained popularity as it provides the rapid on-set of spinal combined with the longer-term facility of epidural while being somewhat more selective with sensory and motor blockade. The technique can be performed through one lumbar interspace by firstly inserting a Tuohy needle into the extradural space then using it as a guide for introducing the smaller gauge spinal needle into the subarachnoid space, referred to as needle-through-needle technique (Carrie *et al.*, 2000). Following injection of analgesic solution and needle withdrawal, a catheter is introduced into the epidural space. The alternative technique involves inserting the needles through separate lumbar spaces. Epidural needles are usually in the range of 16–18 G and spinal needles are much finer, e.g. 26–27 G. This finer gauge and specialised low trauma tips reduce leakage of cerebrospinal fluid (CSF) and in turn post-dural puncture headache (PDPH). Whitacre and Sprotte are the two main needle designs at present.

Both techniques have many plus factors for mother, baby and anaesthetist although in spite of the benefits, there are potential drawbacks. Local analgesic solution toxicity is a continuing danger with epidural as repeated doses via the catheter can lead to accumulation, especially when being used for surgery and continuing post-operative pain relief. Hypotension due to sympathetic blockade is common to both techniques, although there is a much more rapid onset with the spinal route which is a particular danger in obstetrics as beside a primary hazard to the mother, placental perfusion is compromised and can lead to foetal distress (Chamberlain, 1995). Measures to offset this possibility include pre-loading with IV fluids and/or vasopressor drugs such as ephedrine, which can be prepared as an IV infusion, stand-by syringe containing 50 mg in 10 ml, or is sometimes given prophylactically preoperatively via intramuscular injection (Oyston, 2000).

As the subarachnoid space contains CSF and the extradural space is a fluid-free potential space, the properties of the drugs for each differ. To prevent spinal drugs from the natural tendency of rising within the CSF, they have a higher specific gravity. This is created by presenting the drug in dextrose, making it 'heavy', as with heavy marcaine which is 0.5% bupivacaine in 8% dextrose. As the epidural space is fluid-free, 'normal' drug solutions are used. Lignocaine and marcaine of varying strengths and percentages have been popular as well as those containing a vasoconstrictor such as adrenaline. The intention is to obtain adequate sensory nerve analgesia combined with sufficient motor block-ade. More recently ropivacaine and levobupiva-caine have gained popularity. Both are said to be longer acting and particularly with the latter, have reduced motor blockade and toxicity effects (Arias, 2002). The actual drug volume requirement is less with spinal than epidural thus reducing the potential for toxic overdose. Local analgesic can be administered in lower concentrations when used in combination with preservative-free opioids such as fentanyl, sufentanil, morphine as well as pethidine and diamorphine to provide effective, synergistic analgesia while also reducing motor blockade. Nevertheless, they still carry the danger of respiratory depression, nausea and vomiting and urine retention. Both techniques create the desired density of block but attention to spread is also important and an area from nipple to perineum is desirable especially to block peritoneal pain during surgery. The block produced is adequate for surgery and any required sedation is commonly provided by an oxygen 50% and nitrous oxide 50% mix. Continuous spinal using an indwelling catheter has not proven popular, mainly due to the difficulties surrounding threading of a 30 G catheter through a 26 G needle and consequent resistance to injection and flow. Pudendal block is the only other commonly found regional technique and is used for episiotomy but may not provide adequate analgesia for forceps delivery or procedures that involve extensive manipulation (Rudra, 2004).

Opinion and debate continue over patient positioning when performing epidural and spinal, especially for C/S, either lateral or sitting position with legs over the edge of trolley, bed or operating table. Additionally, left or right lateral also insti-gates discussion, initially with regard to unilateral block, however, there are proponents of both left and right lateral. The thinking of the former relates to vena-caval occlusion and the fact that the patient will be in left tilt during surgery is used to support the latter view.

Two uncommon problems associated with regional techniques that the AP should be familiar with are total spinal and blood patch for dural puncture. Total spinal happens when local analge-sic solution spread is too advanced and affects cranial nerves, leading to paralysis of respiratory muscles, loss of consciousness, hypotension and bradycardia. It is more likely to happen during epidural when the needle may inadvertently pierce the dura mater and the large volume of analgesic solution is injected into the subarachnoid space (Carrie *et al.*, 2000). Blood patch is carried out for the relief of post-spinal headache and is an attempt to plug the dural leak with 10–20 ml of the patient's venous blood injected into the extradural space (Smith & Williams, 2004).

There is no one dominant or recognised pain-care regime common to obstetric anaesthesia. Regional analgesia by nature can provide its own pain relief and there is a growing use of PCEA (patient controlled epidural analgesia). The obvious discom-fort and distress of pain to the mother can cause hyperventilation which may lead to maternal hypercarbia, respiratory alkalosis and metabolic acidosis. Consider the already compromised oxygen consumption associated with labour and the need for effective analgesia becomes apparent. Therefore pain control can involve a pre-, inter- and post-operative role for the anaesthetist.

Even though pethidine is not popular with anaesthetists, it persists in the normal delivery setting whereas fentanyl is commonly the drug of choice during surgery although many alternatives, including nubaine and tramadol are not uncommon. Postoperatively, morphine maintains a place whether administered in the traditional intravenous and intramuscular routes or via a titrated PCA system.

It is clear that the obstetric AP has a role within both outlying areas as well as theatres, however, there also exists a diverse level of input by APs throughout different centres. In some it is simply the on-call or stand-by member who attends in the event of an obstetric anaesthetic, whereas in others they have a permanent involvement and profile within the obstetric unit.

The author has worked in many centres in a number of national and international locations and is aware of differing practices so has therefore attempted to limit naming specific drugs, equipment and making reference to particular routines as this can be misleading. The intention has been to present the information in this chapter from the viewpoint, level and need of the post-registration AP. While having to interpret and incorporate this knowledge into their own clinical role, APs must also maintain awareness of personal limitations and be continually mindful of their professional codes, standards and scope of practice (Health Professions Council, 2003).

REFERENCES

Arias, M. G. (2002). Levobupivacaine. A long acting local anaesthesia, with less cardiac and neurotoxicity. *Update in Anaesthesia* (Online) **14**(17). Available at http://www.nda.ox.ac.uk/wfa/html/u14/u1407.0.1htm (Accessed 3 May 2005).

Association of Anaesthetists of Great Britain and Ireland. (2000). Recommendations for *Standards of Monitoring During Anaesthesia and Recovery* (Online). Available at: http//www.aagbi.org/pdf (Accessed 14 April 2005).

Brighouse, D. (2002). Obstetric emergencies. *Anaesthesia and Intensive Care Medicine*, **3**(2), 48–54.

Carrie, L. E. S., Simpson, P. J. & Popat, M. T. (2000). *Understanding Anaesthesia*, 3rd edn. Oxford: Butterworth Heinemann.

Chamberlain, G. V. P. (1995). *Obstetrics by Ten Teachers*, 16th edn. London: Arnold.

Ciliberto, C. F. & Marx, G. F. (1998). *Physiological Changes Associated with Pregnancy*. Available at: www.nda.ox.ac.uk/wfsa/html/uO9003.htm (Accessed 9 March 2005).

Dobson, A. (2004). A critical analysis of caesarean section procedure. *Journal of Operating Department Practice*, **1**(8), 16.

Ducloy, A. & de Flandre, M. J. (2002). Obstetric Anaesthesia – Placental Abruption. *Update in Anaesthesia* (Online), **14**(17). Available at: http://www.nda.ox.ac.uk/wfsa/html (Accessed 5 April 2005).

Faura, E. A. M. (2004). *Anaesthesia for the Pregnant Patient*. Available at: www.daccx.bsd.uchicago.edu/manuals/obstetric/obstetricanaesthesia.html (Accessed 30 March 2005).

Harvey, P. (2005). The role of the ODP in obstetric haemorrhage. *Journal of Operating Department Practice*, **1**(11), 18.

Health Professions Council. (2003). *Standards of Conduct, Performance and Ethics* (Online). Available at: www.hpc.uk.org (Accessed 16 May 2005).

Morgan, B. M. (1987). *Foundations of Obstetric Anaesthesia & Analgesia*. London: Bailliére Tindall.

Nelson, G. L. (1999). Fundamentals of pain relief. In A. Davey & C. S. Ince, eds., *Fundamentals of Operating Department Practice*. London: Greenwich Medical Media Ltd, pp. 245–57.

Oyston, J. (2000). A Guide to Spinal Anaesthesia for Caesarean Section. *Virtual Anaesthesia Textbook* (Online). Available at: http://www.virtual-anaesthesia-textbook.com (Accessed 29 April 2005).

Owen, P. (2002). *Pelvic Arthropathy During Pregnancy*. Available at: www.Netdoctor.co.uk/diseases/facts/pelvicarthropathy.htm (Accessed 26 March 2005).

Rudra, A. (2004). Pain Relief in Labour. *Update in Anaesthesia* (Online), **18**(3). Available at: http://www.nda.ox.ac.uk/wfsa/html (Accessed 9 March 2005).

Ryan, T. (2000). Fundamentals of obstetric and emergency anaesthesia. In *Fundamentals of Operating Department Practice*. London: Greenwich Medical Media.

Simpson, P. & Popat, M. (2001). *Understanding Anaesthesia*, 4th edn. Oxford: Butterworth Heinemann

Smith, B. & Williams, T. (2004). *Operating Department Practice A–Z*. London: Greenwich Medical Media.

Torr, G. J. & James, M. F. M. (1998). The role of the anaesthetist in the management of pre eclampsia. *Update in Anaesthesia* (Online). Issue 9 (4). Available at: http://www.nda.ox.ac.uk/wfsa/html/uO9/uO9/_012.htm (Accessed 19 April 2005).

Tortora, G. J. & Grabowski, S. R. (2003). *Principles of Anatomy & Physiology*. New York: John Wiley & Sons.

Yuill, G. & Gwinnutt, C. (2003). *Postoperative Nausea and Vomiting*. (Online) Issue 17, article 2. Available at: www.nda.ox.ac.uk/wfsa/html (Accessed 21 March 2005).

Wenstone, R. (2000). *Identification and Management of Anaesthetic Emergencies. Fundamentals of Operating Department Practice*. London: Greenwich Medical Media.

USEFUL RESOURCES

Association of Operating Department Practitioners
www.aodp.org

GASNET:
http://gasnet.med.yale.edu/gta/
Health Professions Council
www.hpc-uk.org
Medline/Patient UK
www.patient.co.uk
Association for Perioperative Practice
www.afpp.org.uk
National Electronic Library for Health
www.nelh.uk
Nursing & Midwifery Council
www.nmc-uk.org
Obstetric Anaesthesia & Analgesia. Available at: www.themediweb.net/obstetrics/Anaes%20Considerations.htm
Obstetric Anaesthetic Association
www.oaa-anaes.ac.uk
Royal College of Anaesthetists
www.rcoa.ac.uk
Royal College of Nurses
www.rcn.org.uk

13

Understanding blood gases

Helen McNeill

Key Learning Points

- Understand the sampling methods for arterial blood gases
- Understand and interpret arterial blood gas results. This will include:
  - Oxygen transport in the body
  - Mechanisms of normal acid-base balance
  - Disturbances of acid-base balance
  - Step-by-step guide to arterial blood gas analysis
  - Clinical scenarios

Introduction

Arterial blood gas (ABG) analysis is now common-place in perioperative and acute-care settings and is used to aid diagnosis and to monitor the progress of the patient and the response to any interventions. It is essential that staff working in the perioperative environment understand the key principles of ABG analysis so that results can be dealt with quickly and appropriately, thereby improving the safe management of the patient.

Arterial blood gas analysis is often central to the management of the patient who is either already critically ill or is at risk of deterioration in their condition (Simpson, 2004). Many patients cared for within the perioperative environment will fall into one of these two categories and this makes ABGs one of the most common tests performed in theatres. Jevon and Ewens (2002) also suggest

indications for ABG analysis may include respiratory compromise, evaluation of interventions such as oxygen therapy and respiratory support, as a preoperative baseline and following a cardiorespiratory arrest.

It is imperative to note at the start of this chapter that, just as with any investigation, ABGs must always be interpreted in conjunction with other clinical information about the patient (Adam & Osborne, 1997). A thorough clinical examination and assessment of a patient will present many clues about the physiological status of that individual – ABG analysis just adds another piece to that jigsaw. Additionally, what may be an adequate set of results for one person may be entirely unacceptable for another, depending on their current diagnosis and any pre-existing illnesses.

Table 13.1 shows the basic parameters measured by blood gas analysers and their normal values. To help you understand and interpret these values, this chapter will cover some of the fundamentals of the physiology of acid-base balance, alveolar ventilation and oxygenation. Once you are aware of the related physiology, the interpretation of ABG results will be much easier as you will be able to think more clearly about what could be happening to your patient. This chapter also contains a section on the collection and handling of ABG samples.

It is worth remembering that, as with any skill, to become really good at ABG analysis you must

Core Topics in Operating Department Practice: Anaesthesia and Critical Care, eds. Brian Smith, Paul Rawling, Paul Wicker and Chris Jones. Published by Cambridge University Press. © Cambridge University Press 2007.

Table 13.1 Normal values for arterial blood gases

Parameter	Normal values
pH	7.35–7.45
PaO_2	11–13 kPa (80–100 mmHg)
$PaCO_2$	4.5–6 kPa (35–45 mmHg)
Standard bicarbonate	22–26 mmol/l
Base excess/base deficit	−2 to +2 mmol/l
SaO_2	93–98%

practise! There are some examples at the end of the chapter to get you started, but there is nothing like learning in the real world – so, look at real patients with real ABG results and *apply* what you learn in this chapter to genuine clinical situations. Only then will your learning become embedded and ABG analysis become second nature.

Sampling arterial blood gases

It is important to collect and handle the ABG sample carefully in order to reduce the possibility of inaccurate readings. The relevant local policies and health and safety precautions relating to blood sampling must, of course, be adhered to reduce the risk of needle stick injuries.

There are three possible ways of obtaining an ABG sample:
1. From an indwelling arterial catheter.
2. From an arterial puncture (stab), usually from the radial or femoral artery.
3. Capillary sample from the earlobe.

In the perioperative setting it is likely that most samples will be taken from an indwelling arterial catheter. Such arterial lines are not without risk to the patient and are only appropriate for use in areas where the patients are closely monitored and observed (Woodrow, 2004). It is good practice to ensure that arterial catheters are clearly identified and labelled so they are not mistaken for a venous cannula.

Garretson (2005) suggests that there are three major causes of complications in indwelling arterial catheters: haemorrhage, thrombosis and infection. Accidental removal or disconnection of the catheter are the most common causes of haemorrhage and could lead to significant blood loss if they were to go unnoticed. Vigilance is paramount in prevention of this problem and the catheter should be well secured and the insertion site and transducer line kept visible and directly observed whenever possible.

Thrombosis is rare, but if a clot were to form in the lumen of the catheter this could be flushed into the arterial circulation and compromise the blood flow distal to the catheter site (Garretson, 2005). Correct maintenance of the pressure transducer system will ensure a continuous flush of saline (usually around 3 ml/hour) to help maintain patency of the catheter. The colour, temperature and sensation of the limb should be observed to assess for any signs of compromised circulation. Blanching or discolouration should be reported immediately to medical staff (Moore, 2000).

As with any invasive line, there is a risk of infection with an indwelling arterial catheter if strict hand washing and asepsis are not observed during both insertion and sampling (Moore, 2000). It is also important that the lines and sample ports are kept free from blood and other debris. Signs of infection include localised redness, warmth and discharge at the insertion site and the patient may develop a pyrexia (Garretson, 2005).

Arterial puncture or 'stab' from the radial or femoral arteries is usually the method of choice for sampling if there is no indwelling arterial cannula. Complications can include spasm of the artery, clot formation within the lumen of the blood vessel, haematoma formation and bruising (Williams, 1998). These can potentially compromise blood flow distal to the puncture site; consequently the radial artery is the optimal site as patients usually have a good collateral blood supply via the ulnar artery.

Prior to a radial arterial stab or cannulation, a simple Allen's test can be performed to determine the adequacy of collateral circulation to the hand via the ulnar artery (Moore, 2000).

The Allen's test can be performed by following these steps:

1. Occlude both the ulnar and radial arteries to the hand.
2. Ask the patient to clench their fist several times until their hand goes pale.
3. Release the pressure on the ulnar artery and observe colour of the hand.

If the ulnar artery has a good blood flow the hand should return to the normal colour within 5–7 seconds. Any delay indicates poor ulnar circulation and an alternative site should be used (Moore, 2000).

Arterial puncture can be painful for the patient. Crawford (2004) found that 49% of patients reported a pain score of 5 or more on a visual analogue pain scale of 0–10. Williams (1998) recommends the use of local anaesthesia prior to the puncture. Arterial puncture sites take longer to stop bleeding than venous ones so it is recommended that pressure is applied for at least 5 minutes to reduce the risk of bruising and haematoma formation (Williams, 1998; Crawford, 2004; Woodrow, 2004). Patients with prolonged clotting may need longer than 5 minutes and must be assessed individually.

Capillary samples from the earlobe may be used occasionally, particularly in patients requiring multiple samples who do not have an indwelling arterial cannula. Woodrow (2004) suggests that the difference between the arterial and ear lobe capillary sample is not clinically significant, however, Williams (1998) argues that whilst the $PaCO_2$ does not vary significantly the accuracy of the PaO_2 reading is dependent on good sampling technique from a warmed, vasodilated earlobe.

A heparinised syringe must be used so that the blood does not clot in the tubing of the blood gas analyser and there are many commercially prepared blood gas syringes available that are pre-heparinised. To prevent the exchange of carbon dioxide and oxygen between air and the blood sample all bubbles must be expelled and the syringe sealed with an airtight stopper. As the constituents of blood continue to remain metabolically active for some time after the sample is drawn it is advisable to analyse the blood as soon as possible to ensure accuracy. Many operating departments will have rapid access to an analyser but if the sample needs transporting to a laboratory it should be cooled quickly (Williams, 1998). Cooling the sample has the effect of slowing the metabolism of the blood cells and will prolong the time available for analysis to about 1 hour (Woodrow, 2004). It is common practice to place the syringe into ice to cool the sample but Woodrow (2004) suggests there is anecdotal evidence that this may cause haemolysis and so recommends that iced water is used as long as it does not cause undue delays in transporting the sample.

As the course of treatment a patient receives is often based on the ABG results, it is imperative that all possible measures are taken to optimise the accuracy of the readings. Many modern blood gas analysers automatically calibrate themselves at predetermined intervals and require little in the way of maintenance (Williams, 1998). It is, however, essential that practitioners liaise closely with their hospital laboratory services to ensure that the manufacturer's guidelines and local Trust policies for quality control and health and safety are adhered to.

What can ABGs tell you?

Arterial blood gases will provide a set of values that can be used to determine key aspects of the patient's condition. These values can be broadly categorised into:

1. oxygenation status
2. adequacy of alveolar ventilation
3. acid-base balance.

The oxygenation status of the patient can be determined by looking at the partial pressure of oxygen in arterial blood (PaO_2). Additionally, many machines will also provide a reading of the arterial oxygen saturation (SaO_2) and haemoglobin (Hb) if they have the addition of a co-oximeter.

The adequacy of alveolar ventilation is reflected by the partial pressure of the arterial carbon dioxide level ($PaCO_2$) and provides invaluable information about respiratory function. Examination of the acid-base status will provide useful information about both the respiratory and metabolic components of acid-base balance. Each of these three categories will now be discussed in more detail.

Oxygenation

Often, one of the primary reasons for ABG analysis is to ascertain the oxygenation status of the patient. The body has no means of storing oxygen and so cells are dependent on a continuous supply that meets their metabolic needs. If the supply of oxygen does not meet demand then tissue hypoxia will develop and the vastly inefficient process of anaerobic metabolism will commence, with the resultant production of lactic acid (Fitz-Henry & Lewis, 2001).

There are two sites within the body where oxygen transfer occurs: at the lungs from the alveoli to the haemoglobin in red blood cells, and at tissue level from the haemoglobin to the mitochondria in the tissue cells (Moore, 2000). A significant factor in oxygen transfer is the natural affinity of haemoglobin for oxygen. This relates to how easily oxygen will bind to haemoglobin in the lungs and how readily it will be released to the tissues. Successful oxygen transfer is, of course, also entirely dependent on adequate respiratory and cardiovascular function.

The diffusion of oxygen relies upon the passive movement of oxygen down a partial pressure gradient (i.e. concentration gradient), which allows oxygen molecules to cross the tissue barriers (Leach & Treacher, 1998). As the concentration of oxygen found in the alveoli (P_AO_2) is higher than that of the deoxygenated blood in the pulmonary capillaries, oxygen will diffuse across the alveolar-capillary membrane. This is known as the A-a gradient. Similarly, at tissue level, the concentration of oxygen in arterial blood (PaO_2) is greater than that of the tissue cells, therefore, oxygen will diffuse

from the capillaries into the tissues. The A-a gradient can be manipulated by the administration of oxygen therapy as increasing the P_AO_2 can improve the PaO_2 and SaO_2 and oxygen delivery to the tissues (Treacher & Leach, 1998).

The alveolar-capillary oxygen gradient indicates that the inspired oxygen level must always be higher than the arterial oxygen level. In a healthy subject, the difference between the two is about 10 kPa. This is because at sea level, 1% O_2 is approximately the same as 1 kPa, therefore, a patient breathing room air (21% O_2) should have a PaO_2 of greater than 11 kPa (Resuscitation Council, 2004). This 'rule of 10' provides a useful estimate of what you could expect your patient's PaO_2 to be (Simpson, 2004). Consequently, if you have a patient who is on 40% oxygen you would expect their PaO_2 to be approximately 30 kPa. If the difference between the inspired oxygen and the PaO_2 is greater than 10 this is suggestive of pulmonary disease causing a mismatch between the ventilation of the alveoli and the perfusion of the pulmonary capillaries.

As mentioned at the beginning of this chapter, many blood gas analysers will provide the SaO_2 expressed as a percentage. In terms of oxygenation, it is crucial to remember that saturation measurements do not take into account the haemoglobin level of the patient (Woodrow, 2004). For example, one of your patients could have an Hb of 6 g/dl and another an Hb of 12 g/dl. It is clear that the patient with an Hb of 12 g/dl will have a much greater total oxygen content of the blood than the patient with an Hb of 6 g/dl, even if their SaO_2 was exactly the same.

The oxygen-haemoglobin dissociation curve

The relationship between PaO_2 and SaO_2 is complex and is reflected by the S-shaped oxygen-haemoglobin dissociation curve, illustrated in Figure 13.1.

If you observe the curve in Figure 13.1 it can be seen that one of the most distinctive features is the S-shape, with a steep slope followed by a flattened

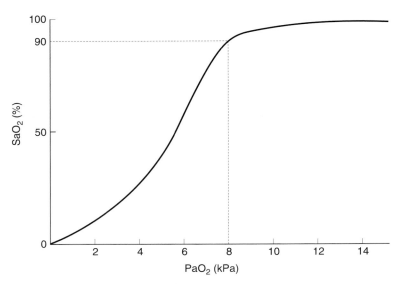

Figure 13.1 Oxygen–haemoglobin dissociation curve.

area at the top. It is useful to note that a PaO_2 of 8 kPa correlates with an SaO_2 of approximately 90% indicating adequate oxygen-carrying capacity if the Hb is normal (Williams, 1998). Additionally, the curve demonstrates why SaO_2 monitoring will not indicate if you are giving your patient too much oxygen, as the PaO_2 will continue to rise even when maximum SaO_2 has been reached.

The S-shape of the curve has other important clinical implications. The oxygen-haemoglobin dissociation curve indicates that, at the upper plateau of the curve, the SaO_2 can be maintained at an acceptable level even in the face of significant alterations in the PaO_2. The area of the curve reflected by the steep slope demonstrates that, beyond a certain point, the PaO_2 will fall precipitously along with the SaO_2. This explains the common scenario whereby a patient apparently 'suddenly' drops their SaO_2. In fact, the change in the patient's condition is often not sudden at all as a gradual fall in PaO_2 is masked until the curve reaches the steep area of the slope, at which point the patient will appear to suddenly deteriorate. Even though monitoring SaO_2 is an invaluable

tool in managing acutely ill patients it is clear that, for the above reasons, it is not a replacement for a complete ABG analysis when assessing oxygenation.

Another clinically significant feature of the oxygen-haemoglobin dissociation curve is that it can shift to the left or the right under certain conditions, reflecting alterations in how readily haemoglobin will bind to or dissociate from oxygen. This has implications for acutely ill patients whose cellular oxygenation may already be critically impaired. When the normal curve is plotted it is assumed that several physiological parameters are within the normal range. These parameters include, amongst other things, the patient's temperature, the pH and the $PaCO_2$ (Moore, 2000). Nevertheless, if these conditions alter, as they frequently do in acute illness, the curve will shift resulting in a change to the affinity of haemoglobin for oxygen.

- **Left shifts of the curve** – alkalosis, a low $PaCO_2$, and hypothermia cause a left shift of the curve resulting in an increased affinity of haemoglobin for oxygen. Oxygen will, therefore, easily bind to haemoglobin in the lungs but because the haemoglobin will not readily unload the oxygen at the tissues, cellular hypoxia may occur despite an adequate PaO_2.

• **Right shifts of the curve** – acidosis, a high $PaCO_2$, and pyrexia cause a right shift of the curve resulting in a decreased affinity of haemoglobin for oxygen. This means that the haemoglobin will readily release oxygen to the tissues but, because of the reduced ability of oxygen to bind to haemoglobin at the lungs, patients may need supplementary oxygen therapy to increase the alveolar-arterial oxygen gradient and maintain an adequate PaO_2 and SaO_2.

Alveolar ventilation

One of the key purposes of ABG analysis is to assess respiratory function and the $PaCO_2$ reading provides invaluable information on this aspect of the patient's condition. Carbon dioxide diffuses across the alveolar-capillary membrane more readily than oxygen and, consequently, changes in alveolar ventilation are promptly reflected by corresponding changes in the $PaCO_2$ (Williams, 1998).

Alveolar ventilation is defined as the movement of air into and out of the lungs (Williams, 1998). The total amount of air moved with each breath is known as the tidal volume (V_T) and is normally 600 ml (Treacher & Leach, 1998). V_T is composed of the alveolar volume (V_A) and the dead-space volume (V_D). The alveolar volume is dependent on the rate and depth of breathing and is absolutely crucial to gas exchange. It is normally 450 ml. The dead-space is about 150 ml and occupies the oropharynx and tracheobronchial tree and does not, therefore, participate in gas exchange (Treacher & Leach, 1998). It is important to note that the V_T must be large enough to overcome the V_D and provide sufficient alveolar volume for gas exchange to take place.

Alterations in alveolar ventilation will have a corresponding effect on $PaCO_2$. Hypoventilation will cause a rise in $PaCO_2$ and hyperventilation will cause a fall in $PaCO_2$. For example, a patient who has had opiates post-operatively may become drowsy and have a reduction in alveolar ventilation due to a fall in the V_T and/or respiratory rate. This will mean that the $PaCO_2$ would become elevated. As you will by now appreciate, the expected fall in PaO_2 that would also accompany hypoventilation could easily be masked by the administration of oxygen therapy making ABG analysis crucial in assessing the effectiveness of gas exchange.

$PaCO_2$ levels also have a fundamental role to play in the control of acid-base balance. This will be looked at in more detail in the next section.

Acid-base balance

Normal cellular function is dependent on the pH being held within an extremely narrow range and the human body has a remarkable ability to maintain this through homeostatic mechanisms. Nevertheless, during acute illness in the perioperative period, disturbances of acid-base balance are common. If the pH becomes either too acidic or too alkaline then the enzymes that govern cellular activity will not be able to function correctly. If the body is unable to correct an abnormality of the pH this may eventually lead to such profound disturbance of acid-base balance that the patient could die (Moore, 2000).

Acids

Acids readily dissociate to release free H^+, which are harmful to the body. Strong acids release more H^+ than weak acids.

Alkalis (bases)

Alkalis (also called bases) combine with free H^+ and help to prevent increases in H^+ levels. A strong alkali will more readily bind to H^+ than a weak alkali.

The pH scale is a measure of the concentration of hydrogen ions (H^+) and ranges between 1 (very strong acid) and 14 (very strong alkali), with 7 being the neutral point in the middle of the scale.

• A pH below 7 is *acidic* and indicates an increasing level of hydrogen ions.

- A pH above 7 is *alkaline* and indicates a decreasing level of hydrogen ions.

The body will always strive to maintain the pH within the very narrow range of 7.35–7.45, which, as you can see, is actually very slightly alkaline as it is above 7. In terms of acid-base balance any reading below 7.35 is seen as acidic and any reading above 7.45 is alkalotic, however, for the purposes of ABG analysis 7.4 is often regarded as the central point when determining acidosis or alkalosis.

Regulation of pH

Acid is a by-product of cellular metabolism. If the body does not excrete this waste product it will accumulate and disturb the delicate balance between acids and alkalis (bases). The body has several complex mechanisms that interact with each other to keep the pH within a normal range. The pH is regulated by three main mechanisms: buffer systems, the lungs and the kidneys, with the latter two both having a vital role in the excretion of acids. Even though the control of pH often seems confusing the huge advantage of such a system is that if one mechanism fails the other mechanisms can try to correct, or *compensate*, for the problem. Understanding this process of compensation is crucial if you wish to be able to correctly interpret ABGs.

Buffers react within seconds to changes in pH and work by removing or replacing hydrogen ions (Martini, 2001). They are the first line of defence against disturbances of acid-base balance; however, buffers do have a limited capacity and are a short-term measure only. There are numerous systems in the body that can buffer acids including haemoglobin, phosphates, plasma proteins and the carbonic acid-bicarbonate system. Haemoglobin is an important buffer as it is involved in the transport of carbon dioxide (as well as oxygen) and can buffer hydrogen ions.

The carbonic acid-bicarbonate system is one of the most important means of regulating pH.

Most of the carbon dioxide (CO_2) in the body is carried within red blood cells where it is converted to carbonic acid (H_2CO_3), which then dissociates into the alkaline bicarbonate ion (HCO_3^-) and the acidic hydrogen ion (H^+). This reaction is reversible according to the needs of the body and can be understood by looking at the equation below.

$$H_2O + CO_2 \leftrightarrow H_2CO_3 \leftrightarrow H^+ + HCO_3^-$$

(water + carbon dioxide ↔ carbonic acid ↔ hydrogen ion + bicarbonate ion.)

The respiratory and renal elements of acid-base balance can also be explained by examining the above equation in more detail. The left-hand side of the equation represents the respiratory element, with carbon dioxide either being excreted or retained by the lungs according to need. The lungs can respond to pH changes within minutes because sensitive chemoreceptors detect alterations in pH of the cerebrospinal fluid and send messages to the respiratory centre in the medulla oblongata. If the pH falls to acidic levels the lungs will increase respiratory rate and depth to 'blow off' carbon dioxide, thereby reducing the amount of carbonic acid in the body. If the pH rises and becomes alkaline, the respiratory rate and depth will reduce and the lungs will retain carbon dioxide. The consequent rise in carbonic acid levels will help restore the pH balance.

The right-hand side of the equation represents the renal element, which is usually referred to as the metabolic component of acid-base balance. The kidneys excrete acidic hydrogen ions as ammonium salts and hydrogen phosphate. Another very important aspect of renal function is the reabsorption and manufacture of the bicarbonate ion by the renal tubules. This process is essential because bicarbonate is normally consumed by neutralising the acids produced by cellular metabolism. The kidneys are much slower to respond to pH changes than the buffers or the lungs and can take from a few hours to a couple of days to resolve an imbalance.

Compensation

The correct function of the buffers, the lungs and the kidneys is vital to maintaining the pH within a normal range. Normal acid-base balance involves not only having a normal pH, but also a normal $PaCO_2$ and HCO_3^- (Cooper & Cramp, 2003). The ability of one system to compensate for another is a critical physiological function that allows patients to survive potentially disastrous changes in acid-base balance. A useful analogy to help you understand acid-base disturbances is to think of it as a carefully balanced set of scales, as outlined in Figure 13.2.

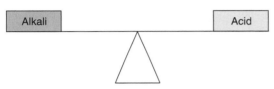

Figure 13.2 Normal acid–base status – the scales are balanced.

Normally, the buffers, lungs and kidneys work together to keep the scales balanced, but during periods of illness, these scales can become disturbed and the balance can be tipped in favour of acidosis or alkalosis.

An alkalosis can be caused by an ***excess of alkali*** or a ***deficit of acid*** as illustrated in Figure 13.3.

Equally, an acidosis can be caused by an ***excess of acid*** or a ***deficit of alkali***, as illustrated in Figure 13.4.

Compensatory mechanisms will work to attempt to rebalance the scales. Therefore, an imbalance caused by a problem with the respiratory component can be compensated for by the metabolic component. Equally, an imbalance caused by a problem with the metabolic component can be compensated for by the respiratory component. Compensation can be either complete, partial or absent.

- Complete compensation – the pH has been returned to within the normal range. It is unusual for compensation to be complete.
- Partial compensation – the body is making attempts to compensate but has not been able to return the pH to within a normal range, usually because the compensatory mechanisms have been overwhelmed.
- Absent – no compensatory attempts have been made. This could occur because the body is unable to compensate. For example, patients who are anaesthetised and are undergoing mechanical ventilation no longer have the ability to adjust their own respiratory rate.

Clinical example of compensation

A patient with chronic obstructive pulmonary disease (COPD) will retain CO_2 due to altered lung function. This tips the scales in favour of an acidosis because of an excess of acid and a subsequent fall in pH. In an attempt to rebalance the scales the kidneys will manufacture and retain additional bicarbonate to compensate and attempt to return the pH to normal.

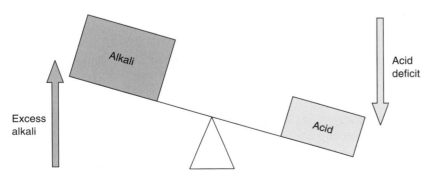

Figure 13.3 Alkalosis – the scales tip due to excess acid or alkali deficit.

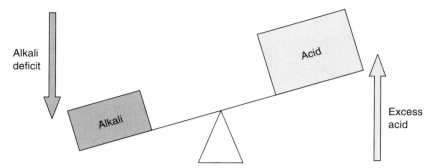

Figure 13.4 Acidosis — the scales tip due to excess acid or alkali deficit.

Disturbances of acid-base balance

This section of the chapter will consider what can go wrong with the normal mechanisms that regulate acid-base balance, since an understanding of this is essential if you are to be able to interpret ABG results. According to Cooper (2004) acid-base disturbances can occur for the following reasons:

- Problems with respiratory function.
- Problems with kidney function.
- Excessive amounts of acid or alkali in the body that overwhelm the normal pH regulation mechanisms.

Disturbances of acid-base balance may be either *respiratory* or *metabolic*, with the term 'metabolic' being used to encompass any disturbance that is not of respiratory origin. These are divided into four categories of acid-base disturbance, which are named after the primary cause of the problem: respiratory acidosis, respiratory alkalosis, metabolic acidosis and metabolic alkalosis.

Respiratory acidosis

Respiratory acidosis results when the $PaCO_2$ levels increase to above the normal upper limit of 6 kPa (hypercapnia) due to decreased alveolar ventilation. Consequently, the levels of carbonic acid rise and the pH falls below 7.35. Gallacher (2004) suggests that the factors that cause alveolar hypoventilation can be categorised into respiratory and non-respiratory:

- Respiratory – e.g. asthma, pneumonia, pulmonary embolus, pulmonary oedema, COPD, airway obstruction, under-ventilation with a mechanical ventilator and chest trauma.
- Non-respiratory – e.g. altered level of consciousness, opiates, sedation, excess alcohol, neuromuscular disorders, pain, spinal cord injury, and electrolyte depletion causing respiratory muscle weakness (especially potassium and phosphate).

Symptoms of respiratory acidosis include: altered mental state, tachycardia, peripheral vasodilation (often causing a flushed appearance and headaches), muscle twitching and cardiac arrhythmias (Moore, 2000).

It is important to note that the respiratory rate in itself is not indicative of hypoventilation, as the depth of breathing is a significant factor in alveolar ventilation (Cooper & Cramp, 2003). It is entirely possible that a patient may have a normal or even elevated respiratory rate but if they have shallow breathing with low tidal volumes, this will cause a reduction in alveolar ventilation. Rarely, hypercapnia can be caused by excess CO_2 production in patients with severe lung disease who are pyrexial or who have had a diet high in carbohydrates (Drage & Wilkinson, 2001).

Respiratory alkalosis

Respiratory alkalosis is the result of hyperventilation causing an abnormally low $PaCO_2$ of below 4.5 kPa (hypocapnia). As a consequence of hyperventilation, carbon dioxide is 'blown off' leading to reduced levels of carbonic acid in the blood and a rise in pH to above 7.45. Hyperventilation is commonly seen in anxiety states or in patients with severe pain, however, it is important to remember that hyperventilation is a sign, not a diagnosis (Cooper & Cramp, 2003). A common cause of hyperventilation is hypoxia, which can cause an increased respiratory drive resulting in a respiratory alkalosis (Drage & Wilkinson, 2001). Conditions that cause hypoxia include shock, pulmonary disease, and early sepsis. Additionally, some neurological conditions including brainstem injury and cerebral haemorrhage can cause hyperventilation. Over-ventilation with a mechanical ventilator can obviously also cause a fall in carbon dioxide levels and a respiratory alkalosis.

Symptoms of respiratory alkalosis include paraesthesia and numbness, impaired consciousness, arrhythmias and seizures.

Metabolic acidosis

Metabolic acidosis occurs when there is a failure to remove or buffer excess hydrogen ions (Gallacher, 2004) and is characterised by a pH below 7.35 and a plasma bicarbonate level below 22 mmol/L. According to Drage and Wilkinson (2001), metabolic acidosis is caused by the following:
- Excess acid production.
- Inadequate excretion of H^+.
- Excessive loss of HCO_3^-.
- Ingestion of acid.

Perhaps the commonest of these is an excess production of lactic acid as a result of anaerobic metabolism. This could be attributable to a very low PaO_2, severe anaemia or hypoperfusion (Drage & Wilkinson, 2001). Hypoperfusion can be localised, such as in an ischaemic bowel, or it can be seen in conditions causing systemic hypotension such as in cardiac arrest, hypovolaemic shock or sepsis. Severe sepsis can also cause mitochondrial dysfunction, which means that cells cannot use oxygen effectively, leading to anaerobic metabolism (Drage & Wilkinson, 2001). Additionally, liver failure can cause a metabolic acidosis due to an accumulation of lactic acid, which the liver normally metabolises (Gallacher, 2004). Another example of an abnormal production of large amounts of acid is diabetic ketoacidosis (DKA). Here, a lack of insulin means the body is unable to use glucose for energy and so instead utilises fats with the resultant production of large amounts of ketone bodies.

Another common cause of metabolic acidosis is acute or chronic renal failure. This leads to inadequate excretion of hydrogen ions and is compounded by insufficient reabsorption and manufacture of bicarbonate ions by the renal tubules. Excessive loss of bicarbonate is a less common cause of metabolic acidosis and may be seen where there are large losses of gastrointestinal secretions from the small bowel. The small bowel secretions are rich in bicarbonate ions (to neutralise stomach acid) and large losses can occur in severe diarrhoea or fistulas. Ingestion of acids as a cause of metabolic acidosis is unusual but it can be seen in cases of poisoning with ethylene glycol (antifreeze) or methanol.

Symptoms of metabolic acidosis include headache, fatigue, reduced level of consciousness and arrhythmias. In spontaneously breathing patients you may also see rapid, deep respirations as the body tries to 'blow off' carbon dioxide to compensate for the increased acid load.

Metabolic alkalosis

Metabolic alkalosis is not seen as often as the other causes of acid-base disturbance (Simpson, 2004) and can be due to either excessive loss of hydrogen ions, excessive reabsorption of bicarbonate or ingestion of alkalis. It will cause the pH to rise above 7.45 and the plasma bicarbonate to become elevated to above 26 mmol/L. Large losses of acidic

Table 13.2 Summary of major causes of acid-base disturbance

Acid-base disturbance	Major causes
Respiratory acidosis ↓ pH ↑ $PaCO_2$	• Inadequate alveolar ventilation • Excess CO_2 production
Respiratory alkalosis ↓ pH ↓ $PaCO_2$	• Hyperventilation
Metabolic acidosis ↓ pH ↓ HCO_3^-	• Excessive H^+ production • Inadequate excretion of H^+ • Excessive HCO_3^- loss • Ingestion of acid
Metabolic alkalosis ↓ pH ↑ HCO_3^-	• Excessive loss of H^+ • Excessive reabsorption of HCO_3^- • Ingestion of alkali

gastric secretions, as seen in conditions causing prolonged severe vomiting or high nasogastric aspirates, are a potential cause of metabolic alkalosis and are often associated with hypokalaemia (Gallacher, 2004). Thiazide or loop diuretics can cause excessive bicarbonate reabsorption in the kidneys because of increased chloride loss in the urine (Drage & Wilkinson, 2001). Additionally, volume depletion can cause a metabolic alkalosis due to an increased bicarbonate ion reabsorption in the kidneys triggered by the renin-angiotensin cycle (Gallacher, 2004). Ingestion of alkalis is unusual although, occasionally, too much alkaline antacid medication can cause a mild alkalosis.

Symptoms of metabolic alkalosis include weakness, confusion and convulsions. In a spontaneously breathing patient, the respiratory system will attempt to compensate and will conserve carbon dioxide by reducing respiratory rate and depth (Gallacher, 2004).

Table 13.2 provides a summary of the four key acid-base disturbances discussed above. Becoming familiar with the clinical conditions associated with these disturbances will help your understanding of and ability to analyse ABGs. It is also worth remembering that patients, particularly if they are critically ill, can have mixed disorders of their acid-base balance that have both a respiratory and a metabolic component.

ABG analysis

Analysis of ABGs is often regarded as being very difficult, however, if you have understood the previous sections of this chapter relating to the physiology you should find this part reasonably straightforward. There are several ways of approaching the analysis of ABGs and it does not matter which one you choose as long as you understand it and follow a logical structure that is thorough, so you do not miss any clues. This chapter will offer a simple step-by-step guide that has an accompanying flow chart (Figure 13.5) to help you ask the right questions. Some clinical scenarios will then allow you to practise your skills in analysis of ABGs.

Before you move on to the step-by-step guide it is worth clarifying the terminology used to describe the parameters that an ABG measures. The normal values are shown in Table 13.1 at the beginning of the chapter.

• **pH** – a measure of the negative logarithm of hydrogen ion concentration. A negative logarithm is just a way of making very small numbers easier to understand.

• **PaO_2** – partial pressure of arterial oxygen. In the UK partial pressure is measured in kilopascals (kPa) although US texts still use mmHg.

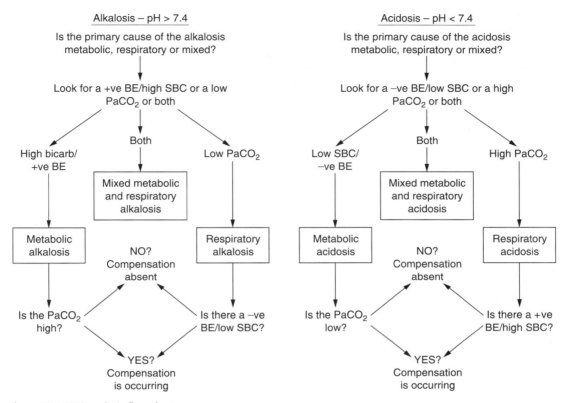

Figure 13.5 ABG analysis flow chart.

- **PaCO$_2$** – partial pressure of arterial carbon dioxide measured in kPa.
- **Standardised bicarbonate (SBC)** – ABG analysers usually measure the SBC in addition to the actual bicarbonate. The SBC is much more useful for the purposes of ABG analysis because it is calculated in such a way as to represent only the metabolic component of bicarbonate. This removes any respiratory influence on bicarbonate levels from the carbonic acid-bicarbonate system.
- **Base excess (BE or BXS)** – this is a useful way of assessing the metabolic component of acid-base disturbances and is an important predictor of the severity of illness. It is a calculated figure that represents the amount of strong acid that

would need to be added to return the pH of the blood sample to 7.4 (Cooper & Cramp, 2003). The number is expressed as either a positive or a negative figure:

- A positive number shows an *excess* of base, therefore, the sample is alkalotic so acid would need to be added to restore the pH to 7.4. This is seen when metabolic alkalosis is the primary acid-base disturbance.
- A negative number shows a *deficit* of base so no acid needs to be added because the sample is already acidotic. This is seen when metabolic acidosis is the primary acid-base disturbance. Many ABG analysers will provide a print out with the base deficit figure shown as a negative BE, however, most people find the

concept easier to understand if they think of this in terms of a base *deficit*, rather than try to comprehend the idea of a 'negative excess'.

The step-by-step guide to ABG analysis

1. **Assess oxygenation**: is the level within the normal range? Note the percentage of inspired oxygen the patient was receiving when the sample was taken: how does this compare to the PaO_2? Also check the Hb and SaO_2 at this point if the machine allows.
2. **Assess the pH**: is it acidic or alkaline? Use 7.4 as your reference point to help you discover whether the pH is moving towards either the acid or alkali side of the scale. If the pH is normal, along with the $PaCO_2$ and SBC, there is no acid-base disturbance. If the pH is normal but the $PaCO_2$ and SBC are not, then complete compensation for a disturbance of acid-base balance has occurred.
3. **Determine the primary acid-base disorder**: the primary acid-base disorder explains the observed pH. Use the flow chart to help you determine which of the four major disturbances of acid-base balance has occurred (respiratory acidosis, respiratory alkalosis, metabolic acidosis or metabolic alkalosis). The $PaCO_2$ will provide clues about the respiratory status and the SBC/BE will tell you about metabolic problems. Remember, it is possible for patients with complex medical conditions to have both metabolic and respiratory disorders simultaneously.
4. **Determine any attempts at compensation**: compensation is usually incomplete and only has a moderating effect on the primary disorder. Again, use the flow chart to help you with this.

Clinical scenarios

Scenario 1

Joe is a 72-year-old man who has undergone an emergency laparotomy for a perforated

diverticulum. There was evidence of faecal contamination of the peritoneum and he had episodes of hypotension intra-operatively, despite being given large volumes of intravenous fluids. He has now been in recovery for 2 hours and is on 40% oxygen. His blood pressure is 118/58 and he is passing adequate urine volumes.

pH	7.18
PaO_2	20.9
$PaCO_2$	3.41
SBC	9.2
BE	−16.4

What do these gases show? Use the step-by-step guide and the flow to help you. Using the information above, what do you think could have caused this disorder?

Scenario 2

Mike is a 28-year-old man who is anxiously awaiting theatre following an open femoral fracture sustained during a climbing accident. He has had opiates for pain and 3 l of crystalloid to manage his hypovolaemia. He starts complaining of feeling light-headed and appears dyspnoeic, despite being on oxygen at 3 L/min.

pH	7.48
PaO_2	14.2
$PaCO_2$	3.8
SBC	22
BE	−1.9

What do these gases show? Use the step-by-step guide and the flow chart to help you. Using the information above, what do you think could have caused this disorder?

Answers

The step-by-step guide and flow chart (Figure 13.5) should have helped you to reach the correct answer but it is just as important that you understand *why* you have the right answer as treatment of acid-base disorders is almost always focused on treating the underlying cause of the problem.

Scenario 1 – Metabolic acidosis with respiratory compensation

The PaO_2 is high so Joe could potentially have his oxygen reduced. The pH is acidotic, but the $PaCO_2$ is low so it is not a respiratory acidosis. The SBC is very low and there is a marked base deficit which both confirm that this is a *metabolic acidosis*. The $PaCO_2$ is low as there is *respiratory compensation* for the metabolic disorder. The information about Joe offers us a few clues about the possible causes of his metabolic acidosis. At first glance Joe's blood pressure looks reasonable, but for someone of his age this may be unacceptably low, so poor tissue perfusion caused by hypotension may be the cause. Additionally, he has been pyrexial for 2 days and had evidence of peritonitis so sepsis could be a factor. Sepsis causes hypotension due to vasodilation, hypovolaemia due to 'leaky' capillaries and problems with cellular uptake of oxygen. Either of these scenarios could cause the tissues to resort to anaerobic metabolism with the by-product of lactic acid.

Scenario 2 – Respiratory alkalosis (uncompensated)

Mike has satisfactory oxygen levels. His pH is high indicating an alkalosis. The $PaCO_2$ is low and the SBC and BE are normal so this indicates a *respiratory alkalosis* with no compensatory changes in the metabolic parameters. It would be easy to write this off as an anxiety or pain problem, but a respiratory alkalosis can also be triggered by tissue hypoxia as the body increases the respiratory rate and depth. It would be important to check Mike's blood pressure and Hb to ensure tissue oxygenation and perfusion were adequate.

REFERENCES

Adam, S. K. & Osborne, S. (1997). *Critical Care Nursing – Science and Practice*. Oxford: Oxford University Press.

Cooper, N. (2004). Acute care: arterial blood gases. *Student BMJ*, **12**, 105–7.

Cooper, N. & Cramp, P. (2003). *Essential Guide to Acute Care*. London: BMJ Books.

Crawford, A. (2004). An audit of the patient's experience of arterial blood gas testing. *British Journal of Nursing*, **13**(9), 529–32.

Drage, S. & Wilkinson, D. (2001). *Acid Base Balance*. World Anaesthesia Online. Available at: www.nda.ox.ac.uk/wfsa/html/u13/u1312_01.htm (Accessed 3 November 2005).

Fitz-Henry, J. & Lewis, N. R. (2001). Anaesthesia explained, Part 3. *Student BMJ*, **9**, 94–6.

Gallacher, S. (2004). Chapter 30: Arterial blood gas analysis. In T. Moore & P. Woodrow, eds., *High Dependency Nursing Care*. London: Routledge pp. 282–9.

Garretson, S. (2005). Haemodynamic monitoring: arterial catheters. *Nursing Standard*, **19**(31), 55–64.

Jevon, P. & Ewens, B. (2002). *Monitoring the Critically Ill Patient*. London: Blackwell Science.

Leach, R. M. & Treacher, D. F. (1998). Oxygen transport – tissue hypoxia. *British Medical Journal*, **317**, 1370–3.

Martini, F. (2001). *Fundamentals of Anatomy and Physiology*. New Jersey: Prentice-Hall Inc.

Moore, T. (2000). Chapter 3: Supporting respiration. In C. Bassett & L. Makin, eds., *Caring for the Seriously Ill Patient*. London: Arnold, pp. 51–79.

Resuscitation Council. (2004). Acid-base balance: interpreting arterial blood gases. In *Advanced Life Support Course Appendices to the Provider Manual*, 4th edn. London: Resuscitation Council (UK).

Simpson, H. (2004). Interpretation of arterial blood gases: a clinical guide for nurses. *British Journal of Nursing*, **13**(9), 522–8.

Treacher, D. F. & Leach, R. M. (1998). Oxygen transport – basic principles. *British Medical Journal*, **317**, 1302–6.

Williams, A. (1998). Assessing and interpreting arterial blood gases and acid-base balance. *British Medical Journal*, **317**, 7167.

Woodrow, P. (2004). Arterial blood gas analysis. *Nursing Standard*, **18**(21), 45–52.

14

Total intravenous anaesthesia

Kevin Henshaw

Key Learning Points
- Understand the flexibility of TIVA to offer more independent control over each component of anaesthesia
- Describe the pharmacokinetic interaction of the drug on the human body
- Understand the pharmacodynamics of the drug on the human body
- Appreciate the movement and elimination of any drug from the body and the dependency on several factors such as age, sex and weight

It is generally accepted that to achieve adequate general anaesthesia, any technique must be capable of providing all the following components (to varying degrees) at any one time:
- A degree of unconsciousness.
- An appropriate level of analgesia.
- Reversible muscle paralysis.
- Suppression of stress response.
- Amnesia.

The following chapter will focus on the most recent, and the relatively new technique of target controlled infusion (TCI) often referred to as total intravenous anaesthesia (TIVA).

TIVA means intravenous (IV) anaesthesia with a complete absence of all volatile agents including nitrous oxide (N_2O).

Traditionally clinicians titrate or infuse IV anaesthetic drugs, observe the clinical effect and then adjust their anaesthetic technique accordingly.

The concentration of inhalational anaesthetic agents can be either increased or decreased in response to the changes in surgical stimuli.

What's so new about TIVA?

For the first time in the history of anaesthesia all the above components of anaesthesia can be controlled *independently*. The flexibility of TIVA allows the clinician to respond rapidly to the individual needs of each patient. The use of rapid onset, but shorter acting drugs, improved cerebral functioning monitors and the availability of TCI devices have all strengthened TIVA and allowed anaesthetists a real alternative to inhalational anaesthesia techniques.

Perioperative practitioners have a professional duty to ensure that we have an understanding and an appreciation of the dangers of all anaesthetic techniques, including TIVA.

Sir Christopher Wren and Daniel Johann Major in 1656 described the earliest recorded use of an IV technique. This technique involved the use of a sheep's bladder and a sharpened quill (Major, 1667). Intravenous solutions of wine, ale or opium were injected into the veins of dogs (the technique was used as part of an overall study of the human circulatory system). As often happens during any experimentation, an incidental observation was made. The observation in this case was

Core Topics in Operating Department Practice: Anaesthesia and Critical Care, eds. Brian Smith, Paul Rawling, Paul Wicker and Chris Jones. Published by Cambridge University Press. © Cambridge University Press 2007.

that the dogs displayed a 'mild inebriation', noted after injection.

In 1664, a German scientist named Daniel Meyer noted that, when needles were inserted into the tongues of dogs following the injection of IV opium, the animals exhibited a 'decreased response to pain'. Unfortunately the link between the injection of IV solutions and analgesia was not recognised on any one of these occasions.

Subsequently, a period of respite followed together with a reduction in the use of IV injections.

It is generally assumed that there was no further research involving IV-related anaesthesia until 1872, when Pierre-Cyprien Ore used IV chloral hydrate as the sole anaesthetic which was given to a total of 36 surgical patients (Sykes, 1960).

Unfortunately, because of the high incidence of mortality linked to Ore's technique, there was little further interest, and the idea of using the venous system to deliver anaesthesia was dismissed until the late nineteenth century.

Recent research into veterinary anaesthesia has discovered that almost half a century before Ore's work was published, M. Dupy, Director of the Toulouse Veterinary School, had begun to use the external jugular veins of horses to administer IV chemical compounds such as alcohol. Dupy noted, among other things, that 'the expired air smelt strongly of alcohol' (Anonymous, 1831). This was the first reference to an IV substance being excreted by the lungs. The doses of alcohol that Dupy used during his experiments were not enough to render the horses unconscious, just to 'stupefy' them. If larger doses of alcohol had been used to induce unconsciousness then the link between IV induction agents and the loss of consciousness may have been established much sooner. The development of IV anaesthesia might then have taken a different course than it did at the turn of the century. As it happened the casual link between loss of consciousness and the IV injection of a drug was overlooked and the significance of studying the effects of IV injections was lost.

Advances in anaesthesia continued with various inhalational agents able to provide all the components of anaesthesia.

The middle of the eighteenth century saw many technological advances around about the same time; these advances helped pave the way for IV therapies.

In 1845 Francis Rynd invented the hollow needle, while the first syringe was invented in 1853 by Charles Gabriel Pravaz. None of these developments were originally designed for IV use. They were later adapted and refined by Alexander Wood who used them for injecting morphine directly into painful joints (Wood, 1855).

The turn of the twentieth century saw something of a renaissance for TIVA with the development of a number of IV anaesthetics including hedonal (Kissin & Wright, 1988), paraldehyde (Noel & Southar, 1913), magnesium sulphate (Peck & Meltzer, 1916) and ethol alcohol (Naragwa, 1921; Carot & Laugier, 1922). Unfortunately the use of any one of these IV anaesthetics can have harmful, if not disastrous side effects. During the same period inhalational anaesthetic agents were becoming increasingly safer and more established among early anaesthetists.

The first barbiturates were synthesised in 1903 by Fisher (Fisher and von Mering, 1903), with the first short-acting, rapid-onset barbiturate (evipan) being developed almost 30 years later in 1932 (Weese et al., 1932).

The next and most influential advancement in IV anaesthesia was the synthesis of sodium thiopentone (pentothal) which was first used in 1934 (Dundee, 1980) by Lundy and Waters (Lundy & Tovell, 1934; Platt et al., 1936).

Originally used as a single 5% infusion, thiopentone was hailed as a wonder drug, the first real IV monoanaesthetic. Unfortunately, the large doses that were necessary to maintain anaesthesia had devastating side effects. The use of thiopentone as a monoanaesthetic reached its peak during the Japanese attack on Pearl Harbor in 1941 and led to the popular myth that more American military personnel were killed by IV thiopentone than were killed as a result of Japanese fire. Regardless of whether there is any truth to this myth, it became clear that thiopentone was not a monoanaesthetic agent, more importantly 5% thiopentone infusions were linked to high mortality rates.

Nevertheless, as an induction agent, the use of a reduced-strength thiopentone (2.5%) quickly became the gold standard that every other induction agent has since been measured by.

The search for a single anaesthetic agent that could independently control all components of anaesthesia began to lose impetus as anaesthesia quickly changed to become a combination of inhalational and IV agents.

The term 'balanced anaesthesia' has come to represent the preferred technique of achieving general anaesthesia by use of a combination of:
- premedication
- IV opioids
- IV muscle relaxants
- inhalational agents
- regional anaesthesia.

Over the last decade the use of IV drugs to induce and maintain anaesthesia has become a real alternative when aiming to achieve balanced anaesthesia.

The arrival of rapid-onset, short-acting opioids such as remifentanil and alfentanil, with advances in infusion pump technology, and an increased understanding of pharmacokinetics has for the first time, allowed for the development of the technique of TCI.

Pharmacokinetics and pharmacodynamics

Pharmacokinetics simply means the movement of a drug in the body. More specifically pharmacokinetics describes the relationship between the dose of a drug and the amount of time taken for the body to metabolise the drug. This relationship can be represented and predicted by the use of complex mathematical models or algorithms.

The concept of pharmacokinetics was first used in anaesthesia during the 1950s when Brodie and Kety first described the process of drug distribution in the body while researching how thiopentone and inhalational agents are metabolised.

They explained the distribution of thiopentone in vivo and the importance of the role played by lean tissue (not fat) in the redistribution of thiopentone in the central nervous system (CNS).

By gradual refinement, physiologic researchers were able to demonstrate the importance of the effect-site concentration of a drug during anaesthesia. The effect-site concentration of a drug is that point at which the clinical effect is seen. In the case of anaesthetic drugs this is when the blood brain barrier is crossed.

When using inhalational anaesthetics the effect-site concentration can be monitored by using capnography. The potency of a defined volatile agent can then be expressed as the minimum alveolar concentration (MAC). Each volatile agent has a potency value which can be expressed numerically as the MAC. The MAC of an inhalational agent is the amount of anaesthetic needed to prevent purposeful movement in 50% of the population at any one time.

The aim of TIVA is to target the effect site and to adjust appropriate plasma drug levels accordingly. The problem with using a TIVA technique in the past was that most IV anaesthetic drugs that are given as a *fixed* rate infusion can take a long time (>12 hours) to plateau. Manual titration meant that too much or too little anaesthetic was being infused leading to pain or awareness or CNS depression and cardiovascular system (CVS) depression. During TIVA it became apparent that a system that could employ a rapid response, calculate and respond to any adverse clinical signs was needed. That system would have to be flexible enough to change the concentration of a drug quickly and be able to recalculate drug concentration levels in the plasma. This system was first demonstrated by Schwilden (Schwilden, 1981) who was able to maintain target plasma levels of a drug by use of a computer controlled infusion pump.

Any system would need to be able to set a target, reach the target and then maintain the correct level of a drug. Such a system became available for clinical use in 1996 with the introduction of the Diprifusor® (Sebel & Lowdown, 1984). The Diprifusor® was the first commercially available TCI device. The introduction of TCIs has allowed anaesthetists to *target* and *maintain* the desired levels of anaesthetic drugs.

As discussed earlier the problem of maintaining target levels was that as soon as any drug is administered the body begins a process of dilution, distribution and elimination. The time period of this process is dependent upon a number of factors such as the patient's age, weight, sex, type of drug, the dose, speed of delivery and how the drug is metabolised. Within the body if the pharmacokinetic behaviour of a drug is known then mathematical calculations can be used to work out exactly how much of the drug is needed to achieve (and maintain) a pre-set target level. When a target level has been set the infusion rate of the drug is then continuously adjusted in order to maintain the desired target level.

Pharmacodynamics can be defined as 'what the **drug** does to the body', in other words, the effects that a drug has on systems of the body. All inhalational agents, for example, have a depressive effect on the CVS.

How are drug levels maintained at the correct level?

TCI devises make use of microprocessors to calculate the concentration of a drug within the plasma. Calculations are constantly used by the microprocessor which have been programmed with an algorithm that uses a bolus elimination transfer (BET) scheme.

The BET model is used to describe the movement of a drug between two theoretical compartments. It is important to emphasise that these compartments are theoretical constructs and *not* real anatomical compartments.

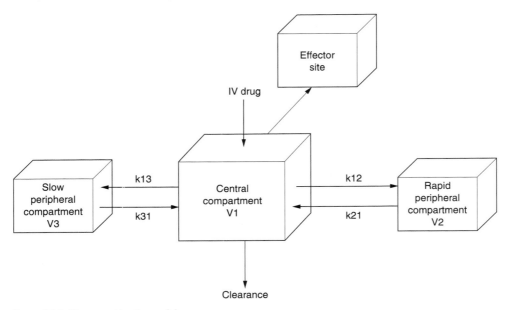

Figure 14.1 Pharmacokinetic model.

The BET scheme was first proposed by Kruger-Theimer (Kruger-Theimer, 1968) and was the first theoretical model to recognise that in order to achieve a steady-state blood concentration of a drug then at least three factors need to be constantly calculated. Any algorithm used by a TCI device must be able to measure:

- The original loading dose of the drug – this determines the first phase of distribution. This is the first phase.
- Any changes to the infusion and be able to compensate for continuous drug elimination. This is phase two of the BET Model.
- An infusion rate that can equilibrate drug concentration in the plasma as the drug is distributed to the peripheral compartment. This is the third and final phase.

After the initial loading dose into the central compartment (phase 1) is given (Figure 14.1), a constant amount of drug begins to be eliminated in a fixed period of time. Therefore, if the elimination times and rates of a defined drug are known then the blood concentration of that drug can be predicted and maintained by either increasing or decreasing the infusion rate to compensate for elimination (phase 2) and equilibration to other compartments (phase 3) (Schwilden *et al.*, 1986).

3-Compartment model

All calculations used by current TCI devices are based on a 3-compartment pharmacokinetic model. The 3-compartment model consists of a hypothetic central compartment (V1), a second compartment (V2), sometimes referred to as 'fast' or 'vessel rich' and a third compartment (V3) commonly referred to as the 'slow' or 'vessel poor' compartment. It is this process of distribution and elimination of drugs between the compartments that forms the basis of all current pharmacokinetic models.

Factors such as the patient's age, weight and sex can all effect the drug distribution between compartments. For this reason it is important

that this information is made available to the perioperative practitioner when practicable. Once good venous access has been established and all of the relevant factors such as age and sex have been entered into the TCI device, then induction can begin.

As the drug begins to move down the concentration gradients between compartments (in an effort to try to achieve equilibrium) and is simultaneously being eliminated from the body, the TCI device calculates the changes between compartments and compensates by either increasing or decreasing the infusion rate in order to maintain the desired target levels.

This ability to adapt infusion rates is the main difference between a standard syringe driver, which will deliver a predetermined amount of drug until the pre-set volume is completed, and a syringe driver that is target controlled and continually adjusts itself to maintain a target dose.

Why use TCI systems?

Advances in computer technology, the development of fast-acting opioid analgesics and muscle relaxants, together with more robust pharmacokinetic models have allowed anaesthetists to target the effector site with the *minimum* amount of anaesthetic drug to achieve adequate anaesthesia.

An important point to remember here is that TCI devices are not computerised anaesthetists. All of the normal clinical observations and decisions regarding the treatment of a patient still need to be made during target controlled anaesthesia. In this sense TCI devices can never replace sound clinical knowledge and experience.

Advantages	Disadvantages
Where the use of high concentrations of oxygen are needed such as: • single lung anaesthesia • hyperbaric medicine	• Increased IV doses of anaesthetic agents are used to compensate for the lack of N_2O

Advantages	Disadvantages
In situations where delivery of inhalational agent may be restricted: • Bronchoscopy • Laryngoscopy • A reduction in atmospheric pollution • A decreased incidence of post-operative nausea and vomiting (PONV) • A reduced trigger for malignant hyperpyrexia	• Designated target controlled infusion devices which may be initially expensive and difficult to use • Difficulty predicting the end of anaesthesia as presently there is no indicator of metabolic clearance of the drug that has been infused. Plasma concentration estimates are displayed but are not a direct measurement of volatile concentration as displayed by end tidal monitors
The use of TCVA in areas where volatile anaesthetics would be contraindicated or difficult to administer. For example: • war zones • lack of anaesthetic equipment, i.e. transfer of the critically compromised patients	• Disconnection, if IV access is lost either through extravasation or mechanical disconnection then anaesthesia is lost. Difficult to detect
Other benefits of TIVA include anaesthesia for surgery where the use of N_2O may be contraindicated. For example: • inner ear surgery • long duration bowel surgery • pneumothorax • air embolism • hepatotoxicity	• A second intravenous infusion line must be used • Delayed recovery if high target plasma levels are maintained for long time periods

Principles of TCIs

As already stated, TCIs use a number of factors to calculate appropriate plasma levels, for example, the body mass index (BMI) of a young, athletic male patient would have a very different pharmacokinetic profile than that of a patient who might be older, more sedentary but may share the same body weight. Depending on which pharmacokinetic model is used (newer TCI devices have a facility to allow selection of specific models) the microprocessor is able to calculate the appropriate target by taking into account BMI, gender and age.

Examples of TIVA in clinical use could be:
• propofol which can be used as both an induction agent and a maintenance drug
• a neuromuscular blocking agent (NMBA) can be used (in conjunction with a peripheral nerve stimulator)
• a short-acting opioid such as remifentanil or alfentanil can be used as a component of analgesia.

At present the only short-acting opioid that has an approved algorithm for TCI is remifentanil. Remifentanil is metabolised anywhere in the body by non-specific esterases and so doesn't rely on hepatic or renal metabolism.

Probably the most well-known TCI device and the most popular for use in Europe is the Diprifusor® which has been available for clinical use since 1996.

The Diprifusor® is only able to use pre-filled glass syringes containing propofol to deliver TCIs. The syringes are single-use only and contain a magnetic strip on the flange of the syringe that 'tells' the microprocessors in the infusion pump that the device is primed with the correct drug and that it is ready to be used. When the syringe is approaching empty the magnetic strip is deprogrammed and an alarm is activated to alert the user that a refill is needed. Once the metallic strip has been deactivated it can no longer be used or refilled.

A common criticism of TIVA is the high capital and running costs incurred when compared to low-flow inhalational anaesthesia. However, since the patent for propofol has expired, newer and cheaper generic propofols have become available and the development of 'Open TCI' devices which can use generic propofol has reduced the total cost of TIVA significantly.

It could be argued that the initial expense of setting up a TCI system can be offset by a reduction in PONV and a reduced stay in the post-operative care unit (POCU). Early discharge and faster patient throughput associated with the use of TIVA are some of the benefits that are thought to offset the initial cost of setting up TIVA regimes. Advocates of TIVA claim that TCIs are best suited to the modern healthcare system with the emphasis on short stay, day case surgery and the growth of endoscopic and invasive radiological procedures. Opponents of TIVA argue that similar results (reduced PONV and faster recovery times) can be achieved using modern volatile agents and improved methods of post-operative analgesia.

Awareness and depth of anaesthesia

At the present time direct measurement of drug concentration at the effect site is not a practical option. Clinical judgement is still needed to assess, and alter drug target levels both pre- and intra-operatively. Most clinicians prefer to see the potency of an anaesthetic agent (the MAC value) and this can be measured reasonably easily by sampling the end tidal volume. This option of not being able to 'see what's happening is not available when using TCIs and is another common criticism of TIVA.

Depth of anaesthesia is a concern for all anaesthetists, but, given the absence of a MAC during TCIs, many anaesthetists see the lack of a numerical indicator as a real disadvantage.

Awareness and recall can and does occur during anaesthesia (even when an adequate MAC is displayed). The widespread use of NMBAs has increased occasions where patients have experienced awareness, pain and even explicit recall during general anaesthesia.

Depth of anaesthesia is notoriously difficult to quantify. Even when adequate MAC levels are displayed studies have demonstrated that recall, learning and even response to commands can still occur during anaesthesia. Patients have been able to obey commands while anaesthetised during surgical procedures for example, but were unable to recall any of the events of the surgical procedure.

Movement is a poor indicator of adequate depth of anaesthesia, as the use of NMBAs prevent the early detection of purposeful movement. Some studies have been able to demonstrate purposeful movement during neuromuscular blockade by isolating the patient's forearms from the NMBAs by use of a tourniquet. Patients were then instructed to move their hands or fingers in response to surgical stimulus. This technique has proved to be a poor indicator of depth of anaesthesia not least of all because patient hand movement during a surgical procedure can be distracting to the surgical staff and a hazard to the integrity of the sterile field. The maximum recommended time for this method is 20 minutes so studies have been limited by time factors.

Adequate depth of anaesthesia has always been a particular concern for users of TIVA as early attempts at providing TIVA consisted of manual infusions that relied on boluses of anaesthetic drugs in response to surgical stimulus. Since the availability of TCIs a smoother and more responsive anaesthetic technique is now available to clinicians.

Depth of anaesthesia monitors goes some way to address these problems and their use in anaesthesia has become more widespread.

The majority of depth of anaesthesia monitors use a variety of electrophysiologic techniques to monitor responses to stimuli. Commonly used monitors in the UK are the bispectral index (BIS) and the auditory evoked potential (AEP).

The perception of auditory stimuli intra-operatively is well documented and AEP monitors use a series of high frequency auditory clicks to stimulate auditory cortical activity which is then measured as a brainstem response. Auditory stimuli are administered through the patient's ears and so are not suitable for surgical procedures that involve accessing the ear, or patients who have pathological hearing disorders.

The bispectral index selectively analyses a number of EEG waveforms and can help to predict movement even in the paralysed patient.

Ultimately the most reliable form of depth of anaesthesia monitor still remains the anaesthetist.

Closed loop systems

Depth of anaesthesia monitors can be used as 'feed back' mechanism for computerised TCI systems. This method has had some limited success when used to control general anaesthesia and sedation. When automatic feedback is used the system is known as closed loop anaesthesia.

Potentially closed loop systems should be able to provide more accurate feedback which can then be used to control the level of anaesthesia. This is already an area where there is a great deal of research in progress and could lead to computer-controlled anaesthesia. Most TCI systems currently in clinical practice rely on an 'open system' which uses clinical judgment to adjust target levels in response to surgical stimulus.

Components of a TCI system

The principal components of a TCI system must contain:
- a means of inputting patient data such as age, sex and weight, and also target drug concentration
- at least one (usually two) microprocessor(s) and an infusion pump
- a display which shows both the targeted and current calculated blood concentration
- a means of displaying the infusion rate
- a means of displaying the amount of drug that has been delivered

- the effect-site concentration (the estimated amount at the effector site in the brain)
- the estimated time needed to lower the target concentration at the effector site.

Future developments

As a result of competition from generic versions of propofol and the introduction of open systems the overall cost and availability of TCI devices have started to come down in price. This reduction in cost of propofol and increased availability has allowed more anaesthetists access to TCI devices. The net result has seen a growth of TIVA which is fast becoming an established technique in today's healthcare setting.

The development of new volatile agents has declined and there is increased pressure from government and regulatory bodies to reduce the amount of pollutants in the atmosphere. This external pressure together with the increased availability of TCI devices is likely to see a further decline in the use of volatile anaesthetics.

The search for a monoanaesthetic continues together with the development of newer, safer IV drugs. In the meantime the newer hypnotic and analgesic drugs with their faster acting and more predictable recovery profiles will enhance anaesthetic practice by allowing the clinician even greater control of the individual components of anaesthesia. Advocates of TIVA claim that the quality and speed of reversal from anaesthesia is greater than with traditional anaesthesia. This is still an area for future research.

A better understanding of pharmacokinetic and pharmacodynamic models has led to the development of more predictable drugs which can be simulated in computer programs.

Finally, the improvements and technological developments associated with drug delivery systems mean that the safety and reliability of TIVA techniques can offer a real alternative to traditional inhalational techniques.

REFERENCES

Anonymous. (1831). Deals with injection of various substances intravenously in horses by M. Dupy. *Lancet*, **2**, 76.

Carot, H. & Laugier, H. (1922). Anaaesthesie par injection intrareineuse d'un produit melange alcool-chloroform-solution physiologique chez le chien. *CRSeances Soc Biol*, 889–92.

Dundee, J. W. (1980). Historical vingettes and classification of intravenous anaesthetics. In J. A. Aldrete & T. H. Stanley, eds., *Trends in Intravenous Anaesthesia*. Chicago: Year Book, p. 1.

Fischer, E. & von Mering, J. (1903). Ueber eine neue klasse von schlafmilteln. *Ther Gengenwart*, **44**, 97–101.

Kissin, I. & Wright, A. J. (1988). The introduction of Hedonal: a Russian contribution to intravenous anaesthesia. *Anaesthesiology*, **69**, 242–5.

Kruger-Theimer, E. (1968). Continuous intravenous infusion and multi compartmental accumulation. *European Journal of Pharmacology*, 317–34.

Lundy, J. S. & Tovell, R. M. (1934). Some of the newer local and general anaesthetic agents: methods of their administration. *Northwest Medicine* (Seattle), **33**, 308–11.

Major, D. J. (1667). *Chirugia infusioria placidis* CL: vivorium dubiis impugnata, cun modesta, ad Eadem, Resposione. Kiloni.

Naragwa, K. (1921). Experimentelle studien uber die intravenose infusionsnarkose mittles alcohols. *Journal of Experimental Medicine*, **2**, 81–126.

Noel, H. & Southar, H. S. (1913). The anaesthetic effects of intravenous injection of paraldehyde. *Annals of Surgery*, **57**, 64–7.

Peck, C. H. & Meltzer, S. J. (1916). Anaesthesia in human beings by intravenous injection of magnesium sulphate. *Journal of the American Medical Association*, **67**, 1131–3.

Platt, T. W., Tatum, A. L., Hathaway, H. R. & Waters, R. M. (1936). Sodium ethyl (α-methyl butyl) thiobarbiturate: preliminary experimental and clinical study. *American Journal of Surgery*, **31**, 464–6.

Schwilden, H. (1981). A general method for calculating the dosage scheme in linear pharmacokinetics. *European Journal of Clinical Pharmacology*, **20**, 379.

Schwilden, H., Strake, H., Schuttler, J. & Lauven, P. M. (1986). Pharmacological models and their uses in clinical anaesthesia. *European Journal of Anaesthesiology*, **3**, 175–208.

Sebel, P. S. & Lowdown, J. D. (1989). Propofol: a new intravenous anaesthetic. *Anaesthesiology*, **71**, 260–77.

Sykes, W. S. (1960). *Essays on the First Hundred Years of Anaesthesia*. 3 vols. Edinburgh: Churchill Livingstone.

Weese, H. & Scharpf, W. E. (1932). Ein neuratiges einschlaffmittel. *Deutsche medizinische Wochenschrift*, **58**, 1205–7.

Wood, A. (1855). A new method of treating neuralgia by direct application of opiates to the painful points. *Edinburgh Medical & Surgical Journal*, **82**, 265–81.

15

Anaesthesia and electro-convulsive therapy

Mark Bottell

Key Learning Points
- Explore the history of electro-convulsive therapy
- Reflect on the clinical conditions about electro-convulsive therapy
- Identify the anaesthetic considerations for the patient
- How to care for the patient having electro-convulsive therapy
- Discuss current standards in electro-convulsive therapy and understand the proposed changes in patient care

The practice of electro-convulsive therapy (ECT) has often created controversy and disagreement. It is a dramatic and alarming form of therapy which is disturbing to watch and equivocal in its effects. It has enthusiasts on both sides, for and against. That it is performed on patients who may be beyond the point of giving fully informed consent only adds to the uneasiness which many feel in helping with these procedures.

ECT has been practised over the years both with and without anaesthesia. The so-called unmodified ECT or that without anaesthesia was commonplace when the treatment was first discovered. The shock given to the patient induced unconsciousness and most of the current passed through the forehead bone.

The main side effect of this treatment was bone fractures because of uncontrolled seizures, mainly due to the lack of any suitable muscle relaxants.

Electro-convulsive therapy has been, for many years, viewed as brutal and barbaric and a treatment used as an abuse as depicted in Ken Kesey's film 'One Flew Over the Cuckoo's Nest'.

Whatever our own perspectives on this practice, it is nevertheless true to say that ECT is now performed all over the world, and there are many practitioners' patients and carers alike, who attest to the benefit of this form of treatment.

How ECT came about, how it became popular with clinicians and specifically, how the patient undergoing ECT should be cared for during the anaesthetic phase will be the subject of this chapter.

How ECT was discovered

Electro-convulsive therapy was first introduced in Italy in 1938. It is reported that physician Ugo Cerletti had observed that the electric shocks passed through the brains of swine queuing for slaughter made the animals docile and manageable. When it was performed on human beings with intractable mental disorder they too became more manageable and even improved in their outlook. How it worked was in many ways as mysterious then as it is now, though one has to say that in the early years its use was considered appropriate in a much wider set of conditions than it is now. Indeed it was used then for a range of conditions for which it would now be considered inappropriate. Nevertheless, half a

Core Topics in Operating Department Practice: Anaesthesia and Critical Care, eds. Brian Smith, Paul Rawling, Paul Wicker and Chris Jones. Published by Cambridge University Press. © Cambridge University Press 2007.

century on, Alan Bennett (2005) indicates some of the benefit that carers still report for intractable depression:

We were told that following a few sessions of ECT, Mam would be more herself, and progressively so as the treatment went on. In the event, improvement was more dramatic. Given her first bout of ECT in the morning, by the afternoon Mam was walking and talking with my father as she hadn't for months. He saw it as a miracle, as I did, and to hear on the phone the dull resignation gone from his voice and the old habitual cheerfulness back was like a miracle, too.

Cerletti specialised in neurology and neuropsychiatry, studying in places such as Paris, Munich and Heidelberg. In 1924, after his appointment as the Head of the Neurobiological Institute in Milan, he took up a post in Bari as lecturer in Neuropsychiatry and in 1928 moved to Rome, where he began to develop ECT practices.

Following his observations on pigs, Cerletti induced grand mal seizures in animals by subjecting them to electric shocks. This built on previous work which had, in the opinion of some therapists, suggested that schizophrenia and epilepsy were antagonistic. In particular, insulin, drugs and even malaria had been used to induce seizures, in the belief that this would abate the delusions of schizophrenia. Nothing however did this as effectually as electric current, especially when it was applied to the brain directly through the temples by electrodes placed on either side of the head.

Cerletti's first promising subject was a 40-year-old man who suffered from schizophrenia. The man came to Cerletti from Milan and could barely speak. The noises emanating from him amounted to gibberish and were incomprehensible, however, after just two treatments, the man was heard to speak clearly and all signs of his former gibberish state had been eradicated. The age of electroshock treatment, as it was then known, was born.

Treatment developed as the years went by and in 1949 Larry S. Goldman introduced unilateral ECT with the electrodes being placed on the right side of the head only. This was done to minimise the side effects and in particular the memory loss, as unilateral ECT has virtually no side effects but is unfavoured by practitioners due to the fact that the response to such treatment takes far longer than with bilateral ECT. Nevertheless, post-ictal excitement in patients who have undergone bilateral or right unilateral treatment is greater than those undergoing left-sided unilateral ECT.

Furthermore, variations of these positions were trialled and bi-frontal ECT was introduced in the early 1970s.

This was basically a modification of bilateral ECT but the electrodes were placed on the forehead, just above the lateral angle of each eye orbit.

It was found to be as effective as bilateral ECT but it needs higher energy doses to induce a seizure and therefore to be of any benefit to the patient's condition.

It is felt that these doses need to be at least five times greater than doses associated with bilateral ECT to be effective.

Pippard and Ellam (1981) describe that the 1970s saw the greatest decline in the use of ECT from an estimated 60 000 in Britain in 1972 to 30 000 in 1979. It is felt that one of the main reasons for this lay in the public's perception of ECT and how it was portrayed in the media and on the big screen in such films as described above.

This all led to people becoming confused about ECT and its uses and calls for a complete ban were common. Also development of drug and therapeutic treatments became more complex and apparent.

The use of ECT was also deemed as being used indiscriminately and utilised as a punishment instead of a therapeutic intervention.

Civil right groups became concerned and the issues regarding people being able to give consent came to the fore.

Nevertheless, despite such concerns it became apparent that a core group of patients did not benefit from any chemical or psychological input and that ECT was the only form of treatment that would benefit such individuals.

The conditions that ECT is used to treat

Electro-convulsive therapy is not only used to treat depression, but has been used to treat obsessive compulsive disorders as well as being used to treat the distressing symptoms which may accompany schizophrenia such as extreme lethargy, manic states and delusional ideas. Nevertheless, its main focus has been on the treatment of the depressed patient, including the debilitating effects of post-natal depression.

The spread of symptoms which ECT is intended to treat indicates that it is best regarded as a form of symptom control rather than as a specific cure. In fact the way that ECT works is still largely mysterious. That it interferes with the deranged brain chemistry of the suffering person illuminates the area hardly at all. The lack of understanding of how the procedure works only heightens the controversy relating to its use. It has been likened by doubters to taking a hammer to a Swiss watch. Its use is illegal in Slovenia.

Yet the ECT aspects of the procedure are, relatively speaking, rather safe. The main danger point comes where the person is given a muscle relaxant to prevent the convulsions which, in previous generations, broke bones and pulled muscles. With the relaxant must also come the anaesthetic agent which is intended to attenuate the horror of losing control of one's muscles and being subject to the current. Both combined present the staff with the dangers inherent in general anaesthesia and muscle relaxation. These risks and how to reduce them will form the rest of the chapter.

Anaesthetic considerations for those undergoing a course of ECT

Electro-convulsive therapy practice has come a long way since the early years of the treatment. The pioneers of the therapy gave no anaesthetic and permitted uncontrolled grand mal seizures. These were dangerous to the patients and traumatic to the staff. Restraining patients often involved enough force to induce injuries and broken bones. One of these events gave rise in law to the case which formed the basis of the Bolam Standard (*Bolam* v. *Friern*, 1958). It was the case that in the late 1940s over 20% of patients treated with ECT had compression fractures of the spine.

As time went on, the treatment was given under a light anaesthetic and by using muscle relaxants such as curare, which was introduced in 1942, and suxamethonium which was introduced in 1951. The two components of the triad of anaesthesia meant the process became much more humane and far fewer injuries were sustained (Powell, 2002).

Calvey and Williams (1997) describe the introduction of methohexitone in 1959 and more recently propofol in 1985. The anaesthetic treatment of patients has become much smoother and again has led to a more benevolent type of treatment. Furthermore the suggestion by Andersen *et al.* (2001) that combining methohexitone or propofol with remifentanil would produce a longer seizure in the patient thus offering a more 'favourable clinical outcome'.

The problem with this approach is that it introduces other risks which are scarcely less serious such as airway protection and all of the range of risks which anaesthesia brings in its wake. Any person who is considered to require ECT has exactly the same anaesthetic risks as anyone who is to have an elective surgical operation.

In order to meet these risks the patient is thoroughly assessed. The patient is seen prior to the first treatment by the anaesthetist and a preoperative assessment is undertaken.

It is generally agreed that preoperative investigations are decided locally, but the recommendation of the ECT Accreditation Service (ECTAS) is that they should include an ASA grade, cardiovascular, respiratory and neurological assessment. ECTAS is composed of doctors who belong to the Royal College of Psychiatrists, Royal College of Anaesthetists and the Royal College of Nursing.

As well as recommending pre-anaesthetic assessment and evaluation measures, ECTAS offers guidance on the number and training of staff required in a centre, on medico-legal matters such as the gaining of consent and follow-up, and on the care of special groups such as children and the elderly.

Today, all patients undergoing ECT are treated as day cases, indeed some patients come in from home to undergo treatment. We can now go on to discuss the care of patients having treatment and will look at this from the perspective of pre-, intra- and post-treatment risks.

The care of a patient pre-, intra- and post-ECT

A person is to having ECT will be assessed prior to treatment by the anaesthetist and any necessary investigations will be carried out. All patients will have a general physical examination and will have blood taken for a full blood count test. The person's medical history will be taken with particular emphasis placed on previous anaesthetic problems, and also any family history of anaesthetic problems. Here special reference will be made to malignant hyperpyrexia, or sickle cell disease in those patients who may be susceptible to those conditions.

It is generally felt that chest X-rays only need to be performed for those patients over 40 years of age and electrocardiograms are only completed on those patients over 65 years or with a current known cardiac complaint.

As with many day cases, patients requiring general anaesthetic must be fasted from midnight the night before treatment. Any cardiovascular or gastrointestinal drugs can still be given at 7 a.m. on the morning of the treatment.

In November 2005 the Royal College of Nursing in conjunction with the Royal College of Anaesthetists issued guidelines on preoperative fasting and stated that the intake of water or other clear fluids, i.e. tea or coffee with no milk can, in adults, be taken up to 2 hours prior to the induction of anaesthesia.

The intake of solids, including milk, is restricted to a minimum of 6 hours before anaesthetic induction. It also states that the chewing of gum should not be allowed on the day of treatment.

Consent issues

One of the biggest concerns involving ECT relates to doubts about the patient's ability to give informed consent. It is fair to say that almost 80–90% of patients who undergo treatment do so freely and voluntarily. Most will be in hospital informally and will give consent voluntarily, much like any individual who is to have a surgical operation. Nevertheless, there will always be a small number of patients who are detained in hospital under the Mental Health Act of 1983, and due to their mental incapacity, will not be able to give informed consent.

These patients will usually be placed on a Section 2 for assessment of mental state for up to 28 days or, more likely, a Section 3, which is for treatment and can last up to 6 months.

Just because this Section 3 is for treatment, it does not mean that the treatment can be given randomly to anyone under the terms of this section. The person may give their consent for this treatment, should their mental state allow. If not, a second opinion will be sought from an independent psychiatrist who is approved by the Mental Health Act Commission. Together with the patient's nurse and one other individual who is involved in the patient's care such as a social worker or occupational therapist, they will assess the patient and a decision will be made. The decision will determine whether the treatment will be of benefit to the patient and whether it is in their best interests. Should it be decided that treatment will aid recovery, then the independent psychiatrist will complete the necessary paperwork and will indicate the maximum number of treatments a patient should have. When this number is complete a further assessment is made if it is felt that more treatments may be needed. This safeguard avoids patients having unnecessary treatments.

A preoperative assessment is made on the ward by the nursing team responsible and two checks are completed to ensure the patient undergoing treatment is the correct person and that all basic tests, such as blood pressure have been performed and are within normal limits.

Patients walk down to the ECT suite with the nurse who will stay with them throughout treatment. Monitoring of blood pressure, pulse, respirations, ECG and pulse oximetry is commenced and the patient's details are checked again by the suite manager.

Electro-encephalogram monitoring is also applied at this point to measure the brain's activity during the seizure; the importance of this procedure will be explained in more detail a little further on.

The patient is then anesthetised usually with an induction dose of propofol at 1.5–2.5 mg/kg or less in those patients who are over 55 years of age. This is not the only substance used. Benbow (2002), describes the virtues of etomidate as an alternative to propofol, especially for those patients whose length of seizure is below 25 seconds (see below). She states that etomidate increased their mean seizure duration by 245%.

Suxamethonium is then given. This is used because of its rapid onset of muscle relaxation and short duration of action. It is given in doses of 1 mg/kg. When fasciculation or twitching of muscles indicates that the suxamethonium is working, the current is applied.

The shock is induced by placing the electrodes from the machine to either side of the head just above the temple area. Jelly similar to ECG or ultrasound jelly is applied to the electrodes to aid contact with the skin. Once the current is passed, the seizure begins. There are various stages of the seizure:

Tonic phase – where muscles become rigid, though this is greatly reduced due to the administration of the muscle relaxant.

Clonic phase – also known as the ictal phase, where there is movement of the arms, legs/feet and facial muscles. Again this is controlled due to the suxamethonium.

Post-ictal phase – when the patient begins to recover and regains consciousness.

The seizure is paramount in the successful treatment of the condition, as the therapeutic effect of the ECT is thought to increase in proportion to the length of the seizures. Many research studies have found that 25 seconds is the optimum time for the seizure to last. If this time is increased, the efficacy of the treatment is not improved.

Electro-encephalogram activity is also monitored. The length of this monitoring should exceed the seizure by 10–15 seconds. Should either the seizure or EEG activity continue after 60 seconds, then the seizure is terminated by the use of intravenous diazemuls given in doses of 10–20 mg at a rate of 0.5 ml every 30 seconds.

During the seizure, the patient's dentures are protected by a bite guard placed between the teeth prior to the seizure taking place.

It was common practice in the early years of ECT to hold and restrain the patients during treatment.

Indeed Jefferies and Rakoff (1983) argue that ECT itself is a form of restraint and describe how patients who did not respond to chemotherapy were given ECT to modify their behaviour.

Such restraint during ECT greatly contributed to the number of fractures that occurred to patients but at the time it was done in the best interest of the patient and with good faith. Nevertheless, it was soon realised that this was not indeed the case and the practice was eventually stopped.

Within a couple of minutes the patient recovers consciousness and is transferred to the recovery suite where they are cared for by a trained recovery practitioner. All vital signs continue to be monitored and, when fully awake, the patient is given the option of a cup of tea or coffee. It is vital that the patient's nurse remains with them. This is to ensure patient safety but also so that, once awake, the person has someone with them who they know and recognise. This will aid orientation to time, place and person.

When it is felt that the patient has recovered enough to return to the ward, he/she is escorted in a wheelchair with their nurse. Back on the ward, the patient is allowed to sleep but is carefully observed until they are fully roused.

Orientation to time, place and person is an important observation on the ward, as one of the most common side effects of ECT is short-term memory loss. A headache is also common. Apart from these, other than feeling a little weak from the anaesthetic, the side effects of treatment are minimal.

The short-term memory loss should disappear within a couple of hours of treatment and the headache can be dealt with by simple paracetamol.

It can be seen that anaesthetic considerations for ECT are relatively simple compared to, for example, those patients undergoing major orthopaedic or cardiac surgery.

Nevertheless, several important elements need to be emphasised.

The majority of patients having ECT will also be on other medications which can influence the seizure threshold. These include diazepam and other benzodiazepines, anti-convulsants, hypnotics, phenothiazines, to name but a few.

From this it can be assumed that the dose of anaesthetic as well as the ECT treatment dose needs to be titrated to enable the optimum seizure in the shortest amount of anaesthetic time.

Airway management of patients is again kept fairly uncomplicated due to the short-term duration of unconsciousness. It is agreed generally that patients can breathe with the use of a facemask whilst asleep. It is always essential however that a supply of laryngeal masks and endotracheal tubes of various sizes are kept close at hand for emergency use.

Oxygen is supplied from wall or cylinder outlets via a Waters or Bains circuit, and as a general rule, an anaesthetic machine is not part of the equipment in the ECT suite. Other essential equipment required is a selection of airways, both oropharyngeal and nasal, laryngoscopes of various types and sizes, gum elastic bougies, intravenous fluids together with the appropriate giving sets and also a defibrillator which is regularly checked and maintained by unit staff.

All actions taken during the ECT session are recorded in the patient's case notes and this includes anaesthetic, ECT stimulus dose and monitoring parameters of the patient during treatment.

In 2005, the Royal College of Psychiatrists issued strict guidelines on the use of ECT and how it will be managed as a practice in the future.

Guidance as to how specific illnesses should be treated using ECT are discussed. Basic requirements in ECT clinics including staffing and training issues are addressed.

Basic good practice guidelines about consent and treatment have now been issued and ECT clinics are now being inspected and audited both internally and externally by health and government bodies including the Mental Health Act Commission and ECTAS.

This inevitably will bring about higher and better maintained standards for the care of those undergoing ECT.

The overall aim is to undoubtedly make treatment more acceptable and to banish the stigma of ECT that still exists today.

Depression and ECT favour no nation, class, gender or religion in incidence or spread. Many famous patients have successfully survived depression having undertaken a course of ECT including Vivien Leigh, Tammy Wynette, Ernest Hemmingway, Lou Reed and Yves Saint Laurent, to name but a few.

It is hoped that this chapter has clarified any points that the reader was unsure of and it is hoped that any of the myths surrounding this 'mysterious' treatment have been addressed.

ECT continues to be used worldwide to treat mental health problems and despite numerous attempts to deny its efficacy, many patients are able to live their lives in a normal manner and can go about their daily tasks, thanks to the benefits of ECT.

REFERENCES

Andersen, F.A., Årsland, D. & Holst-Larsen, H. (2001). Effects of combined methohexitone-remifentanil anaesthesia in electroconvulsive therapy. *Acta Anaesthesiologica Scandinavica*, **45**(7), 830.

Benbow, S. (2002). *Anaesthesia for Electroconvulsive Therapy: a Role for Etomidate*. Available at: http://pb.rcpshych.org/cgi/content/full/26/9/351 (Accessed 23 February 2006).

Calvey, T.N. & Williams, N.E. (1999). *Principles and Practice of Pharmacology for Anaesthetists*, 3rd edn. Berlin: Blackwell Science Ltd.

Jefferies, J.J. & Rakoff, V.M. (1983). E.C.T. as a form of restraint. *Canadian Journal of Psychiatry*, **28**(8), 661–3.

Pippard, J. & Ellam, L. (1981). *Electroconvulsive Treatment in Great Britain 1980*. London: Gaskell.

Powell, J. (2002). History of anaesthesia, lecture handout. *O.D.P. Course Bristol 18.1.02*. Available at: www.john.powell.net (Accessed 23 November 2005).

Royal College of Nursing. (2005). *Perioperative Fasting in Adults and Children – A Clinical Guideline*. Available at: www.rcn.org.uk/publications/pdf/guidelines/Perioperative fasting in Adults and Children – 002779.pdf (Accessed 3 February 2006).

FURTHER READING

Austin, A.T. (1990). Available at: www.23nlpeople.com/electroshock_history.htm (Accessed 23 November 2005).

Cerletti, U. (1970). *Citizens Commission on Human Rights*. (Accessed 16 February 2006.)

Easyweb.easynet.co.uk/simplepsych/ect.html-electroconvulsive therapy in easy to understand English.

ECTAS. (2004). Available at: www.rcpsych.ac.uk/cru/ECTAS Standards (Accessed 23 November 2005).

Hollander, A.B. (2000). *Electro-Convulsive Therapy*. Available at: http://serendip.brynmawr.edu/bb/neuro/neuro00/web2/Hollander.html 3–17k (Accessed 1 February 2006).

The E.C.T. Accreditation Service (ECTAS) Standards for the Administration of E.C.T., 3rd edn, December 2005, at: www.rcpsych.ac.uk/cru.

The E.C.T. Handbook (2nd edn). The Third Report of the Royal College of Psychiatrists' Special Committee on E.C.T., June 2005, ISBN 1904671225.

Van der Schaar, J. (2005). *History of ECT*. Available at: http://www.priory.com/psych/ectolhistory.htm (Accessed 23 November 2005).

www.aagbi.org/guidelines.html. Consent for Anaesthesia (2006).

www.dh.gov.uk/-30k-31mar2006 – D H Home: The Department of Health.

www.medhelp.org/lib/ect.htm-10k – All about E.C.T. – Electro convulsive therapy.

www.nice.orguk/page.aspx?mode±text & 0=20218–40k – The clinical effectiveness and cost effectiveness of electro-convulsive therapy for depressive illness, schizophrenia, catatonia and mania.

16

Mechanical ventilation of the patient

Jill Nolan

Key Learning Points
- To understand the indications for mechanical ventilation
- To appreciate the differing regimes of ventilatory support and their indications
- To be able to describe the patient safety aspects of mechanical ventilation
- To be able to indicate differing approaches to weaning from mechanical ventilation

Introduction

Mechanical ventilation is sometimes used within recovery areas and is commonly used in the intensive care setting to artificially ventilate persons who are unable to breathe spontaneously at all or are unable to provide themselves with adequate spontaneous ventilation to guarantee satisfactory gas exchange.

Post operative patients may occasionally require a short time on mechanical ventilation until they can be safely extubated, whilst those in an intensive care setting often require a longer period of ventilation.

Mechanically ventilated patients may need to be transported to other departments within the hospital, for example, to receive a scan, or to a different hospital for various reasons. Operating department practitioners (ODPs) play an important role in maintaining the safety of these patients

during transfer. So, whilst it is imperative for the intensive care nurse to have a thorough understanding of the principles and mechanics of mechanical ventilation, ODPs and theatre staff must familiarise themselves with these principles to ensure the safest care of their patients.

This chapter will examine issues surrounding mechanical ventilation and the care of patients who are recovering from surgery.

Mechanical ventilation is the artificial control of the breathing cycle by means of a machine (Ashurst, 1997).

Mechanical ventilation has been used for many years. The 'iron lung' was a method of ventilation that was used in the 1950s. It worked by exerting a negative pressure to the patient and was used to treat patients during polio epidemics.

Advances in medical technology over the years have meant that ventilators have changed beyond recognition since this time.

Indications for ventilation

The classical indication for ventilatory support is reversible acute respiratory failure (Tan & Oh, 1997).

Many authors have produced detailed indications for endotracheal intubation and mechanical ventilation. Quite often these can appear exhaustive and complicated for many to understand. Figure 16.1 provides a clear and easy-to-understand list of criteria of the indications for

Core Topics in Operating Department Practice: Anaesthesia and Critical Care, eds. Brian Smith, Paul Rawling, Paul Wicker and Chris Jones. Published by Cambridge University Press. © Cambridge University Press 2007.

- *Protect the airway* – for example, facial trauma or burns, unconscious patient
- *Treat profound hypoxaemia* – for example, pneumonia, cardiogenic pulmonary oedema, acute respiratory distress syndrome
- *Post-operative care* – for example, following cardiothoracic surgery and other major, complicated or prolonged surgery
- *Allow removal of secretions* – for example, myasthenia gravis, Guillain-Barré syndrome
- *Rest exhausted patients* – for example, severe asthma
- *Avoid or control hypercapnia* – for example, acute brain injury, hepatic coma, chronic obstructive pulmonary disease (Shelley & Nightingale, 1999)

Figure 16.1 Indications for endotracheal intubation and mechanical ventilation.

intubation and mechanical ventilation. Many of these indications will apply to post operative patients. These patients will require careful evaluation and re-evaluation in the recovery area, and in some cases may require direct transfer to the critical care unit if their problems are deemed to be longer term.

Patients may require intubation at the onset of anaesthesia. In some patients the circumstances of the initiation of anaesthesia may not be ideal. In emergency surgery for instance, the patient may not have been investigated and/or resuscitated comprehensively.

Also the baseline health state of the patient may not be ideal. The patient may have a degree of lung disease or be in heart failure and may at the outset be unlikely to be liberated quickly from the ventilator at the end of surgery. These patients may need ventilatory support in the recovery area.

Special considerations

The commonest reason for a patient to be artificially ventilated perioperatively is that they cannot protect their own airway or breathe spontaneously due to the administration of anaesthetic and/or muscle relaxants required for the procedure. ODPs and theatre staff will commonly observe patients who are intubated immediately prior to surgery and extubated as soon after as is possible in the recovery area: 'If adequate spontaneous respiration is not established at the conclusion of surgery, the patient may require a period of controlled ventilation in the recovery room' (Eltringham *et al.*, 1998).

It should be remembered however, that many patients transferred to theatre from an intensive care unit may have been ventilated for days or even weeks prior to this transfer.

Types and modes of ventilation

Accepting that a patient may require ventilation in the recovery area, we will now examine how a patient is ventilated. The aim here is to enable the reader to grasp a basic understanding of the modes of ventilation.

Commonly used abbreviations which will be used in this part of the chapter are indicated below. The ability to familiarise yourself with these abbreviations and their meanings will assist you in the understanding of the modes of ventilation.

- ASB – Assisted spontaneous breathing
- BIPAP – Bi-phasic positive airway pressure
- CMV – Controlled mechanical ventilation
- CPAP – Continuous positive airway pressure
- MV – Mechanical ventilation
- NIPPV – Non-invasive positive pressure ventilation
- NIV – Non-invasive ventilation
- PCV – Pressure controlled ventilation
- PEEP – Positive end expiratory pressure
- SIMV – Synchronised intermittent mandatory ventilation
- VCV – Volume controlled ventilation.

Mechanical ventilation can be either invasive or non-invasive. For invasive ventilation, the patient must have an artificial airway in place (either a cuffed endotracheal tube, laryngeal mask or tracheostomy) which will then be connected to a ventilator.

Non-invasive ventilation requires the patient to maintain their own airway and is administered through a tight-fitting mask. Non-invasive ventilation will be discussed later on in this chapter.

Types of ventilation

Ventilators may be pressure- or volume-controlled – delivering either a pre-set pressure or a pre-set tidal volume.

In contrast to the 'iron-lung' ventilator which applied a negative pressure to the thorax, virtually all ventilators used in intensive care units today, apply a positive pressure to the airways and lungs (Lanken, 2001). It is from here the term 'positive pressure ventilation' stems.

Even though negative pressure ventilation strategies are occasionally used in specialist units, this chapter will focus on positive pressure ventilation only.

There are two main types of positive pressure ventilation:

1. Volume-controlled ventilation (VCV) – this forces a pre-set volume of air into the lungs.
2. Pressure-controlled ventilation (PCV) – this inflates the lungs to a pre-set pressure.

The clinical condition of the patient will determine which type is the safest and most appropriate to be applied.

Within these two types of ventilation, different modes may be used. 'The term "ventilator mode" refers to how the machine ventilates the patient' (Urden et al., 1998).

Common modes of ventilation which are used and will be discussed within this chapter are:

- controlled mechanical ventilation (CMV)
- synchronised intermittent mandatory ventilation (SIMV)
- bi-phasic positive airway pressure (BIPAP)
- assisted spontaneous breathing (ASB).

Settings

When considering positive pressure ventilation, the understanding of the settings on a ventilator are of immense importance. Common settings are:

- Mode. CMV/SIMV/BIPAP/CPAP
- FiO$_2$. Fraction of inspired oxygen
- PEEP. This applies a positive pressure to the alveoli and airways to prevent collapse
- Tidal volume. The amount of air that is delivered with each ventilatory breath
- Frequency. The number of breaths the ventilator will deliver per minute
- Pressure support. The ventilator will 'boost' each breath initiated by the patient (makes each breath bigger) which will increase the tidal volume and reduce the effort needed by the patient
- Inspiratory pressure. Air is delivered by the ventilator up to this pre-set airway pressure.

Controlled mechanical ventilation (CMV)

This is a commonly used mode of ventilation for a patient undergoing a surgical procedure (i.e. sedated and paralysed), however it is rarely used within the intensive care setting. This mode provides almost complete respiratory support. The ventilator will deliver a set frequency and tidal volume/airway pressure. This can be very uncomfortable for the patient if they try to initiate breaths of their own as the ventilator breaths will not synchronise with their own. This can cause the patient to 'fight' against the ventilator which will result in inefficient gaseous exchange.

Synchronised mandatory ventilation (SIMV)

This mode of ventilation will deliver a set number of breaths (mandatory) to the patient. It will also allow the patient to initiate breaths on their own between the mandatory breaths but not during them. The ventilator will synchronise these breaths with the machine breaths (unlike CMV), which is a lot more comfortable for the patient.

SIMV can be either volume-controlled or pressure-controlled. If pressure-controlled (SIMV-PCV) is chosen, a pressure limit is set and the mandatory breath will be delivered up to the pre-set pressure limit. If volume-controlled (SIMV-VCV) is chosen, a tidal volume is set and the mandatory breath will be delivered to achieve a set tidal volume.

Bi-phasic positive airway pressure (BIPAP)

This is a form of pressure-controlled ventilation and is sometimes referred to as PCV for this reason. The ventilator will deliver a set number of breaths to a set peak airway pressure. This is achieved by switching between two set continuous positive airway pressure levels at pre-set time intervals. As with SIMV, even though there are a set number of delivered breaths, the patient may also take spontaneous breaths.

In BIPAP mode, however, these spontaneous breaths can be taken anywhere within the ventilatory cycle.

Assisted spontaneous breathing (ASB)

This is used as a weaning mode of ventilation. This mode will not allow the machine to deliver any mandatory breaths therefore it relies on the patient to be breathing spontaneously. As the patient initiates a breath a pre-set pressure (pressure support) will assist the breath. This reduces the effort of early inspiration and makes breathing more efficient. The pressure support can be increased or decreased as required by the patient. Patients may alternate between fuller modes of ventilation to ASB during the weaning process, for example, during periods of fatigue.

Positive end expiratory pressure (PEEP)

'PEEP remains the most frequent intervention used to provide airway pressure therapy for atelectasis, consolidation and pulmonary oedema' (Park & Sladen, 2001).

Positive end expiratory pressure may be used with all forms of ventilation. It applies a positive pressure to the airways during expiration which helps with lung expansion and prevents complete collapse. This facilitates adequate gaseous exchange and prevents hypoxaemia.

Positive end expiratory pressure may be increased or decreased depending upon the clinical need of the patient. There are risks however associated with the use of PEEP. Volutrauma, which is discussed later on in this chapter, can occur as a consequence of overdistension of the airways and alveoli caused by high levels of PEEP. Positive end expiratory pressure will also cause a rise in intrathoracic pressure which can reduce venous return. This can cause hypotension which can be particularly dangerous in the hypovolaemic/inotropic-dependent patient for example.

Non-invasive ventilation

The justification for mechanical ventilation must be considered carefully and non-invasive ventilation (NIV) is a means of avoiding intubation either temporarily, or if successful can be instrumental in eliminating the need for intubation altogether.

Non-invasive ventilation is used in the clinical setting when ventilatory support is required but the need for intubation is not immediate. The use of NIV may hold advantages not only for gas exchange, but also by avoiding mechanical ventilatory induced lung injury, infection and other complications (Barbas et al., 2005).

Bronchard et al. (1995), suggested that not only can NIV reduce the need for intubation but it can also reduce the length of hospitalisation and mortality rate in selected patients with respiratory failure. NIV can also be used to avert reintubation following extubation (Esteban, et al., 2004).

Short term non-invasive ventilation is administered through an occlusive mask that fits tightly over the nose or the nose and mouth. The patient must be co-operative, be able to maintain their own airway and remove their own secretions.

Although NIV avoids tracheal intubation and therefore reduces the complications of artificial ventilation, air leaks are invariably present and the airway is unprotected.

The patient must therefore have the ability to clear his own secretions unless a mini tracheostomy can be performed.

There are disadvantages to NIV however, and these are listed below:

- Tight-fitting mask may be very uncomfortable for the patient.
- Pressure sores may occur particularly on the nose and ears.
- Particularly difficult for patients who suffer from claustrophobia.
- Risk of aspiration of gastric contents, therefore, very important to have a nasogastric tube *in situ* (Woodruff, 2003).

The advantages of NIV are illustrated in Figure 16.2.

Non-invasive ventilation can be divided into two groups:

1. Non-invasive positive pressure ventilation (NIPPV).
2. Continuous positive airway pressure (CPAP).

Non-invasive positive pressure ventilation (NIPPV)

Non-invasive positive pressure ventilation works in the same principle as BIPAP does except the patient must be spontaneously breathing for this non-invasive form. Two set pressures are used – expiratory positive airway pressure (EPAP) and inspiratory positive airway pressure (IPAP) with the application of PEEP.

Evidence now supports the use of NIPPV in selected patients and for facilitating the discontinuation of ventilatory support (Calfee & Matthay, 2005).

Continuous positive airway pressure (CPAP)

CPAP is often confused with NIPPV. It uses a high flow oxygen supply and a valve is applied which creates a positive pressure in the lungs throughout the respiratory cycle. This is measured in cm H_2O and the usual range used is between 5 and 15 cms. This provides a constant positive pressure during inspiration and expiration which 'splints' open the alveoli allowing more effective gas exchange to take place. The result of this is a reduction in the work of breathing.

Recent developments to reduce the discomfort of applying CPAP to a patient have seen the introduction of a CPAP hood. Even though this method of delivering CPAP has been used infrequently in the UK, it has however been successfully used in Italy for 15 years (Patroniti *et al.*, 2003).

The benefits of the hood have been shown to include increased patient comfort, less frequent breaks and skin necrosis of the nasal bridge and the absence of vomiting (Tonnelier *et al.*, 2003).

Weaning

Because mechanical ventilation can have life-threatening complications, it should be discontinued at the earliest possible time. The process of discontinuing mechanical ventilation termed 'weaning', is one of the most challenging problems in any recovery area (Esteban *et al.*, 2000).

Weaning is the gradual withdrawal of mechanical ventilation and the re-establishment of spontaneous breathing.

The length of time spent on a mechanical ventilator varies among patients. Weaning should occur without undue delay, in order to reduce the risk of complications (such as pneumonia and airway trauma) and their associated costs (MacIntyre *et al.*, 2001). For the majority of patients weaning will be an uncomplicated process of stopping sedation, sitting up and

- Avoidance of intubation
- Eliminates the need for sedative agents to be used
- Can reduce the length of stay on a critical care unit
- Admission to a critical care unit may be avoided as CPAP is increasingly being implemented on high dependency units and respiratory wards
- Has less complications than invasive ventilation methods
- Weaning is typically easier than with an invasive method of ventilation

Figure 16.2 Advantages of non invasive ventilation

extubation. To consider a patient for extubation they must be able to cough, clear their own secretions and maintain their own airway. As a rule of thumb, if a patient does not vigourously agree when offered extubation then early extubation should be reconsidered.

It has been recognised that premature weaning can also have undesirable results such as compromised gas exchange and if the patient must be reintubated, difficulty in re-establishing an airway (Lindgreen & Ames, 2005).

Goldhill (2000), produced guidelines for weaning from a ventilator as illustrated in Figure 16.3.

Guidelines for weaning from a ventilator

It must be remembered however, that weaning strategies need to be focused on an individual basis depending upon the patient's clinical condition.

Whichever method is chosen, weaning is an individualised process during which no two patients will follow the same course. Support,

reassurance and observation of the patient's vital signs, especially his/her cardio-respiratory function and appropriate nursing responses are critical to success (Carroll, 1996).

Monitoring and alarms

Monitoring patients who are receiving mechanical ventilation is essential to their safe management. This monitoring takes many forms that anticipate potential problems related to:

- the function of the ventilator
- the ventilator-patient interface
- the patient's physiological status (Lanken, 2001).

Continuous monitoring of the mechanically ventilated patient is essential. The nurse and ODP are responsible for checking and setting the ventilator alarms, which should alert the nurse to changes in the desired parameters. Alarms are usually set with upper and lower limits. However, the importance of not relying on such alarms continuously must be

IF	The patient is stable
	Underlying respiratory failure is improving/resolving
	and there is no upper airway obstruction
	The patient is not receiving sedatives or vasoactive agents
AND	$PaO_2 > 8.0$ kPa and $FiO_2 < 0.4$ and PEEP < 5 cm H_2O and G.C.S. > 13
THEN	Start a 3 minute trial of spontaneous breathing
IF	Resps < 35 breaths/min and tidal volume > 5 ml/kg body weight

CONTINUE

IF	Resps < 35 breaths/min	or
	$SpO_2 < 90\%$	or
	Heart rate > 140 bpm	or
	Heart rate changes by $> 20\%$ of base line	or
	Systolic blood pressure > 200 mmHg or < 80 mmHg	or
	The patient is agitated/sweaty/anxious	

DISCONTINUE

IF	Successful spontaneous breathing for > 1 hour

CONSIDER EXTUBATION

Figure 16.3 Guidelines for weaning from a ventilator.

emphasised. The clinical appearance of a patient is of utmost importance and should not be ignored at any time.

The nurse and ODP must have a clear understanding of the ventilator alarms and their related problems. This is to ensure that any changes to the patient's status may be detected quickly and the appropriate action is carried out.

Figure 16.4 shows examples of ventilator alarms and their relevance which has been adapted from Ashurst (1997).

An alternative method of ventilating the patient, e.g. Waters circuit with an attachable PEEP valve should always be available and kept connected to an oxygen supply.

Monitoring during transport

Consideration needs to be given to the safety of the patient at all times but particularly during the transfer of the patient.

ALARM	PROBLEM
Low airway pressure	Leaks from circuit or tracheal access tube
Low expired minute volume	
High airway pressure	– Coughing and retained secretions
	– Biting on tube
	– Tubing kinked
	– Water in tubing
	– Worsening lung function – risk of barotrauma
Apnoea and low expired minute volume	No spontaneous breathing
Low expired minute volume	Hypoventilation
High expired minute volume	Hyperventilation
High respiratory rate	– Patient agitated/anxious
	– Wrong ventilator mode
	– Patient fighting ventilator
	– Inadequate ventilatory support for spontaneous breaths
	– Not coping with weaning
	– Patient in pain
Oxygen calibration fault	Oxygen cell not calibrated
Oxygen supply	Oxygen supply disconnected

Figure 16.4 Examples of ventilator alarms and their relevance which has been adapted from Ashurst, S. (1997).

Guidelines have been published for the transfer of critically ill adults. These guidelines apply to patients transferred between hospitals and those moved between departments within the same hospital ICS, 2002.

Guidelines produced by the Intensive Care Society in 2001 on the transport of the critically ill patient state that the minimum standards required for all patients are:

- continuous presence of appropriately trained staff
- Continous ECG monitoring
- Non invasive blood pressure measurement (NIBP)
- Measurement of oxbgen saturation (SaO$_2$)
- End tidal carbon dioxide (EtCO$_2$) in ventilated patients
- Temperature (preferably core and peripheral).

Intubated patients should normally be paralysed and sedated. Inspired oxygen concentration may be guided by SpO$_2$ and ventilation by EtCO$_2$.

Following stabilisation on the transport ventilator, at least one arterial blood gas analysis should be performed prior to departure to ensure adequate gaseous exchange.

Sedation

The ability of a patient to co-operate and comply well with ventilation is an important aspect of their treatment. Without this, ventilation may become ineffective and therefore decrease the patient's chances of recovery. The use of sedation in mechanically ventilated patients can help to ensure tube tolerance, patient comfort and reduce levels of anxiety.

Sedation scoring is commonly used to alert the carer to signs of over/under sedation in order to provide optimal care to the patient. Analgesia is also important for the mechanically ventilated patient. All opioid drugs may produce unwanted side effects such as respiratory depression and decreased peristalsis. The respiratory depressant action may be useful in some patients, i.e. those with increased respiratory drive or severe cough reflex, whereas in others it may inhibit spontaneous breathing and prevent weaning from the ventilator (Ashurst, 1997).

Daily sedation breaks are instrumental in not only the patient's ability to wean more effectively but can decrease the incidence of side effects from the prolonged use of sedative agents.

Risks of mechanical ventilation

A host of complications are associated with mechanical ventilation. Figure 16.5 illustrates many of these complications.

A common term used to describe damage caused to a patient by mechanical ventilation is ventilator-associated lung injury (VALI). This can manifest itself in various forms such as pneumothorax or at the most extreme level, multi-system organ failure (Cooper, 2004).

Ranien and Zhang (1999) reported that mechanical ventilation cannot only worsen lung injury but it can actually initiate it.

Dreyfuss and Saumon (1998) characterised VALI by dividing it into four aspects

1. Barotrauma.
2. Volutrauma.
3. Atelectrauma.
4. Biotrauma.

- Problems associated with endotracheal tube
  - trauma
  - obstruction
  - displacement
  - disconnection
- Barotrauma
- Pneumonia
- Surgical emphysema
- Impaired venous return
- Sodium and water retention

Figure 16.5 Problems with endotracheal intubation.

Barotrauma

It is well understood that high airway pressures during positive pressure ventilation may cause lung injury due to over-distenstion and rupture of the alveoli. This can result in pneumothorax or surgical emphysema as the air can track out of the ruptured alveoli and into the interstitial tissues. This can be a result of peak inspiratory pressures or PEEP.

The use of certain methods of ventilation, for example BIPAP can reduce the incidence if not prevent barotraumas, as the pressure exerted on the alveoli is set at a predetermined limit.

Volutrauma

Volume-controlled ventilation – where tidal volumes are set, can cause the patient to be at risk of volutrauma. Large volumes of air can cause over-expansion of the lungs causing injury. The ensuing lung injury manifests itself as pulmonary oedema due to increased alveolar-capillary permeability, possibly due to stress failure and/or inflammatory mediators causing epithelial and endothelial breaks (Cooper, 2004).

Atelectrauma

Atelectrauma has been described as a consequence of continuous alveolar collapse and re-expansion. Slutsky and Tremblay (1999) examined this theory and reported that, 'larger forces are needed to re-open a closed airway and the resultant shear forces at the boundary between aerated and collapsed alveoli could cause stress failure of the alveolar membrane and epithelial disruption'. Steinberg *et al.* (2004), suggested that the application of PEEP may prevent atelectrauma as it reduces end-expiratory alveolar collapse.

Ventilator-associated pneumonia (VAP)

Ventilator-associated pneumonia has been shown to cause both excess mortality and prolongation of hospital and ICU stay. Reduction in the use or duration of mechanical ventilation if possible would reduce the incident of ventilator-associated infection. This reduction in episodes of pneumonia is one of the arguments for increased use of non-invasive techniques for respiratory support in acute respiratory failure (Juniper, 1999).

However, not all patients are suitable for non-invasive ventilation and the risk of infection should be viewed as a complication of mechanical ventilation, rather than a reason for it to be avoided. Infection control issues are paramount when caring for a mechanically ventilated patient and should be considered by all members of the multi-disciplinary team. There are an overwhelming amount of complex considerations needed when caring for the ventilated patient. Examples of these are as follows:
- Nutritional needs
- Elimination
- Hygiene needs, i.e. mouth/eye/personal care
- Suction therapy
- Positioning
- Psychological support
- Family support
- Safety issues
- Physiotherapy.

These are all predominantly nursing-based and have not been discussed within this chapter. Their importance however must not be underestimated and further reading is suggested if the reader wishes to have a concise guide to all aspects of caring for a mechanically ventilated patient.

Conclusion

The care of a patient who is undergoing mechanical ventilation is complex and demanding. In previous years the ability to engage in the care of the mechanically ventilated patient could be left to the staff of the intensive care unit. In our day, the care of mechanically ventilated patients has spread to staff in other acute areas such as in recovery areas. Short bursts of ventilation may be required prior to extubation. The patient may be stabilized in the recovery area prior to transfer to the critical care unit for more long term ventilation. Transfer within the hospital or to another hospital might require that a member of theatre staff be familiar with at least the vocabulary of mechanical ventilation as well as an insight into the care of the patient who is receiving this technique. Good care can make all the difference to these patients who are undergoing, after all, an uncomfortable and frightening form of treatment.

REFERENCES

Ashurst, S. (1997). Nursing care of the mechanically ventilated patient in intensive care: 1. *British Journal of Nursing*, **6**(8), 447–54.

Barbas, C. S. V., de Matos, G. F., Pincelli, M. P., *et al.* (2005). Mechanical ventilation in acute respiratory failure: recruitment and high positive end-expiratory pressure are necessary. *Current Opinion in Critical Care*, **11**(1), 18–28.

Bronchard, L., Mancebo, J., Wysocki, M. *et al.* (1995). Non-invasive ventilation for acute exacerbations of COPD. *New England Journal of Medicine*, **333**, 817–22.

Calfee, C. S. & Matthay, M. A. (2005). Recent advances in mechanical ventilation. *The American Journal of Medicine*, **118**(6), 584–91.

Carroll, P. (1996). Getting your patient off a ventilator. *RN*, **59**(6), 42–7.

Cooper, S. (2004). Methods to prevent ventilator-associated lung injury: a summary. *Intensive and Critical Care Nursing*, **20**, 358–65.

Dreyfuss, D. & Saumon, G. (1998). Ventilator-induced lung injury: lessons from experimental studies. *American Journal of Respiratory Critical Care Medicine*, **157**, 294–323.

Eltringham, R., Casey, W. & Durkin, M. (1998). *Post-Operative Recovery and Pain Relief*. London: Springer-Verlag.

Esteban, A., Anzueto, A., Alia, I., *et al.* (2004). How is mechanical ventilation employed in the ICU? An international utilization review. *American Journal of Respiratory and Critical Care Medicine*, **161**, 1450–8.

Esteban, A., Frutos-Vivar, F., Ferguson, N. D., *et al.* (2004). Noninvasive positive-pressure ventilation for respiratory failure after extubation. *New England Journal of Medicine*, **350**, 2452–60.

Goldhill, D. (2000). Clinical Guideline 2: Guidelines for weaning from a ventilator. *Care of the Critically Ill*, **16**(2), 48–9.

Intensive Care Society. (2002). Guidelines for transfer of the critically ill patient. London: Intensive Care Society.

Juniper, M. (1999). Ventilator-associated pneumonia: risk factors, diagnosis and management. *Care of the Critically Ill*, **15**(6), 198–201.

Lanken, P. (2001). *The ICU Manual*. Paul N. Lanken, C. William Hanson & Scott Manaker, eds. W. B. Saunders Company, p. 13.

Lindgreen, V. & Ames, N. (2005). Caring for patients on mechanical ventilation. *American Journal of Nursing*, **105**(5), 50–60.

MacIntyre, N. R., Cook, D. J., Ely, E. W. Jr., *et al.* (2001). Evidence-based guidelines for weaning and discontinuing ventilatory support: a collective task force facilitated by the American College of Chest Physicians, the American Association for Respiratory Care and the American College of Critical Care Medicine. *Chest*, **120**(6 Suppl), 375S–95S.

Park, G. & Sladen, R. N. (2001). *Top Tips in Critical Care*. G. Park & R. N. Sladen, eds. Miton Keynes: Greenwich Medical Media.

Patroniti, N., Foti, G., Manflo, A., *et al.* (2003). Head helmet versus face mask for non-invasive continuous positive airway pressure: a physiological study. *Intensive Care Medicine*, **29**, 1680–7.

Ranien, V. M. & Zhang, H. (1999). Respiratory mechanics in acute respiratory distress syndrome: relevance to monitoring and therapy of ventilator induced lung injury. *Current Opinion in Critical Care*, **5**, 17–20.

Shelly, M. & Nightingale, P. (1999). *ABC of Intensive Care*. M. Singer & I. Grant, eds. London: BMJ Books.

Slutsky, A. & Tremblay, L. (1999). Multiple system organ failure: is mechanical ventilation a contributing factor? *American Journal of Respiratory Critical Care Medicine*, **157**, 1721–5.

Steinberg, J. M., Schiller, H. J., Halter, J. M. *et al.* (2004). Alveolar instability causes early ventilator–induced lung injury independent of neutrophils. *American*

Journal of Respiratory Critical Care Medicine, **169**, 57–63.

Tan, I. & Oh, T. (1997). *I.C. Manual*, 4th edn. T. E. Oh, ed., Heinemann: Butterworth.

Tonnelier, J. M., Prat, G., Nowak, E., *et al.* (2003). Non-invasive CPAP ventilation using a new helmet interface: a case-controlled prospective study. *Intensive Care Medicine*, **29**(11), 2077–80.

Urden, L., Stacy, K., & Lough, M. (1998). *Thelan's Critical Care Nursing Diagnosis and Management*, 3rd edn., Mosby Inc.

Woodruff, D. (2003). Hospital Nursing – Protect your patient while he's receiving mechanical ventilation. *Nursing*, **32**(7), 321–4.

17

Perioperative myocardial infarction

Maria Parsonage

Key Learning Points

- Appreciate the incidence of perioperative myocardial infarction (MI)
- Understand the enhanced risk of the perioperative MI
- Understand the pathophysiology of the perioperative MI
- Give insight into the management for the high-risk patient
- Understand:
  - ECG changes in MI
  - significance of serum markers in MI
- Issues in the management of perioperative MI

Epidemiology

There are currently around 2.6 million people in the United Kingdom (UK) living with a diagnosis of coronary heart disease (CHD). It is by itself, the commonest cause of death in the UK, with 117 000 deaths that are directly attributable to CHD, of which 38 000 are classed as premature (death before the age of 75). Even though current trends suggest death rates from CHD have been falling since the 1970s, and despite having fallen by a staggering 44% in the last 10 years alone, morbidity from CHD continues to rise. Current data suggest that on average, the incidence of myocardial infarction is as high as 87 000 per annum and for those who have or have had a

diagnosis of angina, up to 2.1 million per annum (BHF, 2005).

Currently, the association between a history of CHD and post-operative cardiac morbidity and mortality is well reported. Historically, healthcare practitioners were certain of the detrimental correlation between heart disease and surgery, however in the early twentieth century, little evidence existed. Shamsuddin and Silverman (2004) identified the Butler *et al.* (1930) paper 'The Patient with Heart Disease as a Surgical Risk' as the first to propose a connection. It was not until the early 1970s however that Tarhan *et al.* (1972) published their paper 'Myocardial Infarction after General Anaesthesia' as the first in a series of landmark papers that formally identified the link. By 1977, Goldman *et al.* (2001) had proposed a *cardiac risk index* for patients undergoing general anaesthesia, which was used exclusively to risk stratify this high-risk group of patients.

By the early 1990s, a confusing collection of risk indices existed, many of which were said to be both expensive and time-consuming. Therefore, in 1996 a 12-member taskforce of the American College of Cardiology and American Heart Association were commissioned to review and update current practice within perioperative cardiovascular evaluation for patients undergoing non-cardiac surgery (Eagle *et al.*, 1996). The guidelines were developed to provide an evidence-based framework for considering the cardiac risk of non-cardiac surgery.

Core Topics in Operating Department Practice: Anaesthesia and Critical Care, eds. Brian Smith, Paul Rawling, Paul Wicker and Chris Jones. Published by Cambridge University Press. © Cambridge University Press 2007.

Perioperative morbidity and mortality

It has been reported that over the past 60 years, mortality due solely to anaesthesia has decreased from approximately 1 in 1500 to 1 in 150 000. In the UK, perioperative death (death within 30 days of surgery) continues to remain a central issue with the number of perioperative deaths reported in the last 10 years remaining constant at approximately 20 000 deaths per annum (Foëx, 2003). The 1999 report of the National Confidential Enquiry into Patient Outcome and Death identified that of the 20 000 annual perioperative deaths, up to 9000 of these deaths were attributable to cardiac causes alone. For each cardiac death there were reported to be between 5 and 20 major cardiac complications, such as acute myocardial infarction, unstable angina, life-threatening arrhythmias or acute left ventricular failure. It is known that the peak incidence of cardiac death in these patients is in the first one to three post-operative days (Landesberg, 2003). Indeed, 60% of the patients who died within 30 days of surgery had evidence of CHD and pre-existing valvular heart disease, hypertensive heart disease, and congestive cardiac failure (NCEPOD, 2000).

Non-cardiac surgery is associated with an increase in catecholamines, which will have an effect on increasing heart rate and blood pressure (Devereaux et al., 2005). It is estimated that as the number of non-cardiac operations performed in older patients with pre-existing cardiovascular disease continues to increase, the number of cardiac complications will concurrently rise. Despite medical advances, it is acknowledged that myocardial ischaemia and infarction remain a major cause of perioperative mortality and morbidity in patients undergoing non-cardiac surgery (Landesberg, 2003).

Pathogenesis of acute coronary syndromes (ACS)

Acute coronary syndromes are characterised quite simply by an imbalance between myocardial oxygen supply and demand (Braunwald et al., 2002). The most common process that encapsulates the pathophysiological events in an ACS is the rupture of an unstable, atheromatous plaque, with subsequent formation of a platelet-rich thrombus leading to occlusion. Nevertheless, it should be remembered that coronary vasospasm and vasoconstriction and increased myocardial oxygen demand are also known to play pathophysiological roles (Cheitlin et al., 2003; Grech, 2003; Grech & Ramsdale, 2003; Lily, 2003).

A mature atheromatous plaque is composed of two main constituents. First, the *lipid-rich core*, which is mainly derived from necrotic foam cells or monotype-derived macrophages, which migrate from the tunica intima and ingest lipids. Second, the *connective tissue matrix*, which is derived from smooth muscle cells that migrate from the tunica media to the tunica intima. It is here where they proliferate to form a fibrous capsule around the lipid core (Grech, 2003).

The initial sequence of atherosclerotic events in acute myocardial infarction is due to an erosion or rupture of the fibrous cap of the lipid-rich atherosclerotic plaque leading to the formation of an intra-coronary thrombosis. These platelet-rich red thrombi result from platelet activation, which is provoked by the exposure of plaque contents, collagen, and other vessel wall components. Further downstream embolisation from this friable coronary thrombus may occur, leading to myocyte necrosis and the subsequent release of cardiac troponins (Cheitlin et al., 2003; Cooper & Braunwald, 2003; Grech & Ramsdale, 2003; Lily, 2003).

In the past, experts believed that the natural course of coronary atherosclerotic plaque development and subsequent occlusion proceeded in a uniform manner, gradually progressing to luminal obstruction and the development symptoms over years. Nevertheless, the recent growth in treatment options for ACSs has increased awareness of the pathophysiological mechanisms, and human angiographic studies now support the concept of a pattern of a discontinuous and unpredictable plaque growth (Yokoya *et al.*, 1999).

Because the entire spectrum of ACSs is believed to arise from the same pathophysiological pathway they refer to any constellation of clinical symptoms that are compatible with acute myocardial ischaemia. These include unstable angina, myocardial infarction without ST elevation (NSTEMI) and myocardial infarction with ST segment elevation (STEMI) on the electrocardiograph (Heeschen *et al.*, 1999; Maynard *et al.*, 2000; Braunwald *et al.*, 2002; Grech & Ramsdale, 2003; Lily, 2003).

Clinical features of perioperative myocardial infarction (PMI)

Chest pain or discomfort is often described as one of the cardinal symptoms of myocardial infarction and it is the assessment of ischaemic chest pain that aids diagnosis and prompts treatment in non-surgical myocardial infarction. It is however known that up to one third of patients do not present with chest pain in the setting of myocardial ischaemia and it has been estimated that as many as 95% of post-operative ischaemic events are due to silent ischaemia and are chest pain-free (Shamsuddin & Silverman, 2004).

The most common cause of PMI is due to an obstructive coronary atherosclerosis in the subendocardial layer, which subsequently narrows the vessel lumen (Samsó, 1999). Even though PMI often follows the same pathophysiological process as that of non-surgical myocardial infarction, it has been identified that the perioperative metabolic and haemodynamic fluctuations that affect cardiovascular homeostasis may precipitate asymptomatic myocardial ischaemia (Devereaux *et al.*, 2005). This then often leads to PMI in those at greatest risk of cardiovascular complications (Eagle *et al.*, 1996).

The effects of tachycardia are a well-known determinant of a reduced myocardial oxygen supply and increased energy demand (Table 17.1).

Table 17.1 Factors affecting myocardial oxygen supply and demand that contribute to perioperative myocardial infarction

Factor	Clinical situation
Myocardial oxygen supply	
Low blood oxygen content	• Severe anaemia, hypoxaemia
Decreased coronary perfusion pressure	• Systemic hypotension – Intra-operative haemorrhage – Fluids deficit – Impaired venous return – Spinal anaesthesia – Tachycardia – Myocardial hypertrophy
Increased blood viscosity	• Hyperviscosity
Coronary artery disease	• Coronary stenosis/spasm/thrombosis • Alteration of platelet and endothelial vasoactive factors
Myocardial oxygen demand	
Tachycardia	• Haemorrhage, light anaesthesia, emergence from anaesthesia, cardiotonic agents (i.e. sympathetic activation)
Increased contractility	• Sympathetic system activation, inotropic drugs, increased preload, increased afterload
Other	• Aortic stenosis/cross clamping abdominal aorta

Source: Samsó (1999).

It has been postulated that silent ischaemia in the perioperative setting is associated with the increased cardiovascular instability shortly after the end of surgery, this being the time categorised by an increase in heart rate, blood pressure, sympathetic discharge and pro-coagulant activity (Lucreziotti *et al.*, 2002; Foëx, 2003). High levels of catecholamines are often present in the perioperative period because of anxiety, surgical stress and pain. Catecholamines are known to increase myocardial afterload, heart rate and blood pressure, cause coronary vasoconstriction and platelet aggregation, which may lead to plaque disruption. Perioperative myocardial ischaemia that peaks during the early post-operative period is significantly associated with acute myocardial infarction and an increased risk of cardiac complications (Landesberg, 2003).

The Foëx (2003) study suggested that ST segment trend monitoring revealed this adversely prognostic, silent myocardial ischaemia in up to 50% of asymptomatic adult surgical patients with post-operative ischaemia and infarction. Asymptomatic, silent perioperative ischaemia may be exposed through continuous cardiac monitoring and electrocardiographic evidence. This suggests that continuous monitoring for myocardial ischaemia is the most reliable method of detection and should be used routinely for those patients at high cardiac risk during surgery.

Perioperative clinical evaluation and risk assessment

Despite optimal perioperative management, some patients will continue to have perioperative infarcts that are associated with a 40–70% mortality (Eagle *et al.*, 1996). The 2002 *ACC/AHA guideline update for perioperative cardiovascular evaluation for non-cardiac surgery* was an update of the 1996 guidelines. Again their aim was to review the current evidence around preoperative evaluation of those patients identified at risk (Table 17.2). Risk was evaluated according to the nature of the surgical illness (acute surgical emergency as opposed to urgent or elective cases). The main focus was to identify those patients with potentially serious cardiac disorders such as CHD, heart failure, symptomatic arrhythmia, presence of pacemakers or internal cardioverter defibrillators, which would imply an increased cardiac risk.

Table 17.2 Clinical predictors of increased perioperative cardiovascular Risk

Major
- Unstable acute coronary syndromes
- Acute MI (within 7 days) or recent MI (>7 days or ≤30 days) with evidence of important ischaemic risk by clinical symptoms
- De-compensated heart failure
- Significant arrhythmias
  - High-grade atrioventricular block
  - Symptomatic ventricular arrhythmias in the presence of underlying heart disease
  - Supraventricular arrhythmias with uncontrolled ventricular rate
- Severe valvular disease

Intermediate
- Mild angina pectoris
- Previous MI by history or pathological Q waves
- Compensated or prior heart failure
- Diabetes mellitus (particularly type 1 insulin dependent diabetes)
- Renal insufficiency

Minor
- Advanced age
- Abnormal ECG (left ventricular hypertrophy, left bundle-branch block, ST-T abnormalities)
- Rhythm other than sinus (e.g. atrial fibrillation)
- Low functional capacity (e.g. inability to climb one flight of stairs with a bag of groceries)
- History of stroke
- Uncontrolled systemic hypertension

ECG, electrocardiograph; MI, myocardial infarction.
Source: Eagle *et al.* (1996).

Electrocardiography (ECG)

In the clinical assessment of chest pain, ECG is an essential adjunct to the clinical history and physical examination. Often, in the early stages of acute myocardial infarction the electrocardiogram may be described as normal. Nevertheless, as is described with the atherosclerotic pathophysiological processes, serial electrocardiograms will reflect progressive, abnormal electrical currents during ACSs and will show evolving changes that follow well-recognised and characteristic patterns (Morris & Brady, 2002).

It is important to understand where the ST segment lies on an electrocardiogram when describing elevation or depression of the ST segment. The QRS complex terminates at the J point or ST junction and represents the period between the end of ventricular depolarisation and the beginning of depolarisation (Meek & Morris, 2002). The ST segment can be identified as the point between the end of the S wave and the start of the T wave. In a normal electrocardiogram, the ST segment should be isoelectric, meaning that it should lie on the same horizontal plane as the TP segment (end of T wave and beginning of next P wave) (Figure 17.1).

In an ST elevation myocardial infarction, the earliest differential electrocardiographic signs are described as a subtle and transient increase in T wave amplitude over the affected area. This will then lead to the straightening and subsequent loss of ST segment angle and as the T wave broadens, the ST segment will elevate further often losing its normal concavity (Figure 17.2). In some cases, the QRS complex, ST segment, and the T wave can fuse to form a single monophasic deflection, called a giant R wave or *tombstone*, which Morris and Brady (2002) identified as a poor prognostic indicator.

As the ST elevation myocardial infarction completes, further changes to the QRS complex include a loss of R wave height and the ultimate development of pathological Q waves on the electrocardiogram. Both of these changes reflect the loss of viable myocardium beneath the recording electrode, with the deep, pathological Q waves representing permanent electrocardiographic evidence of myocardial necrosis.

ST segment depression is the commonest of electrocardiographic changes described in PMI due to the presence of myocardial ischaemia with ST segment elevation being described as relatively uncommon (Landesberg, 2003).

Typically, the first and most subtle changes result from a flattening of the ST segment, leading to a more obvious angle between the ST segment and T wave (Figure 17.3B). The more noticeable and prognostically significant changes of ST segment depression are often described as being either horizontal (Figure 17.3C) or downsloping (Figure 17.3D) depression. Channer and Morris (2002) illustrate that substantial (≥2 mm) and widespread (>2 leads) ST depression is a grave prognostic finding as it implies substantial myocardial ischaemia and extensive coronary artery disease.

Serum markers

Historically, total creatine kinase (CK), aspartate aminotransferase (AST), and total lactate dehydrogenase (LDH) were used as biochemical

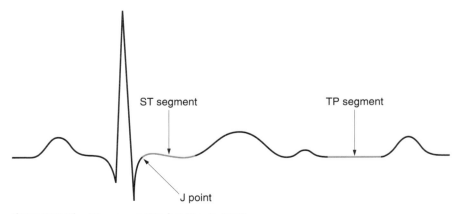

Figure 17.1 The ST segment (Meek & Morris, 2002).

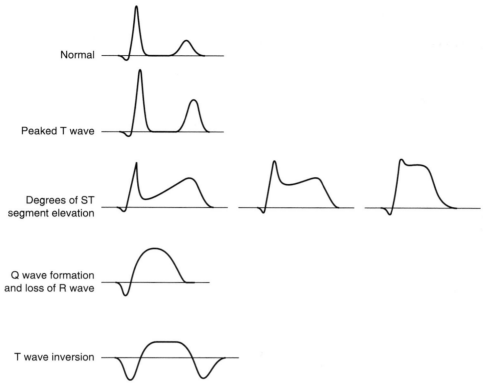

Figure 17.2 Sequence of changes during evolution of STEMI (Morris & Brady, 2002).

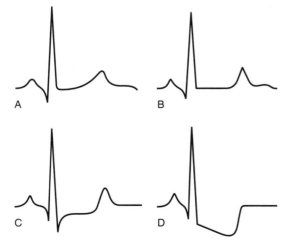

Figure 17.3 ST changes with myocardial ischaemia: (A) normal wave form; (B) flattening of ST segment; (C) horizontal (planar) ST segment depression; and (D) downsloping ST segment depression (Channer & Morris, 2002).

measurements of cardiac necrosis, however, these biochemical markers had poor specificity for the detection of cardiac injury due to their wide tissue distribution. Subsequently, the more specific cardiac biomarkers such as creatine kinase-MB isoenzyme (CK-MB) were used, however their clinical efficacy was limited by their elevation in non-cardiac conditions. Those limitations led to the investigation and clinical development of the highly specific and sensitive cardiac troponins. Considerable research was conducted into their diagnostic capability and potential to allow risk stratification in patients with myocardial ischaemia (Goldman *et al.*, 2001).

Troponin is a complex consisting of three single-chain polypeptides: troponin-I (cTnI), which prevents muscle contraction in the absence of calcium; troponin-T (cTnT), which connects the troponin complex to tropomyosin; and troponin-C, which binds calcium. Together with tropomyosin and under the influence of calcium, they are regulatory proteins of the thin actin filaments of cardiac muscle (Ammann *et al.*, 2004). It is known that cardiac tissue injury can cause these proteins to be released into the peripheral circulation; they will start to rise within 3–4 hours after myocardial damage and remain raised for 4–7 days. The joint European Society of Cardiology, the American College of Cardiology and the American Heart Association have now accepted the measurement of serum troponin as the standard biochemical marker in the diagnosis of ACSs (Braunwald *et al.*, 2002; Ammann *et al.*, 2004).

Even though elevated troponin levels are highly sensitive and specific indicators of myocardial damage, they are not always reflective of acute ischaemic coronary artery disease; these biomarkers reflect myocardial damage but do not indicate its mechanism (Table 17.3).

An elevated value in the absence of clinical evidence of ischaemia should therefore prompt a search for other causes of cardiac damage (Alpert & Thygesen, 2000). Nevertheless, because prognosis appears to be related to the presence of troponins regardless of the mechanism of myocardial

Table 17.3 Causes for detectable serum levels of troponins

Myocardial necrosis Unequivocal	Myocardial necrosis Possible	Myocardial necrosis Unclear
Acute myocardial infarction	Myocarditis	Renal failure
Cardiac surgery	Heart failure	Chronic haemodyalysis
Percutaneous coronary intervention	Rejection of heart transplant	Rhabdomyolysis
Defibrillation	Cardiac contusion	
Radio frequency catheter ablation	Critically ill patients	
Resuscitation		

Source: Goldman *et al.* (2001).

damage, clinicians increasingly rely on troponin assays when formulating individual therapeutic plans (Goldman *et al.*, 2001).

Preoperative management

Recently it has become clear that the management of surgical patients with CHD could be improved by the prophylactic administration of drugs that decrease oxygen demand and improve the distribution of coronary blood flow (Foëx, 2003).

Inhibitors of the enzyme reductase of hydroxymethylglutaryl-coenzyme (HMG-CoA) reductase or *statins* are known to reduce cardiac events and increase survival in patients with both hyperlipidaemia and established CHD. They have been examined recently in the setting of perioperative MI with O'Neil-Callahan *et al.* (2005) suggesting that the use of statins was highly protective against cardiac complications due to a stabilisation of lipid-rich atherosclerotic plaques, however there was no clear statistical data to support this.

It is known that surgical stress has an effect upon platelet activation. Aspirin prevents platelet activation by inhibiting platelet synthesis of cyclo-oxygenase A2 (Madi *et al.*, 2000). Platelet activation is not specifically targeted in perioperative management, and is in fact actively discouraged with patients being instructed to stop their anti-platelets agents prior to surgery. Even though there is much evidence to support the use of aspirin in CHD (ISIS-2, 1988), little evidence exists on the risks and benefits of its use in the perioperative setting.

The mainstay of evidence for reducing cardiac risk is with the use of beta-adrenergic receptor blocking agents. Beta-blockers are drugs that are known to have multiple actions upon the heart. It has long been known that an elevated heart rate is a significant independent predictor of re-infarction and mortality after non-surgical myocardial infarction (Frishman *et al.*, 1984; ISIS-1, 1986). Blockade of beta-1 receptors results in slowing of heart rate, reduction in myocardial contractility, and lowering of systemic blood pressure. In the context of acute myocardial infarction, these effects have been found to be beneficial as they result in a reduced myocardial workload and oxygen demand. The mechanisms by which beta-blockers reduce perioperative complications include a decrease in sympathetic activation, negative inotropy and chronotropy leading to a subsequent decrease in myocardial oxygen demand (O'Neil-Callahan *et al.*, 2005).

The Devereaux *et al.* (2005) systematic review of 22 randomised controlled trials published between 1980 and 2004 examined the evidence for the use of perioperative beta-blockers in non-cardiac surgery. Their review provided encouraging evidence that perioperative beta-blockers may reduce the risk of major perioperative cardiac events, however, caution is advised in that they may increase the risk of symptomatic bradycardia and hypotension.

Current studies therefore suggest that in patients without a contraindication, appropriately administered beta-blockers that reduce an elevated heart rate may reduce perioperative ischaemia and subsequent risk of perioperative MI and death in high-risk patients (Stuhmeier *et al.*, 1996; Oliver *et al.*, 1999). When possible, beta-blockers should be started days or weeks before elective surgery, with the dose titrated to achieve a resting heart rate between 50 and 60 beats per minute. Perioperative treatment with $\alpha2$-agonists may have similar effects on myocardial ischaemia, myocardial infarction, and cardiac death (Eagle *et al.*, 1996).

Post-operative treatment

The aim of the management strategies for the treatment of non-surgical myocardial infarction is to limit myocardial damage and minimise complications (Lily, 2003). These strategies will be dependent upon the type of myocardial infarction diagnosed through ECG changes and will follow two approaches; the *reperfusion approach* is used for ST elevation myocardial infarction through the use of aspirin, thrombolytic therapy or as an alternative, percutaneous coronary intervention (PCI). The aim of the reperfusion approach is to accelerate lysis of the intra-coronary thrombus and restore coronary artery patency to limit infarct size. The *anti-thrombotic approach* that is usually considered for patients without ST elevation on the ECG is through the use of aspirin, heparin, clopidogrel, glycoprotein (GP) II b III a inhibitors and surgical PCI (Connaughton, 2001).

In those patients who experience a symptomatic perioperative ST elevation myocardial infarction, thrombolysis will be contraindicated due to the increased risk of bleeding, however in large infarcts PCI should be considered after assessment of risks versus benefits in an attempt to limit infarct size. The role of prophylactic preoperative coronary intervention in reducing untoward perioperative cardiac complications however remains unclear. As is known, most perioperative infarcts will present without ST elevation on the ECG therefore an anti-thrombotic approach to therapy will usually be taken in order to prevent further propagation of the partially occlusive intra-coronary thrombus (Lily, 2003).

Final diagnosis

In the past, a general consensus existed for the clinical entity designated as myocardial infarction. In studies of disease prevalence by the World Health Organization (WHO), myocardial infarction was defined by a combination of two of three character-istics: typical symptoms such as chest discomfort, enzyme rise and a typical ECG pattern involving the development of Q waves. Current clinical practice however requires a more precise definition of myo-cardial infarction. This led to the publication of The Joint European Society of Cardiology/American College of Cardiology Committee 'Redefinition of Myocardial Infarction'. They redefined the diagno-sis of myocardial infarction as a typical rise and fall in the biochemical markers of myocardial necrosis with at least one of the following: ischaemic symptoms; ECG changes indicative of ischaemia; development of pathological Q waves; or coronary artery intervention (Alpert & Thygeson, 2000).

In the non-operative setting, cardiac troponins play a significant role in the diagnosis of myocar-dial infarction. Even though troponins are accurate in identifying myocardial necrosis, the latter is not always secondary to atherosclerotic coronary artery disease and when establishing the diagnosis of myocardial infarction, cardiac troponins should be used in conjunction with appropriate clinical features and electrocardiographic changes.

A final diagnosis of PMI should be made following assesment of symptoms if present and ECG changes in conjunction with the serial elevation of cardio-specific biochemical markers (Figure 17.4).

In conclusion, the exact mechanism of PMI is not known and most commonly felt to result from both a sudden rupture of an unstable atheromatous plaque and stress-induced myocardial ischaemia.

Myocardial ischaemia commonly starts immedi-ately after the end of surgery, a time characterised by increased heart rate and sympathetic catechol-amine discharge. The ischaemia is often silent and only revealed by electrocardiographic monitoring and the peak incidence of cardiac death being 1–3 days, more commonly in those at high risk of cardiac complications.

Preoperative cardiac evaluation should be aimed at making recommendations concerning cardiac risk in the perioperative period. Guidelines should be based upon the best evidence and patients should be categorised into low-, medium- or high-risk groups along with consideration of the type and urgency of surgery.

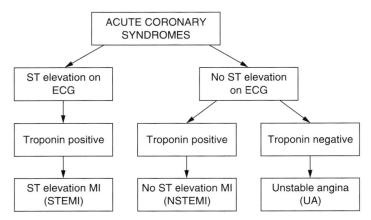

Figure 17.4 Final diagnosis in acute coronary syndromes.

In patients at high risk, post-operative myocardial ischaemia may be prevented through the use of preoperative beta-blockers, thus preventing PMI and other cardiac complications. Further research into the use of aspirin and statins is needed to provide an evidence base into their use in preoperative cardiac risk stratification.

REFERENCES

Alpert, K. & Thygesen, J. S. (2000). Myocardial infarction redefined. *Journal of the American College of Cardiology*, **36**(3), 959–69.

Ammann, P., Pfisterer, M., Fehr, T. & Rickli, H. (2004). Raised cardiac troponins. *British Medical Journal*, **328**, 1028–9.

Braunwald, E. *et al.* (2002). ACC/AHA Guideline Update for the Management of Patients with Unstable Angina and Non-ST Segment Elevation Myocardial Infarction: Summary Article: A Report of the American College of Cardiology/American Heart Association Task Force on Practice Guidelines (Committee on the Management of Patients with unstable angina). *Circulation*, **106**, 1893–900.

British Heart Foundation. (2005). *Coronary Heart Disease Statistics* (on-line). Available at: http://www.heartstats.org/temp/CHDsp2005spcompletespdocument.pdf (Accessed 28 June 2005).

Butler, S., Freeney, N. & Levine, M. A. (1930). Assessment of patients with ischaemic heart disease. *Critical Care Medicine*, **32**(4 Suppl), S126–36.

Channer, K. & Morris, F. (2002). Myocardial ischaemia. *British Medical Journal*, **324**, 1023–6.

Cheitlin, M. D., Sokolow, M. & McIlroy, M. B. (2003). *Clinical Cardiology*, 6th edn. Connecticut: Appleton & Lange.

Connaughton, M. (2001). *Evidence Based Coronary Care*. London: Churchill Livingstone.

Cooper, H. A. & Braunwald, E. (2003) *Acute Coronary Syndromes: A Companion to Braunwald's Heart Disease*. Montreal: Saunders.

Devereaux, P. J., Beattie, W. S., Choi, P. T. L., *et al.* (2005). How strong is the evidence for the use of perioperative β blockers in non-cardiac surgery? Systematic review and meta-analysis of randomised controlled trials. *British Medical Journal*, **331**, 313–21.

Eagle, K. A., Berger, P. B., Calkins, H., *et al.* (1996). Guidelines for the Perioperative Cardiovascular Evaluation for Non Cardiac Surgery. Executive Summary. *Circulation*, **93**, 1278–317.

Foëx, P. (2003). *The Patient with Heart Disease*. (on-line). Available at: http://www.nda.ox.ac.uk/wfsa/html/u17/u1711_01.htm (Accessed 10 May 2005).

Frishman, W. H., Furberg, D. C. & Freidewald, W. T. (1984). Beta-adrenergic blockade for survivors of acute myocardial infarction. *New England Journal of Medicine*, **310**, 830–6.

Goldman, B. U., Christenson, R. H., Hamm, C. W., Meinertz, T. & Ohman, E. M. (2001). Implications of troponin testing in clinical medicine. *Current Controlled Trials in Cardiovascular Medicine*, **2**, 75–84.

Grech, E. D. (2003). Pathophysiology and investigation of coronary artery disease. *British Medical Journal*, **326**, 1027–30.

Grech, E. D. & Ramsdale, D. R. (2003). Acute coronary syndrome: unstable angina and non-ST segment elevation in myocardial infarction. *British Medical Journal*, **326**, 1259–61.

Heeschen, C., Van Den Brand, M. J., Hamm, C. W. & Simoons, M. L. (1999). Angiographic findings in patients with refractory unstable angina according to troponin T status. *Circulation*, **100**, 1509–14.

ISIS-1 (First International Study of Infarct Survival) Collaborative Group. (1986). Randomised trial of intravenous atenolol among 16,027 cases of suspected acute myocardial infarction. *Lancet*, **2**, 57–66.

ISIS-2 (Second International Study of Infarct Survival) Collaborative Group. (1988). Randomised trial of intravenous streptokinase, oral aspirin, both or neither among 17,187 cases of suspected acute myocardial infarction. *Journal of the American College of Cardiology*, **12**(6 Suppl A), 3A–13.

Landesberg, G. (2003). The pathophysiology of perioperative myocardial infarction: facts and perspectives. *Journal of Cardiothoracic and Vascular Anaesthesia*, **17**(1), 90–100.

Lily, L. S. (ed.) (2003). *Pathophysiology of Heart Disease*, 3rd edn. Philadelphia: Lippincott Williams & Wilkins.

Lucreziotti, S., Foroni, C. & Fiorentini, C. (2002). Perioperative myocardial infarction in non cardiac surgery: the diagnostic and prognostic role of cardiac troponins. *Journal of Internal Medicine*, **252**, 11–20.

Madi, A., Plavec, M., Nawaz, D. & Katz, D. L. (2000). Perioperative aspirin can prevent postoperative ischaemia and thrombosis. *Medical Hypotheses*, **55**(2), 164–7.

Maynard, S. J., Scott, G. O., Riddell, J. W. & Adgey, A. A. J. (2000). Management of acute coronary syndromes. *British Medical Journal*, **321**, 220–3.

Meek, S. & Morris, F. (2002). ABC of clinical electrocardiography: introduction II – basic terminology. *British Medical Journal*, **234**, 470–3.

Morris, F. & Brady, W. J. (2002). ABC of clinical electrocardiography: Acute myocardial infarction, Part I. *British Medical Journal*, **324**, 831–34.

NCEPOD. (2000). *Then and Now: The 2000 Report of the National Confidential Enquiry into Perioperative Deaths. The National Confidential Enquiry into Perioperative Deaths.* London: Harvard Associates.

O'Neil-Callahan, K., Katsimaglis, G., Tepper, M. R. *et al.* (2005). Statins decrease perioperative cardiac complications in patients undergoing non-cardiac vascular surgery. *Journal of the American College of Cardiology*, **45**(3), 336–42.

Oliver, M. F., Goldman, L., Julian, D. G. & Holme, I. (1999). Effect of mivazerol on perioperative cardiac complications during non-cardiac surgery in patients with coronary heart disease: the European Mivazerol Trial (EMIT). *Anesthesiology*, **91**, 951–61.

Samsó, E. (1999). *Pharmacological Management of Perioperative Myocardial Ischaemia.* (on-line) Available at:http://www.euroanesthesia.org/education/rc_amsterdam/09rc2.HTM (Accessed 16 July 2005).

Shamsuddin, A. & Silverman, D. G. (2004). Assessment of patients with ischaemic heart disease. *Critical Care Medicine*, **32**(4 Suppl), S126–136.

Stuhmeier, K. D., Mainzer, B., Cierpka, J. *et al.* (1996). Oral dose of clonidine reduces the incidence of intraoperative myocardial ischemia in patients having vascular surgery. *Anesthesiology*, **85**, 706–12.

Tarhan, S., Moffit, E. A, Taylor, W. F. & Giuliani, E. R. (1972). Myocardial infarction after general anaesthesia. *Journal of the American Medical Association*, **220**, 1451–4.

Yokoya, K., Takatsu, H., Suzuki, T. *et al.* (1999). Process of progression of coronary artery lesions from mild or moderate stenosis to moderate or severe stenosis: a study based on four serial coronary arteriograms per year. *Circulation*, **100**(9), 903– 9.

18

Developing a portfolio

Gill Hall

Key Learning Points
- Definition of a professional portfolio
- Structure and purpose of a portfolio
- Collecting evidence for the portfolio
- Uses of a portfolio for professional, personal, employment and educational purposes

When surrounded by subjects that have a specific clinical focus, it is likely that this chapter will be dismissed as being uninteresting and irrelevant. Compared with the obvious relevance of blood gas analysis or while exploring the complexities of neurological trauma, a portfolio's importance for personal and professional development and its significance for influencing patient care is perhaps less than clear. Developing a professional portfolio is often something that practitioners are intrinsically aware has to be done, but is avoided until it becomes necessary. At that point it is at best a chore and at worst a nightmare as it is often difficult to know where to begin, what to include and how it can be structured.

Nevertheless, the portfolio not only provides evidence of growth and achievement over time, it also allows individuals to be reflective and provides a forum to examine and thus improve practice. Practitioners should also consider it to be more than just a 'good idea': it is a 'must' for renewing professional registration with either the Health Professions Council (HPC) or the Nursing and Midwifery Council (NMC).

This chapter therefore aims to outline the main purposes of the portfolio, discuss some of the complexities associated with it and provide a few simple principles that may help practitioners in this task.

Developing a portfolio may be considered by many to be a demanding task. This reluctance may come from a lack of any clear understanding about the role of a portfolio. The purpose of a portfolio can adapt to address different circumstances, which suggests that the content and focus would therefore need to change. This confusion may be reinforced by the fact that there are many different titles, often used interchangeably, to identify the portfolio. For example, some may refer to it as an education profile while others may call it a:
- personal and professional development tool
- student portfolio
- professional portfolio
- portfolio of evidence.

At this stage it may be helpful to view the portfolio as a framework that provides guidance and structure for reflecting, learning and professional development. Irrespective of format or title, one common feature of the portfolio is that it will never be completed, but instead should continue to develop alongside each practitioner within lifelong learning.

As there is no consensus about the design or format of a portfolio, the structure is usually left

Core Topics in Operating Department Practice: Anaesthesia and Critical Care, eds. Brian Smith, Paul Rawling, Paul Wicker and Chris Jones. Published by Cambridge University Press. © Cambridge University Press 2007.

1. Personal Details
   a. introduction
   b. General Education/Academic History
      i.   secondary education with qualifications
      ii. higher education
      iii. other education and training
   c. Professional Education
      i. registerable qualifications
      ii. recordable qualifications

2. Employment History
   a. introduction
   b. ODP/nursing employment
   c. employment outside health
   d. voluntary/community work

3. Continuing Education and Development Profile
   a. details of courses/study days/conferences
   b. clinical supervision notes
   c. appraisals or professional development plans
   d. critical incident analysis
   e. research or project work
   f. publications
   g. unpublished work
   h. lectures/papers/posters presented

4. Additional information
   a. details of innovation in clinical practice – for
      example patient information leaflets, protocols
   b. reflective exercises
   c. assessed work/assignment work

5. Supplementary evidence
   a. letters of thanks from patients/relatives
   b. letters of commendation from managers/
      colleagues

Figure 18.1 Sample structure for a professional portfolio.

to individual choice. A portfolio can simply be an A4 ring-binder with some shop-bought dividers, or alternatively a relatively complex tool presented either as a hard copy or electronically on CD or on the Web. Professional organisations or associations produce many of the latter and include guidance and a concise framework with prepared templates within which to build a comprehensive resource. Irrespective of the choice made there are key sections that may be included (Figure 18.1).

The portfolio as a professional requirement

The portfolio is an essential requirement of any healthcare profession. It plays a vital role in professional registration and ongoing regulation and as such becomes an important area for perioperative practitioners to develop.

Now that all nurses and operating department practitioners are regulated by professional bodies, every practitioner is required to develop a portfolio which will include evidence and data that will be used to prove updates and achievements of clinical skills and knowledge.

These requirements demand that each professional maintains a 'Personal Professional Profile' in which the necessary evidence of updating and achievement is recorded and, where necessary, available for scrutiny and audit by the HPC or the NMC.

Data and evidence collection

From a practical perspective, the portfolio acts as a place where relevant information and evidence can be collected and stored centrally.

For some, portfolio building will have begun at an early stage in their career and will mainly include the education and training related to their initial qualification and registration. For others, portfolio building will only begin post-qualification and is likely to focus on continuing professional development activities. Technically, the portfolio should be a combination of both, thus recording important and significant stages through the individual's professional and personal development, however, depending on circumstances, this may not always be possible.

Irrespective of when the portfolio began, it is likely to contain a wealth of relevant information which may include, for example:

• evidence of attendance at study days
• evidence of attendance at courses/conferences

- transcripts from academic learning, for example, level and credits awarded for successful completion of modules/programmes of study
- certificates of achievement from named awards at, for example, diploma, degree or postgraduate study
- copies of learning outcomes for a study event
- notes associated with study events
- assignment work submitted for assessment
- assignment feedback sheets displaying marks and grades awarded.

In doing so, the information collected within the portfolio will prove the practitioner is keeping up-to-date with developments and innovations in practice. It also summarises and provides that vital evidence of achievements which will fulfil the requirements for professional regulation.

Using the portfolio when applying for a job

Kenworthy and Redfern (2004) view the portfolio as a tool to help nurses record their career and post-registration education and practice. Clearly its use is not only restricted to nurses and can be used by other professions in various ways. They go on to suggest that the portfolio can be a useful resource when applying for a new post or compiling a curriculum vitae (CV). Used in this way the term 'profile' is perhaps more suitable. Brown (1992) contends that a profile is a collection of evidence selected from the personal portfolio and goes on to suggest that it is drawn together for a particular purpose and for a specific audience. The portfolio is then essentially a resource through which the practitioner is able to pick out suitable information and evidence for their job application. This information can then be related to the specific job description and used to show how the individual meets the qualifications and criteria of that post. At different points in a professional career, the evidence used will need to vary, which is why continuous development of the portfolio is worthwhile.

Continuing development of the portfolio, however, requires that it is more than just a store of information. This portfolio needs careful recording and sorting of information to help establish and build a picture of the individual's development. Organising the information into chronological order will provide a logical and systematic representation of how the individual has developed and is a useful aid when putting together a job application or a CV. However, this in itself has limited scope and added information and materials are also required if the portfolio is to reflect the unique nature of each individual practitioner. For this, practitioners could consider including related materials and items of significance, for example, letters of commendation or thanks, copies of patient information leaflets or student study packs they have produced. Practitioners should also provide personal reflections on activities, events or situations. These could relate to particular courses or study events or may focus on situations that arise in and about practice including, for example, a specific moral dilemma, a management situation or the care of a specific patient. In this way the practitioner can look back on what has happened, and consider how that experience will change their practice and what they plan to do to develop or improve it. Using this process, the practitioner might reflect on how these situations, events and activities have influenced that growth.

As a result the portfolio becomes highly personal as it not only represents the achievements in the professional's experience and qualifications but also gives an insight into their thoughts, values and beliefs. From this it becomes clear that the portfolio is more than a receptacle for simply collecting evidence but can become a means of collating and effectively presenting information that specifically reflects the uniqueness of each individual.

Using a descriptive statement which helps to link together the information within a portfolio is helpful, although not always easy to achieve. Therefore, it is suggested that every entry in the

Item Number

Description

Rationale for inclusion

Evidence of:

Reflection/Application to Practice

Conclusions and Action Plan

Figure 18.2 Statement Template.

portfolio should have its own statement attached. The statement need only be brief but should include key pieces of evidence. To standardise the portfolio it may be helpful to use the same format throughout. An example of a template which the practitioner could use for statements is included in Figure 18.2.

As shown in Figure 18.2, the statement identifies the item (for example, the practitioner's experience during a major procedure) and describes what it is about. The rationale provides the individual with an opportunity to discuss why it is included and what it is evidence of. The final section enables the professional to examine how that entry has influenced their practice and what conclusions they have drawn from it. Finally they identify what actions they need to take as a result.

When applying for a job or presenting a CV, the portfolio would enable the practitioner to select information and evidence that best reflects them as an individual and to discuss why and how they meet the job description and person specification. The evidence and statements will also provide examples to highlight particular strengths they have which may be useful in the post while showing what continuing professional development goals the individual has achieved.

Using evidence to claim accreditation for prior learning and experience

Professional regulation has begun to have an impact on many perioperative practitioners. Registration requires evidence of update and achievement within structured professional or academic study. Study opportunities which have been limited in the past are now opening up. This has left high numbers of skilled, experienced individuals eager to move ahead but with little or no previous formalised or academically recognised education and training.

The term 'AP(E)L' is used to describe the assessment of what individuals have achieved through programmes of learning which have not been accredited by national bodies such as universities, or by experience gained in their employment. The development and use of a portfolio to claim accreditation for prior learning (APL) through courses, or accreditation of prior experiential learning (APEL) through employment, is therefore important. The portfolio can therefore not only be used to provide evidence for registration but can help the practitioner to access academic study at a particular level, or to gain exemption from academic study. How does it work?

Accredited Prior Learning focuses on learning achieved through both prior certified learning (APCL) and through APEL which includes courses which have not been academically accredited – for example, study days, in-house courses, conferences, education days and so on. APL also focuses upon experiential learning achieved through employment – for example, while undertaking the role of anaesthetic assistant over a period of time.

For example, a practitioner could make a claim for academic credit for the scope and depth of prior experiential learning while employed as an anaesthetic assistant. The difficulty in doing this is that many practitioners do not have evidence to make this claim. Evidence may include certificates, but is more likely to involve exploring and reflecting on day-to-day situations, working practices and events against specific outcomes of the selected academic programme.

With AP(E)L each individual practitioner makes their own unique claim. The portfolio with its reflective accounts will enable them to show that they have achieved the relevant learning outcomes to the right level. This is done by explanation, discussion and analysis of how they have responded to, dealt with or managed particular aspects of practice. Nevertheless, this is time-consuming and often difficult if the individual has to start from the beginning. The portfolio, with its reflective exercises or reflective journal provides an aid memoir that can offer a useful starting point for claims for APEL.

Performance review and personal development

The professional bodies encourage reflection as a means by which practitioners learn from and in practice, however, reflection on practice can be a daunting prospect for those individuals who have no experience or training in this area. Practitioners often reflect on practice, but not formally or within a recognised framework. There are many reflective models to choose from which provide structure and guidance. Driscoll (2001: 152) believes that 'approaching practice in this way turns routine and everyday practice into potential learning events' and goes on to suggest that this approach could make practice more 'challenging and exciting'.

The practitioner could get this excitement and challenge from looking at practice from a different perspective and actively using events in practice as learning opportunities. Reflecting on them within the portfolio enables the practitioner to question their own practice from a more objective perspective. Rather than criticising, critical reflection will help the practitioner to examine an event or case and identify the positive or negative aspects of the situation. This enables them to identify areas of strength and areas which need improvement.

Thus, reflection can help the practitioner to highlight professional and personal development needs which contribute to performance review. Identifying strengths and highlighting specific areas for improvement can support the individual appraisal and performance review and help develop a personal development plan for the short-, medium- and even long-term. Depending on the areas identified for improvement, individuals may become involved in activities other than formal study, for example, project work, shadowing other staff members, benchmarking and attendance at conferences.

Reflection clearly has a personal focus and is intended to be developed by and for each individual practitioner. This has already been shown to be the case since practitioners can use their portfolio for personal growth in areas such as collecting evidence of personal achievement, identifying strengths and areas for improvement and developing CVs and job applications.

However within its Clinical Governance Agenda, the Department of Health (1998) has integrated personal and professional development of individuals within the area of quality improvement. Thus, each practitioner is also accountable for upholding and improving the practice of their profession as a whole. Continuing professional development is therefore more than simply meeting the personal and professional needs of the individual but also the needs of service and the users of that service. The portfolio plays a pivotal role in guiding practitioners to address service needs and to provide best practice.

Upholding and improving practice is another purpose of the portfolio, not just for identifying personal and professional development needs but also by making links between theory and practice and bridging the theory-practice gap.

In many pre- and post-registration courses, the impetus for students developing a portfolio is, in part, to address the 'theory-practice' divide. Again this focuses on reflection within the portfolio and helps students to make a link between the knowledge they gain in the classroom and the reality of what is experienced in practice. This forms the basis for discussion between the student and their tutor, mentor, peer group and, possibly within the appraisal process, their manager. It may also form the basis of assessed work. This approach is a means of integrating learning with practice and can be seen to be consistent with continuing professional development, work-based and adult learning.

The portfolio as a form of assessment

When designing a programme of study, selecting suitable assessment strategies is an important consideration. Indeed across education as a whole, assessment methods repeatedly come under scrutiny and questions about the reliability and validity of some assessment approaches are still being raised.

In a briefing paper, Baume (2001) criticises conventional assessment methods (such as exams or assignments) used in higher education. He suggests that they may not always be the most effective means of showing to employers what applicants 'can do' as well as what 'they know'. Also he recognises that 'some of the more conventional forms of assessment often test only a narrow range of knowledge and abilities'. Therefore, it is perhaps easy to see why a portfolio as a means of assessment could be a more suitable approach and why portfolios are increasingly used for assessment as well as for personal development.

Baume (2001) outlines how a portfolio can address these and other issues and needs relating to assessment. He states that portfolios can:
- support the development, demonstration and valid assessment of a wide range of personal, professional and academic capabilities, both inside and outside a programme of study
- provide evidence of work done and learning achieved
- show reflection on and analysis of evidence and learning

- support the integration of learning from different parts of the course and beyond.

Portfolios can therefore offer an acceptable and valid approach to assessment, however, students do not always look on them favourably, and may worry about the scale of the task, the workload involved and what they are required to include to pass the course.

These concerns may arise because there is limited evidence available about the use of portfolios as a means of assessment with students appearing to be unclear about how the portfolio can help their learning. This may be compounded because the use of portfolios varies across academic levels, courses and higher education institutions with a lack of any clear consensus or direction for students to work towards.

The portfolio can be used within a course for formative assessment, that is, assessment of progress *during* a period of learning. For example information gathered in the portfolio may be used by the mentor in practice as evidence that the student is achieving a specific skill or learning outcome. Alternatively it can be used as a basis for discussion between the student and the mentor to help the mentor in judging the progress and achievement of the student in meeting the assessment criteria. The portfolio can also encourage the student to gather relevant information to produce a piece of written work that is to be summatively assessed (assessment of progress *following* a period of learning).

Alternatively, several courses are now using the portfolio for summative assessment, or at least part of it, and the portfolios are being submitted, marked and graded against set criteria. As a result it is not surprising that some students seek guidance about their portfolio development or that teaching staff develop guidelines for the students to work in order to meet the specific criteria set.

Within some courses the portfolio presents evidence of achievement of behavioural outcomes or performance competencies of the programme. Sometimes competencies, skill statements or

National Occupational Standards are presented using a checklist or tick box approach. This method reduces workload and the time involved for the assessment, however, it could also reduce the assessor's ability to measure a student's application or understanding of specific areas which results in the assessors setting added assessment work for students. To address this, students produced accounts and reflections which essentially moves the assessment away from simply testing competence in practice towards applying and testing knowledge related to that practice. Corcoran and Nicholson (2004) conclude that portfolios can assess higher order cognitive competencies in practice which academically would relate to such areas as 'critical thinking and synthesis'.

While many students welcome this approach a study by Endacott *et al.* (2004) did raise concerns regarding this issue. It appeared that students believed that they had to tailor their portfolio to meet the requirements of the academic staff who were involved in marking and assessment. Sometimes, assessors in practice seemingly also want to impose criteria or 'place their stamp on' what is included and the way the portfolio is 'presented'. Clearly this could create difficulties and according to the study by Endacott did lead to conflict in students between 'working to maintain their own identity within the portfolio and addressing the requirements set by the lecturer'. This is an interesting dilemma and one not easily resolved. If the portfolio is a personal portfolio then surely the student has ownership of it and what it contains. They also should have control over its appearance and format. Also, if the portfolio is to remain individual, then it should contain reflection that relates specifically to a situation and the individual within that situation and should not be governed, guided or constrained by assessment and lecturer-led criteria. Arguably though, if the student is reflecting appropriately then there would be a focus on analysis, critical examination and objective application of knowledge to a specific situation or scenario. Therefore guidance and

advice could be helpful but would still allow for originality, innovation and creativity within a developing portfolio.

Overall, having considered many aspects of the portfolio, it is perhaps helpful to view it as a 'central store' of information that develops and evolves over time. The portfolio will grow and be amended, and will form a key support for other developments, which is why careful structuring and organisation is important. It is also why this document should remain intact and that copies from it or cross-referencing to it, take place when using the portfolio for other purposes. For example, when submitting a portfolio for a module or course it need not contain all the information discussed within this chapter. Instead it is likely to focus specifically on key objectives and outcomes for the subject being studied. Information about continuing professional development work including critical incident analysis, research, reflective exercise and assessed work may be relevant for inclusion and could therefore be copied. This would be adapted and applied differently within the context of this particular portfolio and added to accordingly in line with the assessment guidance and needs of the specific course being studied.

Some professionals may have several portfolios that they have produced for different purposes. Each is likely to contain some different information but each is also likely to include data and evidence that is common to them all. Each individual will manage this in their own way, but a suggestion is that practitioners each maintain only one portfolio (the central store) with perhaps one or more 'working documents' associated with it. When it has served its specific purpose it is then disassembled and the relevant data and evidence is selected and integrated back into the portfolio.

By now it has become obvious that portfolio development is complex. In its simplest form the portfolio has been described as a loose ring-binder in which information is stored which is easy to understand and even easier to achieve. Now it appears that this ring-binder may also need to be submitted as part of a course and based on what is included, a student may pass or fail the element of study. While this may be true, it is also important to remember that developing a portfolio is a progressive process which reflects each individual's progression and development. Put simply, the content, focus and nature of the portfolio moves in time with the abilities, level and experience of its creator. After all, portfolio development supports independent and lifelong learning and puts students at the heart of the process (Wenzel *et al.*, 1998). A professional development expert has compared a portfolio to a garden. She suggests that it takes planning and hard work, requires weeding out of unnecessary elements, and promotes positive feelings. She rightly goes on to say 'you should be proud to show it off'!

REFERENCES

Baume, D. (2001). *A Briefing on Assessment of Portfolios.* Assessment Series 6. York: Learning and Teaching Support Network.

Brown, R. A. (1992). *Portfolio Development and Profiling for Nurses.* Lancaster: Quay Publishing.

Corcoran, J. & Nicholson, C. (2004). Learning portfolios – evidence of learning: an examination of student perspectives. *Nursing Critical Care*, **9**(5), 230–7.

Driscoll, J. (2001). The contribution of portfolios and profiles to continuing professional development. *Journal of Orthopaedic Nursing*, **5**, 151–6.

Endacott, R., Gray, M. A., Jasper, M. A. *et al.* (2004). Using portfolios in the assessment of learning and competence: the impact of 4 models. *Nurse Education in Practice*, **4**, 250–7.

Kenworthy, N. & Redfern, L. (2004). *The Churchill Livingstone Professional Portfolio.* Edinburgh: Churchill Livingstone.

Wenzel, L. S., Briggs, K. L. & Puryear, B. L. (1998). Portfolio: authentic assessment in the age of the curriculum revolution. *Journal of Nurse Education*, **37**(5), 208–12.

19

Accountability in perioperative practice

Stephen Wordsworth

Key Learning Points

- Recognising the importance of accountability
- Legal, professional and employment areas of accountability
- Accountability in anaesthetic practice

Towards a consensus – recognising the importance of accountability

Patients often see life beyond the operating room door as a mysterious, closed world, viewed only occasionally and with fear. This situation has undoubtedly arisen because of patients' anxiety surrounding surgery and their lack of understanding about what will happen to them once inside the perioperative environment. They are also just as likely to be unaware of who is caring for them, let alone be able to understand the various roles of nurses and operating department practitioners (ODPs) behind the masks.

Anaesthetic practitioners in particular have debated accountability to improve patient care. Sometimes, the real purpose of the discussion may have been for less altruistic reasons, for example to absolve themselves of their responsibilities, or perhaps for one of the professional groups to try to assert a professional dominance. The recent media experiences involving the medical profession (Shipman, Alderhey and Bristol inquiries) would suggest the public are becoming more interested in

seeking redress when their care falls below the standard that they expect. It seems unavoidable that growth in medico-legal litigation and the corresponding litigious culture should extend to other healthcare professions and into all aspects of healthcare practice, including the previously closed world of the operating department.

An accountability matrix

In seeking to show areas of accountability, it is important to understand something of the legal frameworks that exist. In doing so it is also helpful to consider a conceptual model (Figure 19.1) with the

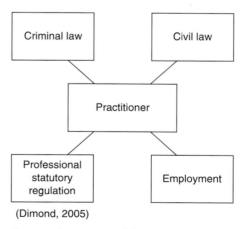

(Dimond, 2005)

Figure 19.1 An accountability matrix.

Core Topics in Operating Department Practice: Anaesthesia and Critical Care, eds. Brian Smith, Paul Rawling, Paul Wicker and Chris Jones. Published by Cambridge University Press. © Cambridge University Press 2007.

perioperative practitioner placed at the centre of an accountability matrix. Examining such a model it is possible to show that lines of accountability radiate out to include criminal and civil legal perspectives, professional statutory regulation, and the responsibilities of the employer and employee.

Accountability and responsibility

Perioperative practitioners sometimes use the term 'accountability' interchangeably with the notion of responsibility leading to confusion in practice. In broad terms accountability may be defined as how far practitioners can be held to account for their actions or omissions. In the legal context this is specifically concerned with potential civil or criminal proceedings to discover why a practitioner acted in a particular way. Equally, practitioners may also be held accountable to codes of conduct or statutory regulations. Perhaps they failed to act, or conversely they have been working outside their contract of employment as agreed with their employer. Perioperative practitioners are held not only accountable for their actions, but also for the decisions that they made that led to any resulting action.

The idea of responsibility places much more emphasis on task, role and action as opposed to the decision-making that should be obvious in those who claim to be accountable. Any anaesthetic practitioner should be able to answer why they acted as they did, what actions they took and be able to justify their reasons.

Sources of the law

In any discussion on the law it is important to note that English and Welsh legal systems differ from those which operate in Scotland and Northern Ireland, although the organisation of the NHS in each country is the same. Perioperative practitioners should also be aware that any discussion on the various sources of the law, or their application to anaesthetic practice should be done so from the perspective of individual patient care. Practitioners should also realise that any practical application of common law in complex issues such as confidentiality, consent and respect, is inevitably going to be affected by several ethical issues. Grubb (2000: 3) makes the distinction that application of medico-legal principles is 'more than the sum of its parts ... defined merely by reference to a set of factual circumstance'. Such legal discussion should now be viewed from the overarching perspective of the Human Rights Act 1998 and the resulting incorporation of the European Convention of Human Rights.

Primary and delegated legislation

Practitioners need also be aware that apart from the Human Rights Act 1998, legislation, such as Acts of Parliament, which have passed through the House of Commons, the House of Lords and have received royal accent by the Queen, are described as *primary legislation*. Such primary sources of legislation include the Abortion Act 1967, Human Organ Transplants Act 1989, Human Fertilisation and Embryology Act 1990.

Common law principles and judicial interpretation

Common law is derived from the work of the courts as a direct result of the practices of the judges in following the decisions of earlier cases. This decision then sets a precedent, which forms the legal rule that will be applied in later cases. In this way Montgomery (2003) points out that common law may be applied to cases which are the same as cases previously heard in court and so the same rules must be applied. In cases which are not identical, judges express themselves in terms of what they would have done if faced with the new circumstances. Where the case is obviously new, judges must develop the law from general principles. Prevalence is always given to statute law over common law principles (Ingman, 2002).

Criminal and civil law principles

Both statute and civil law principles provide the basis of both *civil* and *criminal* principles. Montgomery (2003: 6) suggests that 'civil law governs the relationship between citizens . . . usually resulting in compensation for any injury suffered'. This is in contrast with that of criminal law which concerns society as a whole. Principally, therefore, civil principles set out the legal engagement between the claimant (who seeks compensation), and the defendant (for resulting harm to the claimants interests).

Other distinctions between civil and criminal law exist around the notion of guilt. All common law offences usually require what is called *guilty mind or intention* (mens rea) before a conviction can be secured, however, a criminal conviction is only possible where the principle of a *forbidden act (actus reus)*, is committed with *guilty mind* (mens rea). Put simply, both intention and act need to be apparent. One further difference that is relevant to the perioperative practitioner is that of the burden of proof.

The burden of proof

In order to receive compensation under civil law *plaintiffs* must prove their case on *the balance of probabilities*. Elliot and Quinn (2005) point out that this is a 'lower standard of proof' than the 'beyond reasonable doubt' test used by the criminal courts. Due to the nature of the interpretation of proof it is thus possible in the English legal system to be acquitted in a criminal court but be found to be in breach of civil law.

Criminal accountability in practice

The public glare that would undoubtedly follow a successful criminal prosecution of an anaesthetic practitioner for negligence has not yet appeared. This is in part because of the burden of proof that

is required and because prosecution teams have tended to focus on the more obvious accountability of the medical profession, in this case anaesthetists. This consensus was however put under particular strain in August 2001 when Essex police launched *Operation Orcadian*. This investigation involved 13 separate incidents where blocked anaesthetic tubing led, on one occasion, to the tragic death of a 9-year-old boy. An expert working group set up by the Chief Medical Officer, on behalf of the NHS reported in *Protecting the Breathing Circuit in Anaesthesia* (DoH, May 2004) that: 'The consensus of opinion among the [police] forces initially involved was that the incidents had occurred as a result of criminal acts. The concern was that deliberate acts of sabotage or malicious tampering were carried out by the same person/persons in different hospitals' (page 5).

Mckenna (2002) writing in the *British Medical Journal* reported that the police investigation produced no evidence to show that the series of blockages was because of criminal conduct. In fact it was discovered that intravenous infusion giving set caps, becoming accidentally lodged inside anaesthetic angle pieces, had caused the blockages. Had the allegations in this case been found to be true, the extremity of the situation may have led to a criminal prosecution for murder, as in the Allot and Shipman cases.

The lesser charge of criminal manslaughter is a further possibility following the application of the legal test adopted by the House of Lords in the case of *R* v. *Adomako*. The defendant, who was an anaesthetist, failed to notice that the breathing system had become disconnected. In upholding a previous decision by the Court of Appeal, the House of Lords found that the defendant had been grossly negligent in carrying out his duties. Lord Mackay in his summary simply suggested that 'criminal negligence is when a jury thinks the negligence was criminal'. The implication was that the degree of negligence and legality of a practitioner's conduct is solely down to the discretion of the jury. In practice it is commonplace for all anaesthetic practitioners to be involved in the preparation and checking of anaesthetic equipment, and the reconnection of anaesthetic equipment following the transfer of an anaesthetised patient. Therefore the case has a clear application to the role of the anaesthetic practitioner.

The House of Lords also upheld decisions from previous landmark cases, such as that of *R* v. *Bateman*. Lord Chief Justice Hewart stated that gross negligence is inferred from manslaughter cases that show such a high disregard for the life and safety of others to deserve punishment. This and many other cases point to the fact that the anaesthetic practitioner can be charged with manslaughter because of their own criminal negligence, where their own duty of care, separate from the anaesthetist, also exists. This case outlines further that the anaesthetic practitioner may have shown an *obvious indifference*, or they were aware of a real risk but they chose to ignore it. Secondly, where any attempts to avoid risk were clearly grossly negligent, and finally, where there was inattention or a failure to avert a serious risk that could have been simply avoided (Montgomery, 2003).

Mounting a defence

When faced with such charges, anaesthetic practitioners may well try to argue that overall responsibility rests with the anaesthetist, since the service is still chiefly doctor-led. Such mitigating circumstances can be found in cases involving anaesthetic practitioners, such as *R* v. *Prentice* and *R* v. *Holloway* where the level or lack of supervision by the doctor was called into question.

The anaesthetic practitioner could also sometimes argue that he or she was less than properly supported because current job descriptions and institutional policies may not be in place to match the pace of role development and extensions to some practitioners' scope of practice. A recent initiative such as the developing role of the anaesthesia practitioner (AP) is a case in point. The Royal College of Anaesthetists (RCoA, 2005)

in 'Anaesthesia Practitioners – Frequently asked questions; What will the Anaesthesia Practitioner do?' assert that APs will:

Perform duties delegated to them by their medical anaesthetic supervisor. These will include pre- and post-operative patient assessment and care, maintenance anaesthesia and (under direct supervision) conduct the induction and emergence from anaesthesia. APs will also deputise for anaesthetists in various situations where their airway and venous cannulation skills will assist in patient care and where medically qualified anaesthetists cannot be available.

Only time will define the level of scrutiny the law courts will afford to the AP. In such a case, the concept of *systems failure* may lead to the NHS Trust being criminally responsible for corporate manslaughter, rather than the individual practitioner. So far a jury has not been asked to decide.

Civil negligence and the anaesthetic practitioner

Where some form of malpractice is obvious, most of these cases are concerned with the civil law of negligence. As previously discussed, such litigation seeks not only to provide compensation for victims, but enables practitioners to be held accountable for their actions. In fact Hendrik (2000) identifies several reasons in support of the high number of cases for negligence, including the idea that such litigation acts as an incentive to uphold high standards of care (Philips, 1997).

Nevertheless, in respect of negligence, the law is only concerned with what is expected from the minimum level of competence. Should practice fall below such a standard then a successful negligence claim needs to prove on the balance of probabilities that:
- the defendant (AP) owes a duty of care to the plaintiff
- the defendant breached that duty
- the breach caused the damage (Montgomery, 2003).

The duty of care

The legal precedent of the duty of care was established in *Barnett* v. *Chelsea and Kensington Hospital Management Committee*. This clearly applies to the AP because there is an obvious relationship with the patient, mainly based on the need for care and treatment the practitioner provides separately to that of the doctor. Perhaps this is less obvious in cases where patients are escorted into the anaesthetic room by a parent or by a relative or legal carer. Does the practitioner owe any duty to these people? This is usually established by applying the principle of the 'neighbour test' that was established as a precedent in *Donoghue* v. *Stevenson*. The case demonstrates that a duty is owed to 'anyone who is reasonably likely to be affected by his or her acts or omissions'. This could include failing to warn a patient's escort of the dangers of the anaesthetic room.

Testing for a breach in care

The case of *Bolam* v. *Friern Barnett* established the standard legal test used to prove that a *breach* in a duty of care has occurred. In essence the so-called *Bolam Test* ensures that professionals (practitioners) are judged by the standard of their peers. In so doing the judge's original direction to the jury asserts that '[a doctor] is not guilty of negligence if he has acted in accordance with a practice accepted as proper by a responsible body of medical men ...'. From such case law we can deduce that APs would not be found negligent if they follow a practice that is acceptable to other perioperative practitioners who carry out the same role. Such a test requires expertise from a member of the profession to accept that the defendant's actions were proper. This does not mean the 'expert witness' would have acted exactly the same. Rather, it means the expert witness accepts the legitimacy of the practitioner's actions within a range of acceptable practices. In cases where opinion may differ, the House of Lords, following *Maynard* v. *W. Midlands*, has ruled that it should not choose between different bodies of opinion. So far such case law in the UK has not been applied to health practitioners other than doctors.

The practitioner may develop roles, undertaking the same functions of the anaesthetist, for example, cannulation and intubation. The test for negligence following *Whitehouse* v. *Jordan* would require the same standard as would normally be expected of the averagely competent anaesthetist. Again the emerging role of the AP provides much food for thought in that APs would be expected to perform their duties to the same level as that of an anaesthetist.

The competence of the practitioner is also an important point to consider when proving a breach of duty. In *Jones* v. *Manchester Corporation*, the hospital and the doctor were both found to be responsible in some part. This followed an anaesthetic incident caused by poor supervision provided by a junior doctor, however the lack of competence could not be used as mitigation against the standard of care given, because the junior doctor should have been practising to the same level of competence as an anaesthetist. It has also often been the case, due to the close working relationship with the anaesthetist that some practitioners continue to be involved in carrying out tasks for which they are not qualified. In this situation, failure to refer the patient to someone with the proper skill may itself be a negligent act, as directed in *Wilsher* v. *Essex*.

It is important to remember that in English Law, the most senior member of a clinical team is not necessarily responsible for the actions of the rest of the team. Consider, for example, where a perioperative practitioner is involved in drawing up anaesthetic drugs independently, or at the request of the anaesthetist. This does not make the anaesthetist responsible for any mistakes during this part of the procedure simply because the anaesthetist is ultimately 'in charge' of providing the anaesthetic.

Vicarious liability

In *Cassidy* v. *Minister for Health* it was clear that an operation on a hand had not proved successful, but it was impossible to prove negligence by one individual. The hospital authorities were found responsible given that they had chosen to employ the healthcare professionals. In his summary Lord Denning stated that: 'When hospital authorities undertake to treat a patient, and themselves select and appoint and employ the professional men and women who are to give treatment, then they are responsible for the negligence of those persons in failing to give proper treatment, no matter whether they are surgeons, nurses or anyone else.'

In reality, many perioperative practitioners view the doctrine of vicarious liability as a safety net to enable the plaintiff to receive financial compensation, which under ordinary circumstances could not be met by the individual practitioner.

Was damage caused?

The final aspect of negligence seeks to establish whether the standard of care caused the physical or psychological injuries the victim suffered. If this cannot be proven then the claim will fail. In anaesthetic practice, it seems likely that *causation (i.e that the harm was caused by the anaesthetic technique employed)* is probable, as harm to the patient may be obvious. Proving that harm resulted from the breach in duty also appears to be a simple matter, but the reality is often different. Delays in hearing negligence cases are often cited as being major reasons behind why causation cannot be proven. Hendrik (2000) points out that people involved cannot remember past events with the necessary clarity, and that records are often mislaid. The case of *Whitehouse* v. *Jordan* surrounded a mother's claim that the doctor had been negligent when delivering the baby, eventually leading to brain damage. The evidence was mainly based on the plaintiff's memories of what had happened. This contrasted markedly with the testimony of two expert witnesses whose evidence was based on the medical notes. The doctor concerned could not remember what exactly happened and several witnesses were considered not to be reliable. In the face of such incomplete evidence the plaintiff lost the case.

One aspect of the case that will undoubtedly have specific resonance is the issue over the need to keep accurate records. The AP could do well to remember the mantra that 'if it isn't written down, then it didn't happen'. Also cases can fail at this stage because there may be several possible reasons, or events, contributing to a patient's injury. In practice a patient can receive compensation only when he or she can prove that any injuries were reasonably foreseeable. Such a test tries to show that the original illness or condition has not been cured or that a second or newer injury has been brought about.

Statutory professional accountability

Until recently it could have been argued that professional accountability set apart the nursing and ODP professions, however, the inconsistency has been addressed with the opening of the Health Professions Council (HPC) register for ODPs. The primary aim of both the HPC and the Nursing and Midwifery Council (NMC) is to protect the public and in so doing both organisations are provided, by their respective legislation, with the ability to invoke several sanctions. Both regulators exist because of the review and overhaul of the mechanisms that were in place under the United Kingdom Central Council (UKCC) and the Council for Professions Supplementary to Medicine. The Health Act 1999 created the legislative framework to enact the changes to both regulators. Further detailed rules, which proscribe the mechanisms by which the regulators are to operate within, are set out in the Nursing and Midwifery Order (2001) and the Health Professions Order (2001).

While the functions of the regulators are similar (Figure 19.2), the rules by which the two corporate

Functions of the regulators

NMC	HPC
Keep a register of members admitted to practise	Operate a register
Determine the standards of education and training for admission to practise	Approval of programmes for entry to the register
Give guidance on standards of conduct and performance	Sets standards in: • education and training • standards of proficiency • conduct, performance and ethics • continuing profession development
Administer procedures relating to misconduct, unfitness to practise and similar matters	Intervene if a registrant's fitness to practise may be below standard

Figure 19.2 Functions of the regulatory bodies.

Sanctions of the regulators

Strike from register

Suspension for a specified period
(not exceeding one year)

Impose conditions for which a person must comply
(not exceeding three years)

Caution the practitioner (not for less than one year
and not more than five years)

Refer to another committee

Interim orders

Figure 19.3 Sanctions which can be exerted by the regulatory bodies.

bodies act and their statutory committees are slightly different. The rules also differ in relation to council membership and the functions of non-statutory committees, such as those that operate the financial activities of the two regulators. Nevertheless, the sanctions available to the NMC and HPC are one and the same (Figure 19.3).

Fitness for practice

Where an allegation of fitness for practice is made, both lay and professional 'screeners' are used to find out if the allegation can be heard under the statutory powers; the case can then be referred to a Practice Committee. The first aim is to deal with the allegation through mediation without involvement of the Health or Conduct and Competence Committee.

Dealing with an allegation

For the HPC and NMC, the Investigating Committee will address:
• misconduct
• lack of competence
• a UK conviction for a criminal offence
• an offence committed elsewhere that would constitute a criminal offence in the UK
• physical or mental health
• a determination by a body in the UK under the enactment for regulating a health or social care profession to the effect that his/her fitness to practice is impaired, or, a determination by a licensing body elsewhere to the same effect
• an entry to the register which has been fraudulently gained or falsely made.

Where the Investigating Committee finds that 'there is a case to answer' it has the power to:
• undertake mediation
• refer the case to:
    I. screeners to undertake mediation
    II. the Health Committee
    III. the Conduct and Competence Committee.

Conduct and competence and health committees

Following consultation with other Practice Committees the Conduct and Competence Committee should advise the regulators on:

- performance of the regulating council's function towards standards of conduct, performance and ethics of the registrant/prospective registrant
- requirements relating to good character and health by registrants/prospective registrants
- protection of the public from people whose fitness for practice is impaired.

The regulators will also consider allegations referred by the respective Council, screeners, Investigation Committee and Health Committee. The Conduct and Competence Committee and Health Committee advise on applications for restoration to the register. The latter sits in private but at least one medical examiner must attend; the practitioner can be present and represented legally, or by a friend or counsel. The practitioner may also wish to be represented by their medical advisor. The regulators can call adjournments to provide time to bring witnesses before the committee.

Dual registration

It is the nature of perioperative practice that a significant number of practitioners hold both a nursing and ODP qualification. This typically arose from 'fast-track' National Vocational Qualifications (NVQs) during the 1990s. While this in itself does not infringe either of the regulators' requirements it does have added burdens for the practitioner. Apart from the cost of separate regulation, any allegation will be subject to the independent scrutiny of both regulators. With the impending introduction of the HPC Continuing Professional Development (CPD) policy, re-registration could include added activity to that already required for post-registration and practice (PREP).

When an allegation is made against dual registered practitioners, the public would wish to ensure that both regulators arrive at the same decision and that the same sanctions are applied. This is necessary to avoid incompetent practitioners continuing to work because although they had been removed from one register, they might remain on the other. No doubt in such a case the High Court would want to review the workings of the various statutory committees.

Appreciating employment law

It is important for practitioners to understand their rights as an employee, given the changing nature of NHS culture, driven on by initiatives spearheaded by the 'Modernisation Agency'. Also, many perioperative practitioners are themselves managers in their own right. Like many sources of law the relationship between employer and employee is drawn from many sources. The aim here is merely to raise awareness of some of these issues (Figure 19.4).

The contract of employment

The main method for communicating terms of employment is with a contract of employment. Even though it is not necessarily written down this comes into being at the point where the perioperative practitioner accepts the offer of a post. Up to this point either party may withdraw at any stage.

The sources that are involved in developing the contract can include:

- express terms agreed by employer and employee, such as title of post and salary
- existing express terms, such as those agreed nationally for a particular staff group. These are less obvious now given that Trusts have the ability to negotiate local terms and conditions of employment
- Future terms, such as those agreed under Agenda for Change arrangements but not yet brought into force, or future nationally agreed pay awards
- Implied terms – these place extra obligations on both parties.

Employer	Employee
A duty to take reasonable care of the employee	A duty to obey the reasonable orders of the employer
A duty to pay and provide work	A duty to act with reasonable care and skill
A duty to treat the employee with consideration and support him/her	A duty not to compete with the employer's enterprise
	A duty to keep secrets and confidential information

Figure 19.4 Duties of employers and employees (Dimond, 2005: 216).

The courts have chosen to test such terms in cases where an employer's request is matched by the willingness of the employee. Emergency situations are often cited.

- Custom and practice – concerns work practices and privileges that were not necessarily part of the original contract. It has a much narrower application in law than trade unions sometimes afford it.
- Statutory provision – for example, in The Protection of Children Act 1999 and Sexual Offenders Act 1997, employers can find out if there are grounds for not employing a prospective employee. Statutory employee rights established mainly in the Employment Act 1996, Employment Relations Act 1999 and the Employment Act 2002 includes:
  - protection of wages
  - time off work
  - suspension from work
  - maternity rights
  - termination of employment
  - unfair dismissal
  - redundancy payments.

Breach of contract

Under the implied conditions of the contract of employment, the employer must treat the employee with consideration. If the employer is in breach of this or any part of the contract he or she can pursue a case of constructive dismissal. Conversely, if the employee fails to abide by the contractual obligations, possible sanctions could include more than one aspect of the accountability matrix. This includes not only disciplinary action, but also professional misconduct, and the possibility of being found negligent in law. Several cases have been brought before the Appeal Court following conduct committee findings on employment requirements.

In the case of *Hefferon* v. *UKCC*, the judge found that the decision by the UKCC to remove a practitioner from the register could not be upheld. In not reporting an incident to her superior she had not in fact disobeyed her employers, because under the terms of her employment there was no requirement to do so.

Accountability in summary

It is necessary to accept that accountability is a universally important issue to all perioperative practitioners. Increasingly this is likely to change from coffee room debate to a level of practical experience, particularly as the growth in healthcare litigation grows beyond that aimed primarily at the medical profession. Statutory regulation now encompasses all perioperative practitioners and remaining professional tensions seem increasingly less important in the face of NHS reform and modernisation. Broad principles surrounding legal, professional and employment accountability have been deliberately viewed primarily through the lens of the AP, but can apply to all aspects of peri-operative practice. Nevertheless, the anaesthetic practice has primarily provided some specific examples from the activities of the civil and criminal courts which have a particular, and growing reso-nance. Indeed the very nature on which these legal principles are derived will mean that the broader application to the AP is inevitable, particu-larly where role development is an increasingly likely phenomenon.

The dichotomy between the need to retain public protection may well find conflict with changing employment practices surrounding role develop-ment and the break-up of traditional professional boundaries. In short, practitioners need to under-stand the concept more fully, look to the available evidence and reason how and why this is likely to affect them now and in the future.

REFERENCES

Department of Health. (2004). *Protecting the Breathing Circuit in Anaesthesia; Report to the Chief Medical Officer of an Expert Group on Blocked Anaesthetic Tubing*. London: Department of Health Publications.

Dimond, B. (2005). *Legal Aspects of Nursing*, 4th edn. London: Prentice Hall.

Elliot, C. & Quinn, F. (2005). *English Legal System*, 6th edn. London: Pearson Education, Longman.

Grubb, A. (2000). *Kennedy and Grubb Medical Law*, 3rd edn. London: Butterworths.

Hendrik, J. (2000). *Law and Ethics in Nursing and Health Care*. Cheltenham: Stanley Thornes.

Ingman, T. (2002). *The English Legal Process*, 9th edn. Oxford: Oxford University Press.

Mckenna, C. (2002). Expert panel to look into blocked anaesthetic tubing incidents. *British Medical Journal*, **325**, 183.

Montgomery, J. (2003). *Health Care Law*, 2nd edn. Oxford: Oxford University Press.

Philips, A. F. (1997). *Medical Negligence Law: Seeking a Balance*. Aldershot: Dartmouth Publishing.

Royal College of Anaesthetists. (2005). *Anaesthesia Practitioners (APs) – Frequently asked questions; What will the Anaesthesia Practitioner Do?* Available at: www.rcoa.ac.uk/index.asp?PageID=547 (Accessed 18 October 2005).

The Health Professions Order. (2001). *Health Care and Associated Professions*. No 254. London: The Stationery Office.

The Nursing and Midwifery Order. (2001). *The National Health Service Act 2001*. No 159. London: The Stationery Office.

LIST OF STATUTES

Abortion Act 1967

Employment Act 2002

Employment Relations Act 1999

Employment Rights Act 1996

Health Act 1999

Human Rights Act 1998

Human Fertilisation and Embryology Act 1990

Human Organ Transplants Act 1989

Professions Supplemental to Medicines Act 1960

Nurses, Midwives and Health Visitors Act 1979

Sexual Offenders Act 1997

The Protection of Children Act 1999

LIST OF LEGAL CASES

Barnett v. *Chelsea and Kensington Hospital Management Committee* (1969) 1QB 428, (1968) 1 All ER 1068 (QBD)

Bolam v. *Friern Hospital Management Committee* (1957) 1 WLR 582

Cassidy v. *Minister of Health* (1951) 1 All ER 574

Donoghue v. *Stevenson* (1932) AC 562 HL (Sc)

Hefferon v. *UKCC* (1988) 10 BMLR 1

Jones v. *Manchester Corporation* (1952) 2 All ER 125

Maynard v. *West Midlands Regional Health Authority* (1984) 1 WLR 634

R v. *Adomako* (1995) 1 AC 171, 187B

R v. *Bateman* (1925) LJKB 791

R v. *Holloway* (1993) 4 Med LR 304

R v. *Prentice* (1993) 3 WLR 927

Whitehouse v. *Jordan* (1981) 1 WLR 246

Wilsher v. *Essex Health Authority* (1986) 3 All ER 801

Index